Mucosal Membrane Health

The Key to Preventing Inflammatory Conditions, Infections, Toxicity and Degeneration

By Case Adams, Naturopath

Mucosal Membrane Health: The Key to Preventing Inflammatory Conditions, Infections, Toxicity and Degeneration
Copyright © 2011, 2014 Case Adams
LOGICAL BOOKS
Wilmington, Delaware
http://www.logicalbooks.org
All rights reserved.
Printed in USA
Front cover image: Apttone and Sebastian Kaulitzki

The information provided in this book is for educational and scientific research purposes only. The information is not medical advice and is not a substitute for medical care or personal health advice. A medical practitioner or other health expert should be consulted prior to any significant change in lifestyle, diet, herbs or supplement usage. There shall neither be liability nor responsibility should the information provided in this book be used in any manner other than for the purposes of education and scientific research. While some animal research is referenced, neither the publisher nor author support the use of animals for research.

Publishers Cataloging in Publication Data
Adams, Case
Mucosal Membrane Health: The Key to Preventing Inflammatory
    Conditions, Infections, Toxicity and Degeneration

First Edition
1. Medicine. 2. Health.
Bibliography and References; Index

ISBN-13 ebook: 978-1-936251-31-5
ISBN-13 paperback: 978-1-936251-46-9

Other Books by the Author:

ARTHRITIS – THE BOTANICAL SOLUTION: Nature's Answer to Rheumatoid Arthritis, Osteoarthritis, Gout and Other Forms of Arthritis
ASTHMA SOLVED NATURALLY: The Surprising Underlying Causes and Hundreds of Natural Strategies to Beat Asthma
BREATHING TO HEAL: The Science of Healthy Respiration
ELECTROMAGNETIC HEALTH: Making Sense of the Research and Practical Solutions for Electromagnetic Fields (EMF) and Radio Frequencies (RF)
HAY FEVER AND ALLERGIES: Discovering the Real Culprits and Natural Solutions for Reversing Allergic Rhinitis
HEALTHY SUN: Healing with Sunshine and the Myths about Skin Cancer
HEARTBURN SOLVED: How to Reverse Acid Reflux and GERD Naturally
LIVING IMMUNITY: Supercharging Our Body's Defenses with Probiotics and Other Natural Strategies
NATURAL SLEEP SOLUTIONS FOR INSOMNIA: The Science of Sleep, Dreaming, and Nature's Sleep Remedies
NATURAL SOLUTIONS FOR FOOD ALLERGIES AND FOOD INTOLERANCES: Scientifically Proven Remedies for Food Sensitivities
ORAL PROBIOTICS: The Newest Way to Prevent Infection, Boost the Immune System and Fight Disease
PROBIOTICS: Protection Against Infection
PURE WATER: The Science of Water, Waves, Water Pollution, Water Treatment, Water Therapy and Water Ecology
THE ANCESTORS DIET: Living and Cultured Foods to Extend Life, Prevent Disease and Lose Weight
THE CONSCIOUS ANATOMY: Healing the Real You
THE GLUTEN CURE: Scientifically Proven Natural Solutions to Celiac Disease and Gluten Sensitivities
THE LIVING CLEANSE: Detoxification and Cleansing Using Living Foods and Safe Natural Strategies
THE SCIENCE OF LEAKY GUT SYNDROME: Intestinal Permeability and Digestive Health
TOTAL HARMONIC: The Healing Power of Nature's Elements

Table of Contents

Introduction 1
1. What are Mucosal Membranes? 3
    Where are the Mucosal Membranes? 3
    What are Mucosal Membranes Made of? 4
    What is the Purpose for the Mucosal Membranes? 5
    Where Do the Mucosal Membranes Come From? 7
    Early Mucosal Membranes 9
2. Critical Mucosal Membranes 11
    Airway Mucosal Membranes 11
    The Alveoli Surfactant 14
    The Respiratory Cilia 15
    The Intestinal Mucosal Membranes 17
    Sinus and Nasal Mucosal Membranes 20
    Skin Membranes 27
    Stomach Mucosal Membranes 28
    Intestinal Immunity 29
3. Some Disorders Caused by Weakened Mucosal Membranes 31
    Epithelial Permeability 31
    Allergies and Increased Intestinal Permeability 36
    Asthma and Airway Mucosal Health 37
    Airway Conditions and Membrane Inflammation 42
    What Causes Chronic Cough? 45
    How About the Sore Throat? 45
    Inflammation Overview 46
    Allergies and Airway Hypersensitivity 48
    The GERD Connection: Mucosal Membrane Health 53
4. Our Mucosal Police 61
    The Bad and Not So Bad Microorganisms 61
    Actinomyces sp. 61
    Clostridium sp. 61
    Corynebacterium sp. 61
    Escherichia coli and other Enterobacteriaceae 62
    Enterococcus faecalis (formerly Streptococcus faecalis) 62
    Haemophilus influenzae 62
    Mycoplasmas 62
    Neisseria meningitides 62
    Pseudomonas aeruginosa 62
    Spirochetes 63

Staphylococcus aureus ... 63
Staphylococcus epidermidis ... 63
Streptococcus mitis ... 63
Streptococcus pyrogenes ... 64
Streptococcus pneumoniae ... 64
Streptococcus mutans ... 64
The Good Micros ... 64
Streptococci ... 64
Streptococcus salivarius ... 65
Streptococcus thermophilus ... 65
The Lactobacilli ... 66
Lactobacillus salivarius ... 67
Lactobacillus reuteri ... 67
Lactobacillus acidophilus ... 68
Lactobacillus helveticus ... 70
Lactobacillus casei ... 70
Lactobacillus rhamnosus ... 72
Lactobacillus plantarum ... 73
Lactobacillus bulgaricus ... 74
Lactobacillus brevis ... 75
Gum Disease and Dental Cavities ... 75
Irritable Bowel Syndrome and Crohn's Disease ... 78
Digestive Conditions ... 82
Allergies and Eczema ... 83
Intestinal Permeability ... 87
Polyps, Diverticulosis and Diverticulitis ... 90
Ulcers ... 91
Vaginosis and Vaginitis ... 94
Candida Infections ... 96
Ear Infections ... 97
Respiratory Infections ... 97

5. What Harms Our Mucosal Membranes? ... 99
Synthetic Toxins ... 99
Plasticizers and Parabens ... 100
Foods and Beverages ... 101
Lifestyle Factors ... 101
Heavy Metals ... 102
Water Pollutants ... 102
Toxic Microorganisms ... 105
Pharmaceutical Toxins ... 111

- Chemical Food Additives ... 116
- Air Pollutants ... 119
- Volatile Organic Compounds (VOCs) ... 125
- Synthetic Fragrances ... 127
- Skin Lotion Toxins ... 128
- Household Toxins ... 129
- Asbestos ... 130
- Formaldehyde ... 130
- Other Building Material Toxins ... 131
- That 'New Car Smell' ... 131
- Sick Buildings ... 132
- Occupational Toxins ... 133

6. Rebuilding Mucosal Health ... 137
- Mucosal Herbs ... 137
- Food Choices ... 175
- Dietary Strategies ... 179
- Probiotic Foods ... 180
- Prebiotic Foods ... 192
- Yeasts and Yeast Derivatives ... 194
- Vinegars ... 196
- Antioxidants ... 198
- Greenfoods ... 202
- Mucosal pH Balance ... 206
- Mucosal Fats ... 209
- A Few Mucosal-benefiting Nutrients ... 220
- Methylmethionine ... 224
- Mucosal Hydration ... 225
- Water Therapy ... 226
- Sweating ... 232
- Exercise Strategies ... 232
- Breathing ... 234
- Pollution Control ... 238
- Conclusion ... 249

References and Bibliography ... 251
Index ... 301

Introduction

Our mucosal membranes might be virtually invisible to the naked eye, but they are critical to our health. So much so that many health conditions specifically relate to the health of our mucosal membranes.

Unfortunately, modern medicine has not quite caught on to this fact. While research certainly confirms this, most western physicians ignore the condition of this thin membrane among their patients. While medical schools certainly teach their students about the secretions and membranes of the various epithelial tissues, the fact that these membranes can become damaged has not been on the radar.

In this text, we will lay out the nature of the mucosal membranes, and why they are critical to our health. Some of this information is widely known among healthcare circles. However, much of it is not widely known, even though it is proven science.

One of the reasons our medical institutions have not focused upon the health of our mucosal membranes is that for much of the history of western medicine, the mucosal membranes have been invisible. While doctors have been focused upon the "hard assets" of our anatomy, opening up and dissecting the human body to see the various organs and fluids, the humble mucosal membranes have been out of sight and as such, out of mind.

While the conclusion that faulty mucosal membranes cause serious health conditions might seem alternative to some, the research illustrating these associations has been peer reviewed. It is hard science; most of it double-blind, randomized and placebo-controlled. It is not anecdotal.

After presenting the physiology and the mechanics for the associations between some of the more widespread conditions, this text covers the causes of mucosal membrane damage. This is followed up by strategies to correct damaged or thinned mucosal membranes. Some of these strategies have been confirmed using modern research. Others have been confirmed using clinical evidence, some of this over thousands of years of use among traditional physicians around the world.

While those involved in the research or clinical application may not have realized the mechanisms that produce their therapeutic efforts, we can easily and scientifically connect the mucosal membranes with these mechanisms.

Mucosal health is a gigantic subject. We have abbreviated some of the broad spectrum of consequences simply because an exhaustive discussion of all the disease conditions and disorders related to our mucosal membranes would compare to a significant portion of some of the thickest pathology texts. So I guess we'll have to leave some of this up to the next generation of medical authors.

The text contains a mix of science and practical application. The hope is that the health provider can draw from the science in this text, while the layperson can draw from its practical evidence and application.

In any case, one should consult with their personal health professional before making changes to their diet, lifestyle or supplementation habits.

Chapter One
What are Mucosal Membranes?

Where are the Mucosal Membranes?

The mucosal membranes cover just about every surface of our body that has any contact with the outside environment. Mucosal membranes line the epithelial cells of our skin, nose, throat, mouth, airways, digestive tract, urinary tract, vagina, eyes, ear canal and other surfaces. Some surfaces, such as the skin, have very thin mucosal membranes. Other surfaces, such as the digestive tract and airways, have thick mucosal membranes. Some surfaces are such that they are not typically referred to as mucosal, yet they are still categorized as mucosal membranes, as they are all linked together.

Let's take a moment and review the surfaces that have forms of mucosal membranes, starting from head to toe:

- Scalp
- Ears
- Eyes
- Nasal Cavity
- Sinuses
- Tongue
- Gums
- Oral cavity
- Trachea
- Esophagus
- Airways
- Alveoli
- Stomach
- Intestines
- Colon
- Rectum
- Anus
- Urethra
- Vagina
- Skin

MUCOSAL MEMBRANE HEALTH

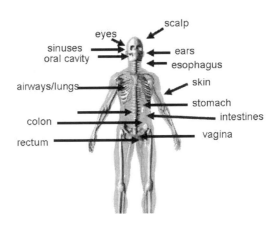

Did we miss anything? Yes. If we include the mucous membranes of many of our inner passageways epithelial cell linings, the list gets longer. These include blood vessel walls, bladder and so on. We can also include here nerve sheath linings, spinal cord lining, vertebral discs and more.

What are Mucosal Membranes Made of?

The mucosal membranes are thin layers of biochemicals produced by the body combined with probiotic bacteria. Most of the body's mucosal membranes are not the same from body region to body region either. Here is a short list of some of the contents of many of these regions:

- glycoproteins
- mucopolysaccharides
- enzymes
- probiotics
- T cells
- B cells
- Immunoglobulin-E
- Immunoglobulin-A

- ionic fluid, which includes ions of bicarbonate, calcium, magnesium, potassium, chloride, sodium and others
- many also contain antioxidant nutrients
- many contain other specialized elements specific to that particular area of the body

What is the Purpose for the Mucosal Membranes?

Each mucosal membrane provides specific functions. However, nearly all of them will also provide common purposes. Let's look at the common functions first:

Transporter Medium

Depending upon the type of mucosal membrane, this ionic fluid provides a transporter medium to escort nutrients and byproducts back and forth between the epithelial cells and the surface of the mucosal membrane. These elements include oxygen, nitrogen, carbon dioxide, hydrogen carbonate and others. In the intestines and stomach, the mucosal membranes also transport nutrients such as proteins, vitamins and others across, between the epithelial cells and the mucosal membrane surface.

Some of these—such as the sodium, bicarbonate and chloride ions—provide the transport mechanisms into the cells and tissues of the skin surfaces. These travel through openings or pores among the cells, attached to nutrients, oxygen and other elements—transporting them in, in other words.

This is critically important in the intestines and the stomach, where the mucosal membranes transport nutrients through the intestinal and stomach wall into the bloodstream.

But this does not mean the other membranes do not provide this service. The oral mucosal membranes also transport certain nutrients through to the bloodstream, especially under the tongue, for example. Also, the skin transports a variety of nutrients through to the epidermal layers of the skin. This also goes for the other membranes as well. Each type of membrane allows certain types of elements in, while blocking others.

Protecting the Cells

Another important function of the mucosal membranes is to protect the cells of the body from toxins, bacteria, fungi, viruses and any number of other elements that can harm the body. We'll focus more on the details of this function later.

Using the mucosal membranes, the body can be choosy about what kinds of elements it will allow into the epithelial cells and tissues. There are countless toxins, microorganisms, debris allergens and other foreigners that the body wants kept out.

So just how does the body keep these invaders from penetrating the body's internal and external surfaces? The short answer is the mucosal membranes. This is why these membranes contain a host of immune cells. These include immunoglobulins such as IgA, B-cells, T-cells and others that are looking to trap foreigners before they get any further. Once they find a foreigner, they will take it apart using one of many immune system strategies.

A Culture for Probiotics

The mucosal membranes also provide mediums—also called cultures—for the survival and sustenance of our body's probiotic species.

The mucous membranes are living structures. Probiotics populate our mucosal membranes, and are an important part of the "wall" of protection provided by these membranes. Tiny protective probiotic bacteria will inhabit all healthy mucosal membranes, including the skin. Like the immune system, these bacteria are trained to protect their territory. If an invading microorganism enters the mucosal membrane, the probiotics will lead an attack on them, with the immune cells in close pursuit.

Epithelial Flexibility

The mucosal membranes give the epithelial cells of the skin, scalp, oral cavity, intestines, stomach and so on their flexibility and their supple-ness. Without this, these tissues could not provide the body with the means to adjust to environmental conditions. It is critical that our skin is supple so that our internal organs and muscles can move from within.

It is also critical that our digestive tract is adjustable so that it can be amenable to swallowing and processing large quantities of food.

As for our airways, they need to be supple so they can expand and contract to inspiration and expiration.

We might compare this to how oil lubricates and protects an engine from overheating and dirt. The function is called viscosity. The mucosal membranes provide viscosity through the biochemicals called mucopolysaccharides and glycolipids. The later contains complexed fats, while the former contains long chain carbohydrates which allow surfaces to glide against each other.

Keeping the Epithelial Region Clean

In a well-maintained car, good motor oil will be circulated through the rods and cylinders. The oil doesn't just allow the steel parts to move with minimal friction: The motor oil also helps keep the engine clean, and prevents dirt and other contaminants from clogging up the system. Imagine what would happen if a car were to run without oil for a few miles? The engine would surely seize up, and likely would break down completely. While this is a crude example, there are several elements that are consistent.

This of course crosses over with the concept of protecting the cells as we just discussed. But killing off invaders is one thing, and keeping the region cleaned is quite another. Remember that our body's immune cells kill off microorganisms and break down toxins within the mucosal membranes. What is the result? A bunch of dead parts of bacteria, viruses, toxins and others floating around the region. Who wants a bunch of dead bacteria parts stuck to their body surfaces?

No one. This is why the mucosal membranes are fluid. Like any fluid body, mucosal membranes have motion and currents. They will thus circulate through the region, dumping out the dead body parts and toxin pieces, all while renewing the area with clean mucosal membrane fluids.

This is what happens when we sneeze, cough, blow our nose, or even breathe or sweat. During these activities, dirty mucosal fluid is being thrown off. In the meantime, the special glands replenish the area with new fluid.

Calming Reactivity

The chemistry of the mucosal membrane also buffers and calms immune response. The mucosal membrane will help transport components such as corticosteroids from the adrenals to squelch inflammatory immune responses among our epithelial tissues. In other words, a healthy mucosal membrane is calming to our digestive tract, airways, skin and so on.

Where Do the Mucosal Membranes Come From?

Later we'll discuss some of the other more specific functions of certain mucosal membranes. For now, let's answer this important question of where the mucosal membranes come from.

The mucosal membrane base fluid, with its glycoproteins, glycolipids and mucopolysaccharides, is secreted from specialized glands within the epithelial layer of cells. In many regions, these glands are called submucosal glands. In other regions, they are named for that particular region. For example in the oral cavity, the sublingual glands, parotid glands and submandibular glands provide saliva along with the mucosal membrane material. In the stomach, pyloric glands and gastric glands provide the fluids that make up the stomach's mucosal membranes. Let's look at a cross section of a couple of types of mucosal membranes to get a clearer picture:

MUCOSAL MEMBRANE HEALTH

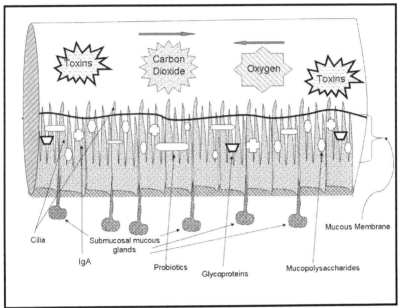

Airway Mucosal Membranes and Cilia

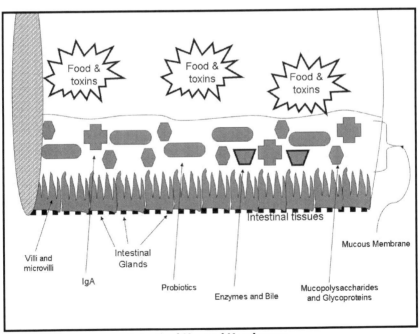

Intestinal Mucosal Membranes

Early Mucosal Membranes

Other than our skin, which has been covered by placenta fluid, our mucosal membranes are raw and not well developed at birth. Gradually, as probiotics begin to colonize the sinuses, mouth and intestines—the mucosal membranes begin to mature. This maturity, as we'll discuss in detail, requires a host of nutrients as well as strong probiotic populations in order to populate the mucosal membranes. As this colonization occurs, the body's epithelial cells and mucous glands provide their balance of chemistry and protective attributes.

This is the basis for the hygiene theory, a product of many studies showing that infants and children that are allowed to roam the floors, parks, soils, and those among larger families have stronger immune systems. This is because all that roaming allows our bodies to collect a variety of probiotic species, which eventually colonize and territorialize our mucosal membranes.

Then there is the transporter mechanism. The mucous membranes utilizes this surfactant quality and the ionic capabilities to transport nutrients among the epithelial cells, allowing them to function efficiently. It also transports toxins out of the area—assuming a healthy mucosal membrane.

Should this transport mechanism not be functioning properly, the region can become laden with a thickened, toxic mucous. Instead of the mucous membranes keeping these surfaces clean, the mucous itself becomes toxic.

This thickened mucous membrane is typical in hyperreactive airway responses among COPD, asthma, and hay fever conditions. In the intestines, the condition produces irritable bowel syndrome, colitis, Crohn's and other intestinal issues. In the lower esophagus and stomach, weakened mucosal membranes produces ulcers and acid reflux. And weakened skin mucosal membranes produce eczema, dermatitis, hives and other skin irritations.

Mucous is secreted by tiny mucous glands that lie within goblet cells scattered throughout these epithelia surfaces. They are called goblets because they are shaped like little goblet glasses, except their upper surface extends through the (internal) surfaces in tiny fingers. In the intestines and airways, they are called microvilli. On skin and other surfaces, they are pores. Yet all these function almost identically with respect to their production of mucous.

The goblet cells and their end points both produce mucin through a process of contraction and glycosylation within the Golgi apparatus of the cells. This glycosylation of proteins produces the glycoproteins that are the mainstay in mucin.

The mucosal goblet cells of the respiratory tract are also similar to the gastric cells of the stomach and duodenum. The difference here is that the gastric cells produce mucous fed by the pyloric glands in addition to the highly acidic gastrin. As we'll be discussing more at length throughout the remainder of the text, this similarity between the goblet cells, the villi and the gastric/pyloric cells facilitates an understanding of the mystery of GERD-related respiratory disorders.

The mucous membrane fluids can also become dehydrated if the ions that open the pores are blocked. Here the pores may be blocked due to an imbalance of ion chemistry in the sub-mucosal membrane. Tests have shown that chlorine and bicarbonate anions stimulate the opening of the pores that bring liquids into the mucous membrane. The mucin proteins produced by the submucosal membrane glands have to be diluted with these ion fluids to give the mucous membrane the right balance of stickiness and fluidity.

However, among dehydrated mucosal membranes, the mucous is thickened and not fluid enough to provide its surfactant and transport functions.

In addition, exposure to toxins, pathogenic microorganisms, cold air and any number of other triggers can stimulate the production of mucous by the goblet cells. In a healthy body, this causes the quick removal of the toxin or invader, as the excess mucous is swept out by the cilia or other drainage facilities of the surface.

However, should the body be immunosuppressed or otherwise overwhelmed by the invasion, the goblet cells will over-produce mucous, which can swamp the epithelial surfaces with dead cell parts and toxins. When these surfaces are drowning in mucous, the removal process is deficient. The lack of mucous transport, combined with the need to remove toxins, produces inflammation as the immune system must engage to remove the toxins.

Chapter Two
Critical Mucosal Membranes

Nearly every epithelial surface of the body is covered by mucosal membranes. We cannot give justice to all of these regions in this text. Instead, here we'll describe the major mucosal membrane areas and summarize some of the similarities of the other regions.

The regions we've chosen to discuss are some of the most critical mucosal membranes in the body. These are the ones, that if not kept healthy, will result in major health consequences.

This is not to say the others are not critical, however. Actually, defective mucosal membranes in any part of the body will result in a diseased condition.

Airway Mucosal Membranes

Mucous membranes cover all of the airways. Airway mucosal membranes contain a thin layer of glycoproteins (mucin), mucopolysaccharides, special enzymes, probiotics, immune cells and ionic fluid.

The ionic fluid provides a transporter medium, which escorts a host of elements back and forth between the airway cells and the surface of the mucosal membrane. These elements include chloride ions, sodium ions, oxygen, nitrogen, carbon dioxide, hydrogen carbonate and others.

These nutrients travel through openings or pores among the cells, transporting them in. In the case of the alveoli, carbon dioxide and other waste products will be transported the other way, from the airway cells to the mucosal membrane surface.

The body is choosy about what kinds of elements it will allow into the bloodstream from the airways. There are countless toxins, microorganisms, debris allergens and other foreigners that the airways need to keep out of the body.

This is where the mucosal membranes come in. The mucosal membranes, along with cilia, work to trap and remove invaders. The mucosal membrane contains IgA, B-cells, T-cells and other immune cells that attach to and break down foreigners before get any further. Once they find a foreigner, they will take it apart using one of many immune system strategies.

One of the most popular strategies is to destroy the intruder using biochemicals that break down the molecular structure of the toxin or microorganism. Once they are broken down, the cilia sweep out the dead body from the nose or mouth to be purged from the body.

Alternatively, the foreigner might be trapped by an immune cell and broken down within the fluids of the body, and escorted out through the body's lymphatic system or bloodstream.

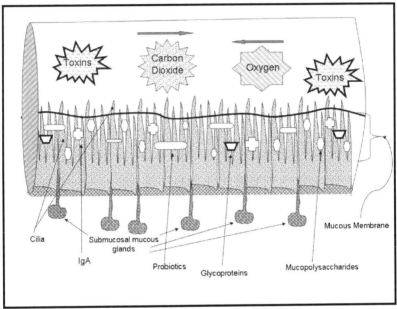

Airway Mucosal Membranes and Cilia

Probiotics are also an important part of this "wall" of protection. Tiny protective probiotic bacteria also inhabit a healthy mucosal membrane. Like the immune system, these bacteria are trained to protect their territory. If an invading microorganism enters the mucosal membrane, they will join the immune system's process of breaking them down to be escorted out of the body. We'll discuss more specifics on the probiotic immune system later.

The bottom line regarding the mucosal membrane is that the health of the fluids of the membrane determines the health of the airways. This is one of the prime reasons the airways become hypersensitive: Their protective coating has been diminished or altered in such a way that allows hostile elements to intrude upon the bronchial epithelial cells—stimulating the immune-inflammatory response that is seen in asthmatic episodes.

The chemistry of the mucosal membrane also buffers and calms immune response. The mucosal membrane will help transport components such as corticosteroids from the adrenals to squelch inflammatory immune responses. In other words, a healthy mucosal membrane is *calming* to the airways.

MUCOSAL MEMBRANE DISORDERS

The mucosal membranes within the respiratory tract are raw and not well developed at birth. Gradually, as probiotics begin to colonize the airways—along with the sinuses, mouth and intestines—the mucosal membrane begins to mature. This maturity, as we'll discuss in detail, requires a host of nutrients as well as strong probiotic populations in order to populate the mucosal membranes. As this colonization occurs, the body's epithelial cells and mucous glands provide a balance of chemistry.

We might compare this to how oil lubricates an engine. In a well-maintained car, good motor oil will be circulated through the rods and cylinders. The oil doesn't just allow the steel parts to move with minimal friction: The motor oil also helps keep the engine clean, and prevents dirt and other contaminants from clogging up the system. Imagine what would happen if a car were to run without oil for a few miles? The engine would surely seize up, and likely would break down completely.

While this is a crude example, there are several elements that are consistent. The lubrication ability of the mucous membrane allows the airways to remain flexible and responsive. This is accomplished by what is called the surfactant quality of mucous. This effectively reduces the surface tension of the epithelial cells.

Then there is the transporter mechanism. The mucous membrane utilizes this surfactant quality and ionic capabilities to transport nutrients among the airways epithelial cells, and the functional structures of the airways. It also transports toxins out of the area—assuming a healthy mucosal membrane.

Should this transport mechanism not be functioning properly, the respiratory airways will become laden with a thickened, toxic mucous. Instead of the mucous membrane keeping the area clean, the mucous itself becomes toxic to the airways, because it has not only thickened, but it has also become full with toxins.

This thickened mucous membrane is typical in hyperreactive asthma lung responses. They are also typical in hay fever, sinusitis, colds, bronchitis and pneumonia.

Mucous is secreted by tiny mucous glands that lie within goblet cells scattered throughout the epithelia of the bronchi, sinuses and other parts of the airways. They are called goblets because they are shaped like little goblet glasses, except their upper surface extends out in tiny fingers called microvilli. In fact, goblet cells within the airways are practically identical with the villi and microvilli of the intestines. They function almost identically with respect to their production of mucous.

The goblet cells and villi both produce mucin through a process of contraction and glycosylation within the Golgi apparatus of the cells. This glycosylation of proteins produces the glycoproteins that are the mainstay constituents of mucin.

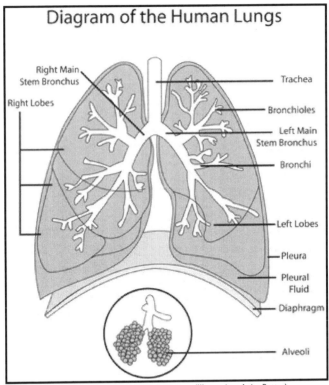

(Illustration: Anita Potter)

Oxygen is by far the greatest nutrient of the body. Oxygen is vital to the immune system and the operation of every organ and tissue system. Oxygen also helps provide an environment among the blood and tissues less hospitable to bacterial or viral invasion. With a poor supply of oxygen—whether caused by poor breathing habits, restricted airways, or contaminated air—the body operates at less than maximum efficiency, leaving our bodies subject to tissue damage resulting from acidosis.

The Alveoli Surfactant

The alveoli also maintain a special membrane. This is a special surfactant that helps transport oxygen and carbon dioxide across the alveoli tissue-blood barrier. This surfactant, produced by alveoli cells, provides hydrostatic surface that attracts water on one side and repels it on the other. This enables a process called *adsorption,* and promotes the transfer of gases between the alveoli membranes.

The key principle of this surfactant is the ability of oil to be separated from water. Special proteins made of lipids and phosphorus; called phospholipoproteins, enable this function. The core ingredient of the membrane is a phosphatidylcholine called dipalmitoylphosphatidylcholine. Phosphatidylcholine is also a key component of nerve cell membranes as well.

The bottom line is that alveoli are lined with these specialized cells, maintaining a semi-permeable surface—one that lets certain gases and fluids in, but theoretically keeps out toxins, bacteria and other intruders. This protection is accomplished by two components: a series of ion pores or channels, and the ionized surfactant containing hydrostatic phosphorlipoproteins.

However, during an inflammatory response, or a decrease in oxygen availability, this surfactant can thicken. This thickening can severely restrict the exchange of oxygen and carbon dioxide in the alveoli. An ongoing thickening can collapse the alveoli. This sometimes occurs in emphysema as well as asthmatic remodeling.

A longer-term result of thickened surfactant is the reduction of pulmonary capillaries. With reduced exchange, capillaries began to disappear.

This combination of thickened alveoli surfactant, and the resulting loss of alveoli surface area combined with capillary reduction, puts significant stress upon lung capacity. This can result in an increased need to breathe faster to prevent unconsciousness and brain damage.

Another mechanism that can take place within the alveoli is increased permeability among the pores. This can allow unwelcome toxins into the bloodstream. We'll discuss this increased permeability in more detail later.

We'll leave this important subject for now by adding that the health of the airway mucous membranes and alveoli surfactant directly relates to diet, stress, toxin load, exercise and the health of the immune system.

The Respiratory Cilia

The bronchial epithelial cells of the airway passages are also equipped with microscopic hairs called cilia (see previous and next drawing). The cilia act like tiny brooms: They undulate towards the exits—the sinuses, mouth and pharynx. The little hairs "sweep" out the mucous, together with toxins and dead cell parts caught in the mucous membrane.

The ciliary hairs lining the airways beat rhythmically with the expansion and release of the lungs. This expansion and contraction increases the mucous surfactant as well.

Should toxin particles remain airborne, they will also likely be moved out through breathing and rhythmic ciliary hair undulations in healthy airways.

The membrane and ciliary hair move in slow waves—very similar to what we see among kelp beds as they move with undulating ocean waves. This wave-like action of the ciliary hairs acts as an effective transport system.

This transport mechanism—the clearing of toxins and cell parts out of the area by the cilia—is called the *mucociliary clearance apparatus*. This is a self-cleaning system of the airways: Should these 'automatic sweepers' become caught in the thick mucous of a toxin-rich and/or ionically imbalanced mucous membrane—they become ineffective.

The mucociliary clearance apparatus explains how we will gather an accumulation of phlegm within the throat and sinuses. Most of us clear our throats or blow our noses without a second thought. Little do we realize that much of that phlegm is the result of the cilias' self-cleaning undulations that sweep out toxins and mucous. This sweeping mechanism also helps prevent polluted air and particles from being absorbed into our blood. Those particles not tossed out with the breath or mucous get phagotized (broken down) and swept out. Or they may be transported to the blood or lymph and escorted out of the body through the colon, urinary tract or sweat glands.

However, should the mucosal fluid not be healthy and ionically balanced, thickened mucous will build up within the mucosal membrane. This will overwhelm and in effect *drown* the ciliary hairs—making them far less effective for removing toxins and toxin-rich mucous.

The cilia are stabilized by being seated in a thin pool of thicker mucous, with another layer of thinner mucous on top. The thinner mucous towards the surface of the mucous membrane allows the hairs to undulate faster near and at the surface of the mucous membrane.

It is essential that these cilia are healthy, vibrant, and free of toxin-debris. This is why, as we'll explain, that tar and soot from smoking and pollution can wreck such havoc on the lungs. The tops of the cilia—and mucous—become jammed up in this gummy residue.

Cilia must also have a warm temperature in a moist atmosphere. Should cold, dry air get into the passages where these sensitive airway cilia dwell, they may shut down or become uncoordinated. The ultimate temperature for productive cilia is about 98.6 degrees F with 100% relative humidity. This doesn't mean that outdoor temperatures must be that. A temperature of nearly 100 degrees F with 100% humidity would be practically unbearable.

Rather, the cilia are kept warm and moist by the combination of body heat, the warming of the air as it travels through the sinus turbinates, and the secretion of warm mucous in the airways. Without healthy mucosal membranes, the cilia will also become damaged.

Inflammation, Breathing and Atmospheric Pressure

A worsening of asthma and hay fever has been linked with what is termed *airway remodeling*. This is when the lungs become altered due to a continuing inflammatory event. Chronic allergic rhinitis has been shown to cause upper airway remodeling (Salib and Howarth 2003).

Healthy lung capacity is critical to immune function.

The average lung capacity of an adult is about 6,000 cubic centimeters. When we breathe unconsciously while relaxed, we might breathe 500 to 700 cc in and out. Typically, about 1,200 to 1,500 cc will be left in the lungs during this breathing. If we should completely exhale, we have the capacity to move out 4,800 to 5,200 cc of air.

These numbers indicate that we can utilize our lungs better than we typically do. With better breathing, we will not only bring more oxygen into the bloodstream. We will also push out more stale, acidic carbon dioxide as we exhale. This lowers the carbolic acid and carbon dioxide levels in the bloodstream, allowing more oxygen to associate with hemoglobin. By bringing in more oxygen, more acidified H+-hemoglobin is replaced with oxygenated, alkalized hemoglobin.

The Intestinal Mucosal Membranes

Lining our intestines are walls that keep the contents of our intestines from pouring into our bloodstreams without control. These walls are very complex. They have various layers, made of different materials and densities. This is called the intestinal brush barrier.

In total, the brush barrier is a triple-filter that screens for molecule size, ionic nature and nutrition quality. Much of this is performed via four mechanisms existing between the intestinal microvilli: tight junctions, adherens junctions, desmosomes, and colonies of probiotics. The tight functions form a bilayer interface between cells, controlling permeability. Desmosomes are points of interface between the tight junctions and adherens junctions keep the cell membranes adhesive enough to stabilize the junctions. These junction mechanisms together regulate permeability at the intestinal wall.

The top layer of the intestinal brush barrier is a complex mucosal layer of mucin, enzymes, probiotics and ionic fluid. It forms a protective surface medium over the intestinal epithelium. It also provides an active nutrient transport mechanism.

This mucosal layer is stabilized by the grooves of the intestinal microvilli. It contains glycoproteins, mucopolysaccharides and other ionic transporters, which attach to amino acids, minerals, vitamins, glucose and fatty acids—carrying them across intestinal membranes. Meanwhile the transport medium requires a delicately pH-balanced mix of ionic chemistry able to facilitate this transport of useable nutrient.

Furthermore, the mucosal layer is policed by billions of probiotic colonies, which help process incoming food molecules, excrete various nutrients, and control pathogens.

MUCOSAL MEMBRANE HEALTH

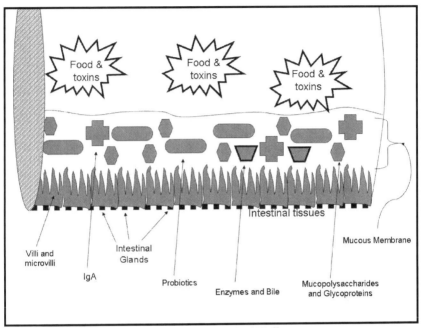

The Healthy Intestinal Wall

This mucosal brush barrier creates the boundary between intestinal contents and our intestinal cells. Should the chemistry of the mucosal layer become altered, its protective abilities become compromised. Its ionic transport mechanisms become weakened, allowing toxic or larger molecules to be presented to the intestinal wall—the microvilli junctions.

This contact of elements not normally presented to the intestinal wall can irritate the microvilli, causing a subsequent inflammatory response. This is now considered a contributing cause of IBS.

The breakdown of the mucosal membrane causes it to thin. This depletes the protection rendered by the mucopolysaccharides and glycoproteins, probiotics, immune IgA cells, enzymes and bile. This thinning allows toxins and macromolecules that would have been screened out by the mucosal membrane to be presented to the intestinal cells.

This mucous membrane thinning, intestinal cell irritation and inflammatory immune response cause desmosomes and tight junctions to open. These gaps now allow larger macromolecules to enter the tissues and bloodstream. These can include large food proteins, endotoxins from pathogenic yeasts and bacteria, and many other substances that have no business in the body.

The Intestinal Defense

The consensus of the research is that the gastrointestinal tract, from the mouth to the anus, is the primary defense mechanism against antigens as they enter the body. The mucous membrane integrity, the probiotic system, digestive enzymes, and the various immune cells and their mediators work together to orchestrate a "total defense" structure within the mucosal membrane. However, should this barrier be weakened or become imbalanced, hypersensitivity can result. The weaknesses in the barrier can be influenced by a number of factors, including toxins, diet, genetics, and environmental factors (Chahine and Bahna 2010).

In other words, poor dietary choices, toxin exposures and environmental forces related to lifestyle and living conditions can wear down and thin this mucosal membrane. Once the membrane is damaged, the intestinal cells become exposed to the foods and toxins we consume.

The intestines also have a microscopic barrier function. The tiny spaces between the intestinal epithelial cells—composed of villi and microvilli—are sealed from the general intestinal contents with what are called tight junctions. As we discussed earlier, should the tight junctions open up, this barrier or seal will be broken.

This results in increased intestinal permeability, as we've mentioned before.

When tight junctions are open—as they are normally in the bladder or the colon—the wrong molecules can cross the epithelium through a transcellular pathway. Researchers have found more than 50-odd protein species among the tight junction. Should any of these proteins fail due to exposure to toxins, the barrier can break down, giving access to what are called macromolecules—molecules that are larger than nutrients that the intestinal cells, liver and bloodstream are accustomed to. Once these macromolecules access the intestinal tissues, they can stimulate an immune response: an inflammatory reaction.

The epithelial mucosal immune system has two anti-inflammatory strategies: The first is to block invaders using antibodies, probiotics and acids. This controls microorganism colonies and inhibits new invasions. The body's immune response counteracts local and peripheral hypersensitivity by attempting to remove them before a full inflammation attack is launched. This is referred to as oral tolerance when it is stimulated in the intestines.

The biochemical constituents of the mucosal membrane (glycoproteins, mucopolysaccharides and so on) also attach and escort nutrients across the intestinal barrier, while resisting the penetration of unrecognized and potentially harmful agents. Intestinal permeability allows molecules that are normally not able to cross the intestines' epithelial barrier access to the bloodstream.

When the intricate balance between the intestinal epithelial layer is destroyed by exposure and inflammation, abnormal protein antigens gain access to the intestinal subepithelial compartment. Here they stimulate the release of immune cells and degranulation (Yu 2009). This produces what is commonly known as an allergic response.

Let's examine the research supporting these conclusions:

Louisiana State University researchers (Chahine and Bahna 2010) found that the intestinal wall uses specific immunologic factors to defend the body against antigens. They showed that integrity of the mucous membrane lining of the intestine is critical. A defective lining, on the other hand, leads to allergic responses and hypersensitivity reactions, according to their research. They named the cause of these *"defects in the gut barrier."*

Hungarian researchers (Kovács *et al.* 1996) tested intestinal permeability among 35 food allergic patients and 20 healthy controls. Intestinal permeability was determined using EDTA. Of the 35, increased intestinal permeability was determined in 29 of the food allergy patients. Of these 29, 21 volunteers were tested for intestinal permeability five years later. IgA antibody titers were increased, among wheat, soy and oat antigens. Significant correlations between intestinal permeability and IgA antibody titers was found, especially against soy and oat proteins.

French researchers (Bodinier *et al.* 2007) studied wheat proteins with patients with intestinal permeability syndrome. They compared the translocation of native wheat proteins with those in a pepsin-hydrolyzed state. They found that the native wheat proteins were crossing the intestinal cell layer, and were able to associate this with their allergic responses.

Hospital Saint Vincent de Paul researchers (Dupont *et al.* 1991) pointed out in their research that the extent of intestinal permeability depends upon the molecule size and the state of the intestinal mucosa. Some intestinal *"porosity,"* as the researchers put it, is normal. However, when macromolecules that were normally not allowed to enter the bloodstream gained entry—primarily protein macromolecules—this stimulated the immune system, according to their research.

Sinus and Nasal Mucosal Membranes

The sinuses and nasal region contain mucosal membranes that are very similar to the airways. In many ways they are even stronger and more resilient than the lower airway mucosal membranes. This is because they have more contact with the environment.

These mucosal membranes are exposed to colder and warmer air, more viruses, bacteria, viruses, pollens, molds and other possible irritants. Therefore, these membranes contain more sticky glycoproteins and mucopolysaccharides than the airways.

These areas also contain more probiotics and more immune cells in the sinuses, nasal cavities. This also goes for the oral mucosal membranes.

The nasal cavity contains a labyrinth of various canals and chambers that allow any air we breath to have plenty of contact with the mucous membranes and cilia of the nasal cavity. Here the air is warmed and humidified as we breathe in. The mucous membrane-lined passageways of the nasal cavity, along with the larynx and pharynx warm and moisten the air. They are our body's natural humidifier system.

It was only recently that researchers became aware that these various chambers housed more than mucous membranes and immune cells: They also hosted legions of probiotic colonies.

These probiotic colonies are saturated throughout the mucous membranes of a healthy person. Here they not only help identify invaders, but they launch their own attacks against invading bacteria, viruses and fungi. They will also translocate between different nasal cavities, the mouth, the pharynx and other regions of the respiratory system.

The ribs, or *concha*, of the nasal region also house olfactory bulbs. The bulbs are also positioned at the top of the sinus cavity on either side of the septum. They sit at the epithelium mucosa surface, where nerve fibers connect to the bulbs. These nerve fibers sense the waveform and polarity of odorous molecules traveling in the air as they interface with the mucosa of the nasal cavity. These 'odor-packets' traveling within and around gas and air molecules stimulate the nerves in the olfactory bulbs.

These olfactory nerve bulbs, collectively called the *vomeronasal organ* or VNO (also *Jacobson's organ*), may be stimulated on a more subtle level by pheromones. Pheromones carry and exchange information through the environment between living organisms. Pheromones have been shown to stimulate sexual and reproductive responses among animals, plants and insects. There is some debate as to whether humans also exchange pheromones. While humans have anatomical VNOs—known for pheromone exchanging in animals—significant nerve conduction has yet to be confirmed physically. The assumption has been that without obvious VNO nerve pathways there would be little chance of information conduction to responsive endocrine or cognitive mechanisms.

Consideration might be given to the work of a well-respected rhinologist Dr. Maurice Cottle. Dr. Cottle, known for his contribution towards the development of the electrocardiogram, invented a diagnostic machine in the mid-twentieth century called the *rhinomanometer*. Dr. Cottle wrote two books on the subject of rhinomanometry, and was a professor and head of Otolaryngology at the Chicago Medical School. Dr. Cottle was able to diagnose a number of ailments in other parts of the body simply by measuring the swelling or shrinking of the tissues and the airflow through the VNO.

The delicate turbinate membranes are more than mucous membranes: They are erectile, with thousands of tiny receptors. They respond to stimulation just as do other erectile regions. The turbinate erectile receptors respond to and coordinate airflow with the rest of the body. Clinical evidence demonstrated that Dr. Cottle's machine could accurately diagnose coronary heart disease, for example.

In reviewing the connection between oral bacteria and cardiovascular disease, we find that the inflammatory response stimulated by pathogenic bacteria through the NK-kappa mechanism could also be at the root of the phenomena Dr. Cottle observed. An inflamed turbinate and sinus area would likely be the result of an imbalance of pathogenic and probiotic bacteria, causing not only cardiovascular inflammation as has been shown in modern research, but the swelling of nasal membranes like the turbinates. This indicates a possible connection between turbinate responses and the body's various probiotic communications.

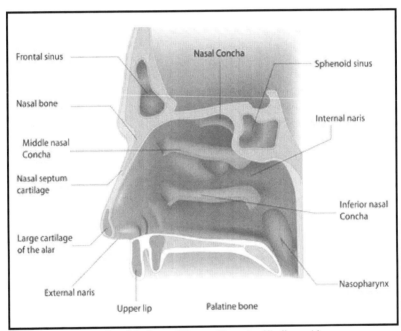

The Nasal Cavity and Sinuses (Illustration: Miro Kovacevic)

We can see the nasal concha and the turbinate regions from the rendering above. At the nasal entry, we see the atrium, then the middle and inferior meatus, separated by the concha inferior. Above these two chambers lie the septum meatus and then the sphenoidal sinus. These different passageways provide plenty of traps and filters to catch foreign particles and microorganisms. They also provide many warm and moist nesting areas for our probiotics.

Once foreigners such as pollens are trapped, these colonies of probiotics—along with our immunoglobulins and various immune cells—corner them and break them apart. This requires a vibrant, active immune system and strong probiotic colonies residing without the mucosal membranes that line these cavities.

Within the mouth, we also find various chambers and traps. The entire oral cavity is lined with mucous membranes that help trap microorganisms. Instead of cilia, however, the mouth has teeth, gums, and a big wet, scaly tongue to trap and block particles and microorganisms. Once trapped, these foreigners can be taken apart or controlled by probiotics and immune cells in a healthy body. Take a look at all these crevices:

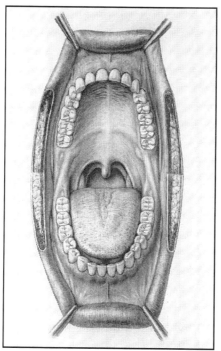

The Oral Cavity

Along with probiotic colonies, all of the oral, nasal and pharangeal mucosal membranes house immune cells and immunoglobulins Here we find legions of IgA and B-cells—along with IgE to a relative degree. These scan and identify particles and microorganisms that might slip past our probiotics and enter the body. When they discover potentially harmful organisms or toxins, they lock onto them in an attempt to break them apart and rid them from the body before they can penetrate our tissues.

Thus, we find, between the probiotics and immune cells, a 'drag net' of sorts within the oral and nasal cavities.

Under the tongue are salivary glands. They produce amylase. Amylase is an enzyme that breaks down starches into simple sugars. This is one reason the body is driven to eat starches. Taking our time and chewing a little more liquefies our food and mixes them with important mucus and enzymes. The mouth contains several parotid glands, located in the jaw behind the ears. As we chew, the parotid glands are stimulated, releasing B-cells and T-cells into the blood, mucous and lymphatic pathways. This gives the oral cavity and mouth more protection against foreigners that might try to slip in through our drag net.

Nasal Neuropeptides and the Stuffy Nose

The mechanisms for the stuffy, runny and blocked nose have eluded many physicians and researchers over the years. Here the mucous membranes have become thick and sticky, and the nasal passages become swollen. Recent evidence points to a collection of neuropeptides located among the sensory, sympathetic and parasympathetic nerves. These include tachykinins, substance P, neurokinin A, calcitonin gene-related peptides (CGRPs), vasoactive intestinal peptides (VIPs), and neuropeptide Y (NPY). These are primarily sensory neuron peptides.

Some of these are interactive. Substance P, for example, increases vascular permeability. Vascular permeability opens the tissues to a greater release of immune factors that cause inflammation. Substance P also stimulates the release of inflammatory factors. This has been seen following the binding to the neurokinin-1 receptor (NK-1R). Together, these responses increase swelling and restrict airflow.

Tachykinins are sensitive to allergen exposure, and they can stimulate the release of substance P. The other neuropeptides like VIPs and CGRPs can act similarly, but stimulating inflammation and vascular permeability.

MUCOSAL MEMBRANE DISORDERS

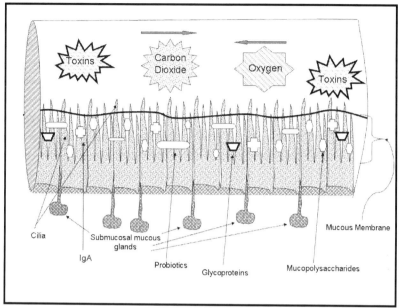

Nasal Mucosal Membranes

Probiotics are also an important part of this "wall" of protection. Tiny protective probiotic bacteria also inhabit a healthy nasal mucosal membrane. Like the immune system, these bacteria are trained to protect their territory. If an invading microorganism enters the mucosal membrane, they will face the immune system's process of breaking them down to be escorted out of the body.

The bottom line regarding the mucosal membrane is that the health of this membrane is crucial to the health of the sinuses. This is one of the prime reasons the airways become hypersensitive in the first place: Their protective coating has been diminished or altered in such a way that allows potential allergens to intrude upon the epithelial cells—stimulating the inflammatory response relating to IgE.

A healthy chemistry among our mucosal membranes buffers and calms immune response. Healthy mucosal membranes contain circulating IgAs that prevent foreigners from accessing our tissues and becoming marked as toxins or allergens by the immune system.

The mucosal membrane will also help transport components such as corticosteroids from the adrenals to squelch inflammatory immune responses. In other words, a healthy mucosal membrane is *calming* to the sinuses.

At birth, the mucosal membranes within our airways are raw and not well developed. Gradually, as probiotics begin to colonize the airways—along with the sinuses, mouth and intestines—the mucosal membrane begins to mature. This maturity, as we'll discuss in detail, requires a host of nutrients as well as stimulated probiotic populations in order to populate the mucosal membranes. As this colonization occurs, the body's epithelial cells and mucous glands provide a balance of chemistry.

We might compare this to how oil lubricates an engine. In a well-maintained car, good motor oil will be circulated through the rods and cylinders. The oil doesn't just allow the steel parts to move with minimal friction: The motor oil also helps keep the engine clean, and prevents dirt and other contaminants from clogging up the system. Imagine what would happen if a car were to run without oil for a few miles. The engine would surely seize up, and likely would break down completely.

While this is a crude example, there are several elements that are consistent. The lubrication ability of the mucous membrane allows the airways to remain flexible and responsive. This is accomplished by what is called the surfactant quality of mucous. This effectively reduces the surface tension of the epithelial cells.

Then there is the transporter mechanism. The mucous membrane utilizes this surfactant quality and ionic capabilities to transport nutrients among the airways epithelial cells, and the functional structures of the airways. It also transports toxins out of the area—assuming a healthy mucosal membrane.

Should this transport mechanism not be functioning properly, the respiratory airways will become laden with a thickened, toxic mucous. Instead of the mucous membrane keeping the area clean, the mucous itself becomes toxic to the airways, because it has not only thickened, but it has also become full with toxins.

This thickened mucous membrane is typical in hyperreactive inflammatory conditions that include hay fever, sinusitis, colds, bronchitis, asthma and pneumonia.

Mucous is secreted by tiny mucous glands that lie within goblet cells scattered throughout the epithelia of the bronchi, sinuses and other parts of the airways. They are called goblets because they are shaped like little goblet glasses, except their upper surface extends out in tiny fingers called microvilli. In fact, goblet cells within the airways are practically identical with the villi and microvilli of the intestines. They function almost identically with respect to their production of mucous.

The goblet cells and villi both produce mucin through a process of contraction and glycosylation within the Golgi apparatus of the sells. This glycosylation of proteins produces the glycoproteins that are the mainstay in mucin.

As mentioned earlier, the mucosal goblet cells of the respiratory tract are also similar to the gastric cells of the stomach and duodenum. The difference here is that these produce mucous fed by the pyloric glands in addition to the highly acidic gastrin. As we'll be discussing more at length throughout the remainder of the text, this similarity between the goblet cells, the villi and the gastric/pyloric cells facilitates an understanding of the mystery of GERD-related allergic asthma.

The mucous membrane fluids can also become dehydrated if the ions that open the pores are blocked or nutritionally unavailable. Here the pores may be blocked due to an imbalance of ion chemistry in the sub-mucosal membrane. Tests have shown that chlorine and bicarbonate anions stimulate the opening of the pores that bring liquids into the mucous membrane. The mucin proteins produced by the submucosal membrane glands have to be diluted with these ion fluids to give the mucous membrane the right balance of stickiness and fluidity.

In dehydrated mucosal membranes, the mucous is too thick and not viscous enough to provide its surfactant and transport functions.

In addition, exposure to allergens, toxins, cold air and any number of other triggers can stimulate the production of mucous by the goblet cells. In a healthy body, this stimulates the quick removal of the toxin or invader, as the excess mucous is swept out by the cilia.

However, should the body be immunosuppressed or otherwise overwhelmed by an invasion, the goblet cells will over-produce mucous, which can swamp the cilia along with dead cell parts and toxins. When the cilia are drowning in mucous, they cannot do their job. The lack of mucous transport, combined with the need to remove a toxin, is typically accompanied by the constriction of the airways, which may protect the airways from more toxins, but also further prevents the toxins in the mucous from being cleared out.

This combination of nasal airway constriction and mucous overload is the mainstay of the allergic rhinitis episode.

This link between the health of the mucosal membranes of the sinuses and airways was illustrated in research from Britain's National Heart and Lung Institute and the Imperial College and Royal Brompton Hospital (Niimi *et al.* 2004). Here 50 patients with chronic coughing, concurrent with asthma, postnasal drip, rhinitis and gastroesophageal reflux related to the coughing were studied. The pH and chloride levels of their condensed breathing were measured. The researchers found that compared with healthy subjects, all of these coughing patients had significantly lower pH levels, indicating an acidic condition among their mucous membranes, along with lower chloride levels. The researchers concluded: *"The epithelial lining fluid of patients with chronic cough has a reduced pH and reduced chloride levels which could contribute to the enhanced cough reflex."*

Skin Membranes

The skin maintains a very thin yet active mucosal membrane. The skin is composed of layers of epidermis cells, also called epithelium. The top layer—or strata—is the corneum. Under the stratum corneum lie the dermal layer cells.

This skin's mucosal membrane is produced by a combination of glands that secrete substances that combine to form an acidic pH that will repel microorganisms and toxins. It also serves to keep the skin moist, flexible and supple. The glands responsible for this membrane include the apocrine and eccrine sweat glands, the sebaceous glands, and the hair follicles.

The sebaceous glands produce a substance called sebum, which is deposited into the hair follicles. These draw the sebum up and onto the skin surface. The sebum also lines the hair. Sebum is an oily, waxy substance. Sebum is what typically makes the skin and the hair feel oily.

Apocrine sweat glands produce a fluid that provides moisture and protection to the skin surface. Most apocrine sweat glands feed into the hair follicles. The fluid has no odor until it comes into contact with the bacteria on the surface of the skin.

The skin's microorganisms are quite hardy. There are several species that typically dwell on the skin, including *Corynebacterium diphtheriae, Pseudomonas aeruginosa, Staphylococcus aureus, Staphylococcus epidermidis* and *Saccharomyces boulardii.* Some of these can cause infections should they grow to large colonies, but when they are balanced by other species and the skin's pH, they actually serve to protect the body from other invaders.

Some of these bacteria also produce the odor from sweat. Sweat produced by the sweat glands is typically odorless when it arrives on the skin. But once on the skin, the microorganisms begin to eat it, and the odor is their waste products.

A number of studies have shown that supplementing with probiotics can help.

For example, researchers from Italy's University G. D'Annunzio (Di Marzio *et al.* 2003) applied sonicated *Streptococcus thermophilus* cream to the forearms of 11 patients with atopic dermatitis for two weeks. This led to a significant increase of skin ceramide levels, and a significant improvement of their clinical signs and symptoms—including erythema, scaling and pruritus.

Stomach Mucosal Membranes

The stomach is also lined with a mucosal membrane. This is often overlooked by physicians and others who diagnose gastric complaints and ulcers. The stomach's cells, often called gastric cells or stomach mucosa, are epithelial cells like many others around the body.

These mucosa cells have pits that are also called gastric pits. The pits have pores in them, which secrete acids and enzymes. There are several glands that produce these acids and enzymes.

The gastric glands of the parietal cells of the stomach produce gastrin, an acid primarily consisting of hydrochloric acid (HCl).

Special glands intertwined among stomach cells secrete a mixture of biochemicals. This blend is composed primarily of hydrochloric acid, pepsin, rennin and a special mucus—made primarily of mucopolysaccharides. To varying degrees, the stomach also secretes lipase, a fat-splitting enzyme. The enzymes pepsin and rennin break down proteins, preparing them for intestinal assimilation.

Healthy gastric juice is critical. Its pH must range from about 1 to 3. Hydrochloric acid (HCL) is the main component for pH control. An acidic pH is critical to sterilize our food. Without enough HCL, we run the risk of allowing various unwanted bacteria into the stomach and intestines. One of these is Helicobacter pylori. Recent research has connected H. pylori overgrowths in the stomach to a majority of ulcers.

Intestinal Immunity

The intestines utilize non-specific, humoral, cell-mediated and probiotic immunity to protect intestinal tissues from larger peptides, toxins and invading microorganisms. This is all packaged nicely into the mucosal membrane that lines the intestines—also referred to as the intestinal brush barrier.

The intestinal brush barrier is a complex mucosal layer of mucin, enzymes, probiotics and ionic fluid. It forms a protective surface medium over the intestinal epithelium. It also provides an active nutrient transport mechanism. This mucosal layer is stabilized by the grooves of the intestinal microvilli. It contains glycoproteins, mucopolysaccharides and other ionic transporters, which attach to amino acids, minerals, vitamins, glucose and fatty acids—carrying them across intestinal membranes. Meanwhile the transport medium requires a delicately pH-balanced mix of ionic chemistry able to facilitate this transport of useable nutrient. The mucosal layer is policed by billions of probiotic colonies, which help process incoming food molecules, excrete various nutrients, and control pathogens.

The brush barrier is a triple-filter that screens for molecule size, ionic nature and nutrition quality. Much of this is performed via four mechanisms existing between the intestinal microvilli: tight junctions, adherens junctions, desmosomes, and colonies of probiotics. The tight functions form a bilayer interface between cells, controlling permeability. Desmosomes are points of interface between the tight junctions, and adherens junctions keep the cell membranes adhesive enough to stabilize the junctions. These junction mechanisms together regulate permeability at the intestinal wall.

This mucosal brush barrier creates the boundary between intestinal contents and our bloodstream. Should the mucosal layer chemistry become altered, its protective and ionic transport mechanisms become weakened, allowing toxic or larger molecules to be presented to the microvilli junctions. This contact can irritate the microvilli, causing a subsequent inflammatory response. This is now considered a contributing cause of IBS.

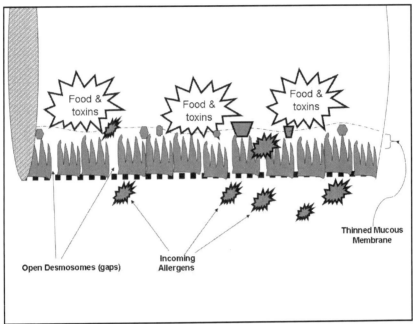

The Unhealthy Intestinal Wall

The breakdown of the mucosal membrane causes it to thin. This depletes the protection rendered by the mucopolysaccharides and glycoproteins, probiotics, immune IgA cells, enzymes and bile. This thinning allows toxins and macromolecules that would have been screened out by the mucosal membrane to be presented to the intestinal cells.

This mucous membrane thinning, intestinal cell irritation and inflammatory immune response cause desmosomes and tight junctions to open. These gaps allow food macromolecules to enter the tissues.

Chapter Three
Some Disorders Caused by Weakened Mucosal Membranes

Epithelial Permeability

When the mucosal membranes become defective, the epithelial cells become directly exposed to numerous toxins, microorganisms and allergens. This exposure in turn will irritate and damage these epithelial cells. This is the central mechanism involved in so many conditions related to the digestive tract, the airways, the sinuses, the skin, the vagina and even many internal epithelial regions including the urinary tract and others.

As the epithelial cells become exposed to foreigners, they will typically become damaged. This damage consists typically of the cell membranes of these cells being corrupted. This corruption results in an increase in permeability—which allows the wrong things through the cell membrane. This in turn inflames the cell, and the immune system (T-cells) marks that cell as damaged, and launches an inflammatory attack against the cells that have been so damaged.

This in turn produces inflammation among those cells, the immune system works to actually destroy and remove those cells so they can be replaced by new (hopefully undamaged) ones.

This process, by the way, has been labeled as autoimmunity. Autoimmunity is described as the body's immune system "attacking its own cells." While this is true from a functional basis, it is only because these cells have been damaged through exposure to toxins, microorganisms and/or allergens. In other words, the immune system is not launching an inflammatory response against cells of the epithelial region just because it doesn't like those cells or something. No. The cells have been damaged, and need to be removed from the body.

The result of this inflammatory process is that the spaces in between these epithelial cells—which are supposed to protect the internal tissues and bloodstream from intruders—open up. When they open up, gaps are created. These gaps allow the entry of microorganisms, toxins and allergens into the body's tissues, causing the body to launch a systemic inflammatory response against these intruders.

These systemic inflammatory responses—and the incoming toxins themselves—produce a variety of conditions, including allergies, asthma, arthritis and others.

This permeability among the epithelial layers can occur within the linings of the mouth, the sinus cavity, the airways, the stomach, the urinary tract, the intestines and other areas. In the nasal and sinus cavity, the result is often allergies to pollens, molds and other foreigners. In the airways, the result is often COPD, asthma and other lung conditions. In the intestines, the result is often intestinal permeability, with the inflammatory condition resulting in IBS, Crohn's, polyps and other intestinal conditions.

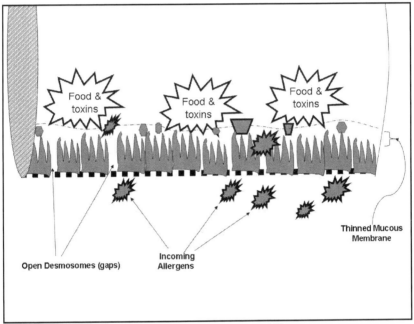

Increased Intestinal Permeability

Increased intestinal permeability has specifically been linked with a variety of disorders.

French researchers (Heyman and Desjeux 2000) found that not only can intestinal permeability cause various disorders, these conditions in turn can worsen intestinal permeability. The researchers found out that as undigested food antigens are transported through the intestinal wall, the immune system launches an inflammatory response. Intact proteins and large peptides, they pointed out, stimulate inflammation among the mucosa of the intestinal wall. IFN gamma and TNF alpha are cytokines that are often part of this inflammatory response. These two—IFN gamma and TNF alpha—also so happen to increase the further opening of the tight junctions.

Researchers from Brazil's Federal Fluminense Medical School (Soares *et al.* 2004) studied the associations between IBS and food intolerance. The researchers used 43 volunteers divided into three groups: an IBS group, a dyspepsia group, and a group without gastrointestinal difficulties. All test subjects were given skin prick tests for nine food allergens. The IBS group presented the highest level of positive allergen responses. The researchers concluded that, *"The higher reactivity to food antigens in group I compared to groups II and III suggests that intestinal permeability may be increased in patients with IBS."*

Researchers (Forget *et al.* 1985) tested intestinal permeability using EDTA in ten normal adults, eleven healthy children, seven children with acute gastroenteritis, and eight infants with eczema. They found significantly greater intestinal permeability among those with either gastroenteritis or eczema.

Researchers from Paris' Cochin-St Vincent de Paul Hospital (Kalach *et al.* 2001) studied 64 children with cow's milk allergy symptoms, and found that higher intestinal permeability levels were also associated with anemia.

Researchers from London's Middlesex Medical School tested intestinal permeability among eight patients with food-intolerance using EDTA testing. While fasting levels were normal, after they ate the sensitive foods, permeability levels changed some, but not that significantly.

Researchers from Paris' Saint-Vincent de Paul Hospital (Barau and Dupont 1990) tested intestinal permeability using the lactulose and mannitol test with 17 children with irritable bowel syndrome (IBS). Of the 17, nine tested positive to IgE food allergies. Among these, permeability levels increased when the children were given foods they were sensitive to, illustrating the link between IBS, food allergies and intestinal permeability among many IBS sufferers.

Russian researchers (Sazanova *et al.* 1992) studied 122 children, four months old to six years old with food intolerances. Symptoms included atopic dermatitis among 52 children, and chronic diarrhea among 70 children. They found antibodies to food antigens among all the children. They also found chronic gastroduodenitis (duodenum and stomach inflammation) among every child with atopic dermatitis and among 95% of those with chronic diarrhea. They observed that lactase deficiencies and microorganism growth in the duodenum increased the levels of intestinal permeability and subsequent allergy response.

Inflammation coordinates the various immune players into a frenzy of healing response. This is a good thing. Imagine for a moment cutting your finger pretty badly. First you would feel pain—letting you know the body is hurt. Second, you will probably notice that the area has become swollen and red. Blood starts to clot around the area. Soon the cut stops bleeding. The blood dries and a scab forms. It remains red, maybe a little hot, and hurts for a while. After the healing proceeds, soon the cut is closed up and there is a scab left with a little redness around it. The pain soon stops. The scab falls off and the finger returns to normal—almost like new and ready for action.

Without this inflammatory process, we might not even know we cut our finger in the first place. We might keep working, only to find out that we had bled out a quart of blood on the floor. Without clotting, it would be hard to stop the bleeding. And without some continuing pain, we would be more likely to keep injuring the same spot, preventing it from healing.

Were it not for our immune system and inflammatory process slowing blood flow, clotting the blood, scabbing and cleaning up the site, our bodies would simply be full of holes and wounds. Our bodies simply could not survive injury.

The probiotic system and immunoglobulin immune system work together to deter and kill particular invaders—hopefully before they gain access to the body's tissues. Should these defenses fail, they can stimulate the humoral immune system in a strategic attack that includes identifying antigens and recognizing their weaknesses. B-cells and probiotics coordinate through the stimulation of immunoglobulins and CDs.

This progression also stimulates an activation of neutrophils, phagocytes, immunoglobulins, leukotrienes and prostaglandins. Should cells become infected, they will signal the immune system from paracrines located on their cell membranes. Once the intrusion and strategy is determined, B-cells will surround the pathogens while T-cells attack any infected cells. Natural killer T-cells may secrete chemicals into infected cells, initiating the death of the cell.

Leukotrienes immediately gather in the region of injury or infection, and signal to T-cells to coordinate efforts in the process of repair. Prostaglandins initiate the widening of blood vessels to bring more T-cells and other repair factors (such as plasminogen and fibrin) to the infected or injured site. Histamine opens the blood vessel walls to allow all these healing agents access to the injury site to clean it up.

Prostaglandins also stimulate substance P within the nerve cells, initiating the sensation of pain. At the same time, thromboxanes, along with fibrin, drive the process of clotting and coagulation in the blood, while constricting certain blood vessels to decrease the risk of bleeding.

In the case where the pathogen is an allergen, the inflammation response will also accompany an H1-histamine response. As mentioned earlier, histamine is primarily produced by the mast cells, basophils and neutrophils after being stimulated by IgE antibodies. This opens blood vessels to tissues, which stimulates the processes of sneezing, watering of the eyes and coughing. These measures, though sometimes considered irritating, are all stimulated in an effort to remove the toxin and prevent its re-entry into the body. As histamine binds with receptors, one of the resulting physiological responses is alertness (also why antihistamines cause drowsiness). These are natural responses to help the body and mind remain vigilant in order to avoid further toxin intake.

At the height of the repair process, swelling, redness and pain are at their peak. The T-cells, macrophages, neutrophils, fibrin and plasmin all work together to purge the allergen from the body and repair the damage.

As macrophages continue the clean up, the other immune cells begin to retreat. Antioxidants like glutathione will attach to and transport the byproducts—broken down toxins and cell parts—out of the body. As this proceeds, prostaglandins, histamines and leukotrienes begin to signal a reversal of the inflammation and pain process.

One of the central features of the normalization process is the production of bradykinin. Bradykinin slows clotting and opens blood vessels, allowing the cleanup process to accelerate. A key signalling factor is the production of nitric oxide (NO). NO slows inflammation by promoting the detachment of lymphocytes to the site of infection or toxification, and reduces tissue swelling. NO also accelerates the clearing out of debris with its interaction with the superoxide anion. NO was originally described as endothelium-derived relaxing factor (or EDRF)—because of its role in relaxing blood vessel walls.

The body produces more nitric oxide in the presence of good nutrition and lower stress. Probiotics also play a big role in nitric oxide production in a healthy body. Lactobacilli such as *L. plantarum* have in fact been shown to remove the harmful nitrate molecule and use it to produce nitric oxide (Bengmark *et al.* 1998). This is beneficial to not only reducing inflammation: NO production also creates a balanced environment for increased tolerance.

Low nitric oxide levels also happen to be associated with a plethora of diseases, including diabetes, heart failure, high cholesterol, ulcerative colitis, premature aging, cancers and many others. Low or abnormal NO production is also seen among lifestyle habits such as smoking, obesity, and living around air pollution.

The intestinal cells are often damaged first by other toxins, resulting in an inflammatory cascade. Once the intestine's cells are damaged, macromolecules/allergens can enter the system through the damaged intestinal wall.

Thus IIPS is usually the result of two events: The first being an inflammatory process responding to an injury to the cells of the intestinal wall. These cells can be damaged by an assortment of toxins, poor dietary choices, microorganism pathogens, stress, smoking, alcohol, pharmaceuticals and toxins. Food macromolecules or allergens can also produce this damage to the cells of the intestinal walls.

Once the cells of the intestinal wall are damaged, the immune system will launch an inflammatory injury response through the T-cell system as described earlier. The T-cells will "repair" the problem by killing off these intestinal cells. This is often described as an autoimmune issue, but in reality, the T-cells are responding to real damage of toxins to these cells. They are not confusing "self" with "non-self."

While this damage and response is active, the intestinal cell wall barrier is altered. This alteration creates further increased intestinal permeability. Now large molecules (macromolecules) and/or allergens may readily enter the tissues and bloodstream, stimulating the IgE-histamine allergic immune response and/or other physiological and immune responses that produce allergies and other types of inflammation.

Allergies and Increased Intestinal Permeability

Once permeability is increased in the intestinal tract, there is no telling what the immune system will begin responding to. At this point it is likely that the immune system is greatly burdened by the many strange and different molecular structures now gaining entry into internal tissues and the bloodstream. What is known is that once permeability is increased, a self-perpetuating cycle of increased permeability and immune response produces more intestinal dysfunction and more immune response (Heyman 2005).

Researchers from Ontario's McMaster University (Berin *et al.* 1999) studied the role of cytokines in intestinal permeability. They found that interleukin-4 (IL-4) increased intestinal permeability and increased horseradish peroxidase (HRP) transport through intestinal walls. They found that IL-4 was inhibited by the soy nutrient genistein, and anti-IL-4 antibodies also reduced the HRP transport. The researchers concluded that: *"We speculate that enhanced production of IL-4 in allergic conditions may be a predisposing factor to inflammation by allowing uptake of luminal antigens that gain access to the mucosal immune system."*

Research has indicated that CD23 encourages the transport of intestinal IgE and allergens across intestinal epithelium. This opens a gateway for antigen-bound IgE to move across (transcytose) the intestinal cells. This sets up the immune response of histamine and atopic environmental conditions (Yu 2009).

Researchers from the University of Cincinnati College of Medicine (Groschwitz *et al.* 2009) determined that mast cells are critical to the regulation of the intestinal barrier function. The type and condition of the mast cells seems to affect the epithelial migration through intestinal cells.

Researchers from the Cincinnati Children's Hospital Medical Center (Forbes *et al.* 2008) found that interleukin-9 appears to help stimulate, along with mast cells, increased intestinal permeability. The researchers found that this *"IL-9- and mast cell-mediated intestinal permeability"* activated conditions for food allergen sensitization.

French INSERM researchers (Desjeux and Heyman 1994) concluded that increased protein permeability in milk allergies follows what they called *abnormal immunological response*. This abnormal immune response, they observed, leads to general mucosal and systemic inflammation.

Asthma and Airway Mucosal Health

The medical term for asthma is *airway hyperresponsiveness* or *bronchial hyperresponsiveness*—also abbreviated as AHR or BHR. Here the airways, which include the lungs and bronchi, become inflamed and irritated, producing airway hypersensitivity. This causes the airway passages that bring air in and out of our lungs to narrow. In minor responses, this produces what some describe as *wheezing*. In more severe episodes, an extreme shortness of breath becomes evident.

The narrowing of the breathing passages is predicated by *bronchoconstriction*. Bronchoconstriction is characterized by a contraction of the smooth muscles surrounding the breathing passages. This contraction is driven by acetylcholine receptors that lie on the smooth muscle fibers. Once these receptors are switched on, the muscles contract and clamp down on the airways. This narrows the breathing passages.

At the same time, mucous builds up in the airways. This mucous becomes thicker and gummier. This inhibits the draining of the mucous membranes in the airways, further reducing the airway passages.

In severe cases, this inflammatory narrowing of the breathing passages can bring about an extended period of chest tightness and gasping for air while struggling to breathe. This is often referred to as a *bronchospasm*. This can become a life-threatening situation, which is often treated with epinephrine and other anti-inflammatory medications.

As we'll discuss in more detail later, this inflammatory narrowing is a reactionary event, which can come from environmental exposures, something consumed, exercise or even stress. The frequency and severity of these bronchospasms depends largely on the underlying condition, as we'll describe shortly.

In general, there are two broad categories of asthma. These are related to their pattern of response to triggers. The first is called *intrinsic* and the other is called *extrinsic* asthma. However, these categories are rather superficial, as we'll describe further.

Atopic Extrinsic Asthma

Extrinsic asthma is also called *atopic* because it is typically triggered by environmental or allergen factors, which provoke a type of immune system response.

Atopy is used frequently among doctors and scientists to describe food allergy responses. What does atopy mean? Atopy is derived from the Greek word meaning *"unusual"* or *"not ordinary."* Atopic is used to describe the condition where a person is reacting to a substance in a manner unrelated to the form of contact with the substance.

For example, a normal response to breathing in some dust is to sneeze. This response is normal for removing dust. But if suddenly, rashes break out all over the body, even on the legs, the reaction becomes more than a normal physiological response: It becomes atopic.

An atopic response is also an extraordinary response with symptom severity outside the realm of typical responses for such an exposure. In the case of atopic asthma, the immune system is triggered by antigens that engage antibodies such as immunoglobulin E (IgE). This engagement with IgE produces what is called a *mediated response*.

This type of IgE response is outside the ordinary IgA response, which expels foreigners before they penetrated the body's tissue systems. The allergen interacts with IgE, and the body produces inflammatory mediators such as histamine, prostaglandins and leukotrienes. These stimulate the inflammatory response, resulting in a constriction of airways and a thickened mucous membrane.

Nearly half of asthmatic responses are considered atopic. For example, researchers from the National Institute of Allergy and Infectious Diseases (Gergen *et al.* 2009) used the National Health and Nutrition Examination Survey (2005-2006) to determine the incidence of IgE-related asthma. Using this huge database of thousands of asthmatics, they found that IgE-related atopy was present in 42.5% of current asthmatics.

Atopy can also cause a variety of other hypersensitivity symptoms, including hives, rashes, itchiness and sinus congestion. Atopic reactions are typically seen among the epithelial layers and mucosal membranes. These are expressed as asthma, allergic rhinitis, conjunctiva rhinitis, and even eosinophilic esophagitis.

Again, these responses are all outside of what would be expected in a healthy immune system. For example, dust or smog might cause sneezing or mild coughing in a normal immune system, while a hypersensitive response can invoke asthma symptoms.

As we'll investigate further, extrinsic asthma is typically triggered by pollen, dust, molds, animal dander, cigarette smoke, smog, food and airborne chemicals. We'll discuss these triggers in more detail later.

Intrinsic, Non-Atopic Asthma

Intrinsic asthma is also called non-atopic because the defect in the airways and immune response already exists. In other words, there is an internal defect that triggers the asthma response, rather than an external allergen that stimulates a mediated release of inflammatory factors. In the intrinsic model, the airways, nervous system and bronchial muscles are in one way or another functionally damaged, and this weakened physiology facilitates the hypersensitive response.

Note that this intrinsic response can still be triggered by environmental elements— such as dust, smog and chemicals—that also can produce allergens and stimulate the atopic response. Exercise, infections and emotional issues can also trigger the intrinsic asthmatic episode. A pure intrinsic response, however, does not usually accompany the degranulation of mast cells related to IgE.

In other words, the intrinsic asthmatic response works much like a reflex. Reflexive actions by the respiratory system are usually categorized as sympathetic. This is because the body's nervous system and adrenal system is responding to a perceived threat with a fight-or-fight type of response. The sympathetic nervous system responds out of proportion to the threat because the physiologies of the airways, immune system and nerves have become dysfunctional.

We might compare this with how small dogs tend to bark the loudest. Why do they need to bark so loud? Because they need to compensate for their lack of size. In the same way, a part of the body that is under duress will respond more urgently because it is more vulnerable.

Mixed Asthma Response

Of course, there may be dysfunctional physiology and an atopic, allergenic response at the same time. This is referred to as mixed asthma because the physiology of the airways, nervous system and adrenal system are damaged and hyperresponsive, while the immune system is sensitized to allergens such as pollens, dander, dust mites and so on.

This mixed response, in fact, can produce more severe and lasting asthmatic responses. The body must recover from both the sympathetic response and the immunologic response. One physiology may recover first, leaving the others to recover later. As leukotrienes might be cleared, the airway smooth muscles may not be ready to relax, for example.

Regardless of the nature of the asthmatic hyperresponse, the basic mechanics of airway hyper-responsiveness indicate an inflammatory response caused by derangements of the immune system, nervous system, adrenal system and/or respiratory system. Something stimulates the hypersensitive asthmatic response because the body feels that it is threatened. When this "something" comes into contact with the body's cells, the body responds with hypersensitivity.

Once the immune system considers any trigger a threat, it stimulates a process to remove or escape that situation. Normally this process is invisible and automatic. We might clear our throat, yawn, sneeze or blink a few times, and that's that. However, if the immune system is damaged, weakened, imbalanced and otherwise overactive, the same trigger can provoke a response out of proportion with what would ordinarily be required to remove such a trigger from the body. Furthermore, once the element or condition is seen as a threat, the immune system will respond similarly every time it comes into contact with that substance or situation—until something changes.

The healthy body is a smart ecosystem. Ordinarily the body can handle challenges without hyperreactivity. A healthy body will respond to such a challenge by either correctional purging or adaptation. A hyperreactivity response simply means that the body has no other reasonable means for responding to the challenge. It cannot adequately purge or correct the challenge; and it cannot adapt to the challenge.

A healthy immune system is designed to do either and sometimes both. This is why we cough and our eyes water when exposed to smoke. It is also why we sneeze when we accidentally inhale pepper or dust.

This means that something else is going wrong. The immune system, nerves, adrenals and airways are responding abnormally. And because there is something wrong, the body responds inappropriately.

Let's discuss the various conditions that have been called asthma:

Exercise-Induced Asthma

Exercise-induced asthma (often abbreviated as EIB—exercise-induced bronchospasm), is the narrowing of the breathing airways following or during exercise. EIB is usually a temporary event that may last from a half-hour to an hour or two. EIB often occurs during or following vigorous exercise.

A more common and mild form of EIB is exercise-induced wheeze, or EIW. While some may question why wheezing after exercise is of any concern (is it not normal to wheeze after vigorous exercise?), the amount of wheeze seen in EIW is considered more than typical.

In fact, we know that asthma is quite common among athletes. For example, University of Iowa researchers (Weiler *et al.* 1998) found that over 16% of Olympic athletes were either diagnosed with asthma, had used an asthma drug, or both. More than one out of ten Olympic athletes was taking an asthmatic medication during the 1996 Olympic Games.

Occupational Asthma

Occupational asthma is bronchial hypersensitivity related to environmental exposures found in workplaces. Industries or workplaces that have reported frequent bronchial hyperresponsiveness include chemical manufacturing, oil refining, natural gas production, metal fabrication, hospitals, automobile manufacturing, pharmaceutical manufacturing, fur and clothing manufacturers, and plastic producers. These exposures can produce asthma among both workers and their families. This is especially the case with pregnant mothers.

Environmental Asthma

This type of airway hyperresponsiveness is quite similar to occupational asthma, in that environmental exposures are also direct triggers. However, this type of BHR includes exposure to cigarette smoke, household dust and mold, animal dander, furniture and carpet materials, homebuilding materials and others. Even an automobile's interior can contain asthma triggers such as formaldehyde.

In reality, most allergies that are not of the first two categories are environmentally triggered. Sensitizations to environmental exposures such as these are found in a majority of asthma and allergy sufferers. The physiological mechanisms of asthma are unique. But there is no escaping that these environmental toxins relate to asthma.

This case is bolstered by the fact that many asthmatics had allergies earlier in life. In multiple studies, many asthmatic children had food or dust mite allergies as infants. We'll connect these issues as we explore the underlying causes for asthma.

Refractory Asthma

A persistent and severe case of asthma that cannot be adequately 'controlled' or maintained by typical medications is called refractory. The term 'refractory' means something that cannot be controlled by the typical control measures. In this case, the 'control' measures used as a baseline are pharmaceutical medications.

Many refractory asthma cases are found to be related to stubborn sinus infections and subsequent sinusitis diagnoses. Subsequently and for reasons we will explore further, this type of asthma will often respond to antibiotics, but not steroids.

Allergic Asthma

This category—the epitome of atopic asthma—has redundancies with other asthma types, but is nevertheless identified specifically by researchers. For many asthma sufferers, allergies to pollens, dust, foods and other allergens are intimately involved in their asthma episodes. For others, there may be a co-existing condition of asthma and allergies. Yes, an allergic trigger may also be independent of a co-existent asthma disorder.

Food Allergy Asthma

University of Colorado medical researchers (Liu *et al.* 2010) determined from the 2005-2006 National Health and Nutrition Examination Survey data that about 2.5% of the U.S. population has a clinical food allergy. Furthermore, they determined that food allergy significantly increases the risk of contracting asthma. They called food allergies, *"an under-recognized risk factor for problematic asthma."*

Food allergy asthma is actually a subclass of allergic asthma. For many asthma sufferers, food allergies appear to be the basis for their asthma. For others, it appears they are independent conditions. We'll focus on this later.

Researchers and Poland's University of Łódź (Krogulska *et al.* 2007) studied 304 asthma patients between the age of five and eighteen years old. Of the 304 asthmatics, 9.8% also had food allergies, as established by double-blind placebo-controlled food challenge (the gold standard).

Researchers from the University of Delhi (Kumar *et al.* 2006) studied IgE levels in 216 asthmatic patients with an average age of 32 years old. Of the 216, they found that 172 had elevated serum IgEs—indicating allergic asthma. Of the total, 11% of the asthma patients were sensitized to rice, 10% were sensitized to black gram, 10% had IgEs specific to lentils while 9.2% were sensitive to citrus (some had multiple sensitivities).

French researchers (Moneret-Vautrin *et al.* 1996) found that asthma was preceded by food allergies in 8.5% of asthma cases. Preceding allergens outside of foods included feathers and latex. Each of these has also been shown to cross-react with foods should a person become airway-sensitized to the protein allergen.

Researchers from Poland's Medical University of Lodz (Krogulska *et al.* 2010) studied 54 children with food allergies and 62 without food allergies. Using methacholine provocation to test forced expiratory volume (FEV1), they found that the food allergic children had greater levels of bronchial hyperreactivity. Among the non-asthmatic children in the study, bronchial hyperreactivity was evident in 47% of the children with food allergies and only 17% of those without food allergies. Furthermore, bronchial hyperreactivity was found in 74% of those children who suffered from moderate anaphylactic reactions, and bronchial hyperreactivity existed among all of the children who had severe anaphylactic reactions.

Airway Conditions and Membrane Inflammation

The mucosal goblet cells of the respiratory tract are quite similar to the gastric cells of the stomach and duodenum. The difference here is that these produce mucous fed by the pyloric glands in addition to the highly acidic gastrin. As we'll be discussing more at length throughout the remainder of the text, this similarity between the goblet cells, the villi and the gastric/pyloric cells facilitates an understanding of the mystery of GERD-related asthma—and the mechanisms for asthma in general.

The mucous membrane fluids can also become dehydrated if the ions that open the pores are blocked. Here the pores may be blocked due to an imbalance of ion chemistry in the sub-mucosal membrane. Tests have shown that chlorine and bicarbonate anions stimulate the opening of the pores that bring liquids into the mucous membrane. The mucin proteins produced by the submucosal membrane glands have to be diluted with these ion fluids to give the mucous membrane the right balance of stickiness and fluidity.

In dehydrated mucosal membranes, the mucous is thickened and not fluid enough to provide its surfactant and transport functions.

In addition, exposure to allergens, toxins, cold air and any number of other triggers can stimulate the production of mucous by the goblet cells. In a healthy body, this stimulates the quick removal of the toxin or invader, as the excess mucous is swept out by the cilia.

However, should the body be immunosuppressed or otherwise overwhelmed by the invasion, the goblet cells will over-produce mucous, which can swamp the cilia along with dead cell parts and toxins. When the cilia are drowning in mucous, they cannot remove it. The lack of mucous transport, combined with the need to remove a toxin, is typically accompanied by the constriction of the airways, which may protect the lungs from more toxins, but also further prevents the mucous from being cleared out.

There are various negative consequences of having poorly oxygenated blood and/or highly acidic, carbon dioxide-rich blood. Poorly oxygenated blood can cause or contribute to brain fog, poor memory, fatigue, restlessness, nervousness, anxiety, indigestion, and cardiovascular diseases such as *cor pulmonale,* hypertension, atherosclerosis and angina. Poorly oxygenated blood can lead to low healing response, poor sleep, and increased inflammatory response—all of which are linked to a poor immune function, hypersensitivity and allergic rhinitis.

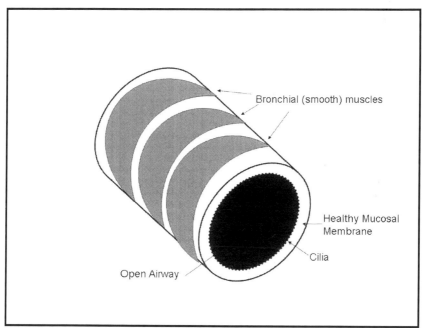

Healthy Bronchial Airways

The inside lumen (or opening) of the airways in a healthy person allows air to pass through unobstructed. In a person with asthmatic hypersensitivity, the walls of the airways are in an inflamed condition. The airway walls are thus irritated easily. In this condition, even the slightest trigger can set off a full blown airway inflammatory response—asthma.

During an inflammatory asthma response, the smooth muscles that wrap around the airways contract, effectively clamping down the airways and reducing airflow. In addition, the airway walls become thicker and fill with mucous. In this state, it becomes difficult to breathe, simply because the airways are nearly closed or constricted. This constricted state produces the characteristic wheezing. This constricted state also further irritates the airways, stimulating the coughing response.

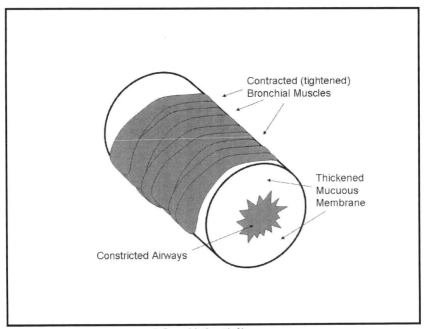

Inflamed Asthmatic Airways

The evidence of bronchial asthma as an inflammatory response is overwhelming. Leucocytes such as eosinophils, mast cells and neutrophils all release inflammatory mediators during asthmatic hyperreactivity. This is the first and primary indication that asthma is an inflammatory condition.

Inflammation also involves reactive oxygen species. Indications of this during asthmatic hypersensitivity include higher levels of superoxide anions and thiobarbituric acid-reactive products (TBARs), as well as hydrogen peroxide. One of the main inflammatory byproducts of superoxide reactions is hydrogen peroxide (H_2O_2).

Research has illustrated that asthmatics generate more hydrogen peroxide when they breathe out than normal people. In one study, asthmatics breathed out 26 times the levels of hydrogen peroxide as healthy subjects did. They also found that TBAR levels among asthmatics were 18 times the levels of healthy subjects (Antczak *et al.* 1997).

Inflammatory eosinophils—evidenced by higher eosinophil cationic protein (ECP) levels—are also significantly higher in asthma. ECP can damage microorganisms such as viruses and bacteria, along with our body's cells. ECP damages cells by forming pores in the cell membranes, which produce a type of cell membrane damage called *permeability alteration*.

Research has indicated that ECP builds up in the airways of asthmatics. While ECP is a defense measure in the case of infection, an overload of ECP as occurs in repeated asthma episodes damages the epithelial cells of the bronchial passages and alveoli. This damage contributes to what is called airway remodeling.

The build-up of ECP is simply part of an inflammatory process that occurs as part of an immune response: A deranged immune response that medical researchers call hyper-reactivity.

What Causes Chronic Cough?

Irritated sites in the airways and lungs stimulate coughing, but this is also attenuated by a neural cough center located within the brainstem and within the cerebral cortex, where coughing is often initiated, suppressed or modified by consciousness. The cough reflex is, as put by Dr. John Christopher, *"a result of nature's effort to expectorate mucous from the lungs, after which breathing becomes easier."*

In other words, the stimulus for chronic coughing is the build-up of mucous in the airways. While incidental coughing might follow the inhalation of some smoke or other toxin, a chronic cough is stimulated by a build-up of thickened mucous in the airways.

And why is there this build up of mucous? Because the immune system is undergoing the inflammatory process by flushing out broken-down cells, broken down toxins, and even live infections. This thickened mucous is like the composition of flushed toilet water after a bowel movement: *it is full of crap.*

How About the Sore Throat?

This is an easy one. The sore throat is simple. Our pharynx and larynx and esophagus are all lined with mucosal membranes that protect the cells from foreigners, including microorganisms, toxins, acidic foods and enzymes, and allergens.

When the mucosal membranes in this region become degraded, they cannot protect our cells any longer. This exposes our epithelial area to toxins, microorganisms and other foreigners. This often produces an inflammatory response by the body, which reddens the area and the area becomes sore.

The instigators of the defective mucosal membrane in a sore throat can be many. These can include all of the elements we'll discuss in the next chapter and more. Often, it is as simple as a microorganism that has become attached to the mucosal membranes. The body launches an immune response to rid the body of the invader. This process can thicken the mucosal membranes, and this thickened membrane can prevent a good clearing of the broken down invader parts. It becomes hard to clear this out, and the toxins in the membranes begin to irritate the cells.

Alternatively, the mucosal membrane can be thinned by a poor diet and overuse of NSAIDs. This can cause toxins to overload our thinned mucosal membranes, irritating the cells of our throat region.

Often the sore throat is a sign of an oncoming cold or flu because the overloading of the virus causes the thickening of the mucosal membranes as the body works to remove the infective agent. This is a healthy response and we should not dread the sore throat. Rather, we should see it as a sign that the body's immune system is on full alert and is actively removing invaders.

Inflammation Overview

Perhaps we should review the process of inflammation a bit more.

Inflammation simply coordinates the various immune players into an organized healing response for damaged cells and tissues, or to remove invading foreigners. Inflammation is our body's clean-up crew, and it is often directed at those cells that make up our epithelial cells and tissues.

The epithelial cells are the front line (behind the mucosal membranes) that guard our body's internal cells. When they are damaged, the immune system gets busy to heal the problem. In other words, inflammation is a good process—and not the villain most people make it out to be.

Imagine for a moment cutting your finger pretty badly. First you would feel pain—letting you know the body is hurt. Second, you will probably notice that the area has become swollen and red. Blood starts to clot around the area. Soon the cut stops bleeding. The blood dries and a scab forms. It remains red, maybe a little hot, and hurts for a while. As the healing proceeds, the cut is soon closed up, leaving a scab with a little redness around it. The pain soon stops. The scab falls off and the finger returns to normal—almost like new and ready for action.

Without this inflammatory process, we might not even know we cut our finger in the first place. We might keep working, only to find out that we had bled out a quart of blood on the floor. Without clotting, it would be hard to stop the bleeding. And without some continuing pain, we would be more likely to keep injuring the wound, preventing it from healing.

Were it not for our immune system and inflammatory process slowing blood flow, clotting the blood, scabbing and cleaning up the site, our bodies would simply be full of holes and wounds. Our bodies simply could not survive injury.

The probiotic and immunoglobulin immune system work together to deter and kill particular invaders—hopefully before they gain access to the body's tissues. Should these defenses fail, they can stimulate the humoral immune system in a strategic attack that includes identifying antigens and recognizing their weaknesses. B-cells and probiotics coordinate through the stimulation of immunoglobulins and clusters of differentiation (CDs).

This progression also stimulates an activation of neutrophils, phagocytes, immunoglobulins, leukotrienes and prostaglandins. Should cells become infected, they will signal the immune system using paracrines located on their cell membranes. Once the intrusion and strategy is determined, B-cells will surround the pathogens while T-cells attack any infected cells. Natural killer T-cells may secrete chemicals into infected cells, initiating the death of the cell.

Leukotrienes immediately gather in the region of injury or infection, and signal to T-cells to coordinate efforts in the process of repair. Prostaglandins initiate the widening of blood vessels to bring more T-cells and other repair factors (such as plasminogen and fibrin) to the infected or injured site. Histamine opens the blood vessel walls to allow all these healing agents access to the injury site to clean it up.

Prostaglandins also stimulate substance P within the nerve cells, initiating the sensation of pain. At the same time, thromboxanes, along with fibrin, drive the process of clotting and coagulation in the blood, while constricting certain blood vessels to decrease the risk of bleeding.

In the case where the pathogen is an allergen, the inflammation response will also accompany an H1-histamine response. As mentioned earlier, histamine is primarily produced by the mast cells, basophils and neutrophils after being stimulated by IgE antibodies. This opens blood vessels to tissues, which stimulates the processes of sneezing, watering of the eyes and coughing. These measures, though sometimes considered irritating, are all stimulated in an effort to remove the toxin and prevent its re-entry into the body. As histamine binds with receptors, one of the resulting physiological responses is alertness (also why antihistamines cause drowsiness). These are natural responses to help the body and mind remain vigilant in order to avoid further toxin intake.

At the height of the repair process, swelling, redness and pain are at their peak. The T-cells, macrophages, neutrophils, fibrin and plasmin all work together to purge the allergen from the body and repair the damage.

As macrophages continue the clean up, the other immune cells begin to retreat. Antioxidants like glutathione will attach to and transport the byproducts—broken down toxins and cell parts—out of the body. As this proceeds, prostaglandins, histamines and leukotrienes are signaled to reverse the inflammation and pain process.

One of the central features of the normalization process is the production of bradykinin. Bradykinin slows clotting and opens blood vessels, allowing the cleanup process to accelerate. A key signalling factor is the production of nitric oxide (NO). NO slows inflammation by promoting the detachment of lymphocytes to the site of infection or toxification, and reduces tissue swelling. NO also accelerates the clearing out of debris with its interaction with the superoxide anion. NO was originally described by researchers as endothelium-derived relaxing factor (or EDRF)—because of its role in relaxing blood vessel walls.

The body produces more nitric oxide in the presence of good nutrition and lower stress. Probiotics also play a big role in nitric oxide production in a healthy body. Lactobacilli such as *L. plantarum* have in fact been shown to remove the harmful nitrate molecule and use it to produce nitric oxide (Bengmark *et al.* 1998). This is beneficial to not only reducing inflammation: NO production also creates a balanced environment for increased tolerance.

Low nitric oxide levels also happen to be associated with a plethora of conditions, including diabetes, heart failure, high cholesterol, ulcerative colitis, premature aging, cancers and many others. Low or abnormal NO production is also seen among lifestyle factors such as smoking, obesity, and environmental air pollution.

Allergies and Airway Hypersensitivity

There are several kinds of hypersensitivity responses within the body. These might sound similar but they are actually different in many ways and yet share a common trait. Let's review these and find the common trait:

Atopic Hypersensitivity

This response occurs when IgE antibodies bind to an allergen. Antigens include air pollutants, pollen, dust mite allergens, and dander. An allergen can also be any food the immune system has become sensitized to. When this binding between an antigen and IgE takes place, the bound IgE will set off the release of inflammatory mediators from white blood cells called mast cells, basophils and/or neutrophils. The mediators released by these immune cells include histamine, prostaglandins and leukotrienes. Depending upon the location and type of mast/basophil/neutrophil cells, these mediators can spark an inflammatory response within the airways, and/or other tissues, including the sinuses, skin, joints, intestines and elsewhere.

This response can be further broken down into two stages: sensitization and elicitation.

MUCOSAL MEMBRANE DISORDERS

Sensitization: The allergen sensitization process takes place when a potential antigen happens to come into contact with a type of immune cell called a progenitor B-cell. As part of their immune system responsibilities, these B-cells will break apart the allergen proteins into smaller parts—often called *epitopes*. These will become attached to hystocompatibility complex class II complex molecules.

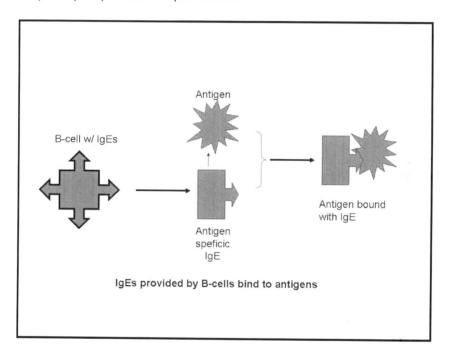

IgEs provided by B-cells bind to antigens

The T-cell hystocompatibility complex is transferred onto the surface of the B-cell, which binds to a particular allergen. Once upon the B-cell surface, T-helper cells take notice of this foreign particle stuck to the B-cell. The T-helper cell cytokine CD4 receptors trigger a response, and this stimulates the production of the IgE immunoglobulins. These particular IgE immunoglobulins are now sensitized to the particular epitope of the antigen in the future.

Elicitation: Once sensitized, the IgE associates with the specific IgE receptors that lie on the surface of the neutrophil, basophil or mast cells. Within these cells are packages called granules.

The granules are stock full of a variety of inflammatory mediators. The most notorious of these in asthma are leukotrienes as we've mentioned. As the allergen-specific IgEs connect with the IgE receptors on these immune cells, the immune cells will release the inflammatory mediators including leukotrienes and histamines into the bloodstream and lymph. This is what drives much of the symptoms of an allergic attack, including but not limited to hives, asthma, uritica, sinusitis and others.

The below diagram illustrates elicitation:

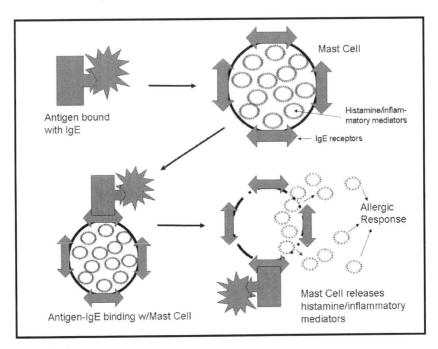

Cytotoxic Responses

In this type of immune response, antigens have penetrated the tissues, and the immune system is on a state of alert as it responds to kill these cells. This typically takes place through an antigen binding to IgG or IgM immunoglobulins in a delayed immune and inflammatory response. This response can happen concurrently to allergic responses; though it is most often a delayed response. It is this type of response that can cause an asthmatic episode that lasts over several days.

Should the red blood cells be involved in the antigen absorption, hemolysis (the destruction of red blood cells) and anemia (a lack of red blood cells) may result. These can in turn cause more severe asthmatic hypersensitivity responses.

Systemic Inflammation Responses

Systemic and chronic inflammation creates hypersensitivity of the airway passages due to the immune system being stressed and on high alert status. In this situation, the immune system is overloaded by infection(s), chemical toxicity, or a diet that constantly exposes the body to toxins. One or a combination of these effects generally produces a whole-body diseased state. In such a state, the body will overreact to an exposure to stress in the airways. These triggers can be as simple as exercise, cold air, smoke or fragrance.

This type of systemic inflammatory status is evidenced by high C-reactive protein in the body. CRP levels are easily determined through blood analysis. We'll discuss some of the research that illustrates this later.

Immune Complex Responses

Here the allergen-bound antibody complex actually penetrates cell tissues and injures them. This can occur within the airway epithelial cells, intestinal cells, liver, or virtually anywhere around the body. Here the damage to the cells immediately stimulates the inflammatory response, regardless of whether there is an allergen trigger involved or not. Whatever is damaging the cells is considered a direct threat.

In some instances, these immune complexes can severely change alveoli permeability, vascular permeability and/or intestinal permeability, producing imbalances in respiration, circulation and digestion—sometimes even simultaneously.

This type of response is also often a delayed response, occurring hours or even a day or two after exposure to an asthma trigger.

This alerted immune complex condition will also stimulate mast cells, basophils and/or neutrophils, resulting in continued degranulation of histamine, prostaglandins and leukotrienes, which in turn produce ongoing asthmatic hypersensitivity.

Delayed T-Cell Responses

While the immune complex response may generate an immediate T-cell response once cells and tissues are damaged, a delayed T-cell response will occur over a period of time—as T-cells continue to destroy damaged airway cells. Here airway epithelial cells become damaged, and the T-cells are removing those damaged cells with an inflammatory response.

This type of response is the driving factor behind airway remodeling. In airway remodeling, the epithelial cell network that lines the airways become inflamed, damaged and chronically irritated. They are swollen and hyperreactive on an ongoing basis, in other words.

This same general condition can exist within the epithelial layers of many parts of the body. On the skin, this is seen as eczema. In the intestines, it is seen as colitis or Crohn's disease. In the sinuses, it is called sinusitis. In the urinary tract, it is called interstitial cystitis. In the stomach and lower esophagus, it is called GERD.

This response is also often attributed to autoimmunity, which is explained as the immune system attacking healthy cells. This notion is incorrect, however, because the immune system is not attacking healthy cells. The immune system is removing cells that have been damaged. Once these epithelial cells are damaged, T-cells stimulate the immune response to clear out the damaged cells. In other words, it is an inflammatory immune response to cellular and tissue toxicity.

Airway Remodeling

Once asthma has taken hold of a person—especially a young person—the airways may undergo what is often described as "permanent" remodeling. In airway remodeling, the bronchi and their mucosal membranes undergo structural changes. This typically means that the walls of our airways—made up of epithelial cells and cilia—become thicker. The smooth muscles surrounding our airways also become dense and thick—much as weight-lifting muscles can thicken. Our mucous membrane chemistry also changes, and the vascular-capillary system around our airways changes.

Airway remodeling is the primary reason given for the irreversibility of asthma. This is despite the fact that airway remodeling often is reversed, and many children with remodeled airways outgrow asthma. The basis for this is that epithelial cells live for a few weeks and then die, to be replaced by newly divided epithelial cells. Cells are also constantly recycling nutrients and fluids. This means that while the DNA of the new cells may respond similarly for a few generations, should the conditions change for these cells (including nutrition, mucous membrane health, environmental conditions and so on) they will adapt to the new conditions and gradually become healthy cells.

Other Responses

There are numerous other physiological mechanisms that can result in an asthmatic response. For example, a cold or flu may spark an inflammatory response by stimulating any number of inflammatory mediators, including prostaglandins, serotonin, platelet-aggregating factor, kinins and others. Fungal and bacterial infections can also stimulate the asthmatic response by sparking an extended period of airway inflammation.

In fact, many asthmatics will experience a combination of these mechanisms at the same time. Or an asthmatic might experience an asthma episode from one mechanism at one time, and have an episode caused by another mechanism another time. The point is that the airways of an asthmatic may become hypersensitive to any number of stressors that overload the body's defense mechanisms. Worse, once a mechanism results in an episode, a metabolic pathway (or release) is created, and the body will be more likely to have that same response in the future when the same stressor is faced.

The bottom line, as we'll prove in Chapter Four, is that the asthmatic is experiencing a defective immune response with an extended period of inflammation. This in fact is the common feature of all the types of hypersensitivity responses discussed here.

Before we go further, let's review the essential elements of the immune system and inflammation to get a clearer understanding of these mechanisms. This will allow the reader to better understand the asthma research.

Should the mucous membrane thin, these mechanisms become irritated, producing an inflammatory immune response that causes the desmosomes and tight junctions to open. These gaps allow toxins and food macromolecules to enter the blood, producing systemic inflammation.

The GERD Connection: Mucosal Membrane Health

A healthy stomach is critical to the health of the body. A healthy stomach means we'll be getting better nourished—to train, build muscle and maintain endurance. A healthy stomach means our food gets prepared for maximum absorption. Imagine only assimilating a small portion of the many healthy (and expensive) foods and supplements we buy. Sadly, this is the case for many of us.

A healthy stomach also means the freedom from heartburn and ulcers. Some reports state that almost a quarter of us will experience heartburn at some point. Nearly one in ten of us will get an ulcer. Some say these reports are conservative, as many cases go unreported. Then there is indigestion. Most of us experience this occasionally, if not daily.

The esophagus is the staging area for our food. If we masticate our food well enough, our food will pass through the esophagus to the stomach within ten seconds. At the bottom of the esophagus is a valve called the esophageal sphincter. This valve lets food into the main stomach while keeping acid and food from backing up into the esophagus. An unhealthy sphincter doesn't close tightly enough—causing heartburn as acids and food irritate the sensitive mucous membranes of the esophagus. If the food delivered to the sphincter comes in too fast and rough, strain will be put on the cricopharyngeus muscle. When this supporting muscle loses tone, the valve weakens.

This is not the only cause for heartburn. As food is dropped into the stomach, it undergoes intense churning and breakdown by the stomach's digestive juices. Special glands intertwined among stomach cells secrete a mixture of biochemicals. This blend is composed primarily of hydrochloric acid, pepsin, rennin and a special mucus—made primarily of mucopolysaccharides. To varying degrees, the stomach also secretes lipase, a fat-splitting enzyme. The enzymes pepsin and rennin break down proteins, preparing them for intestinal assimilation.

As mentioned earlier, healthy gastric juice maintains a pH between about 1 to 3. Hydrochloric acid (HCL) is the main component for pH control. An acidic pH is critical to sterilize our food. Without enough HCL, we run the risk of allowing various unwanted bacteria into the stomach and intestines. One of these is *Helicobacter pylori*. Recent research has connected H. pylori overgrowths in the stomach to a majority of ulcers.

The common premise is that heartburn means too much acid in the stomach. The typical response is to take antacids. This may provide a short fix for those with esophagus sphincter leaks. For many others, antacids don't help the pain at all. Here the sphincter isn't the problem. In this case, antacids may make matters worse, because they drive the pH of our stomach's mucosal membranes too high. When the pH is too high, our food won't get broken down right. The enzymes will be compromised. The stomach and the rest of the body will be left open to bacterial infection.

Acid-blocking medications further exasperate the problem in many cases. While these may be helpful for temporarily easing pain or helping ulcers heal, they also can create the reduction of the very digestive juices we need to break down our foods for intestinal absorption. They also cut back HCL production, again allowing bacteria to grow among our stomach's mucosal membranes.

The other problem that can occur is that the gastric secretions may have reduced mucus content. Mucus lines the stomach cells, buffering them from the harsh stomach acids. Sometimes a burning stomach is the result of too little mucus lining. This is often the case for those who do not drink enough liquids, or those under greater stress. When the body is stressed, it focuses its energies upon muscle and nervous activity, depleting the resources of the gastric glands.

The Asthma and GERD Relationship

Many asthma sufferers also suffer from gastroesophageal reflux (also called GER or when referred to as a chronic disorder, GERD). Researchers are increasingly realizing that asthma's association with GERD is not merely a coincidence: The two disorders are somehow connected. However, the question that has not been answered is: Why are they connected? Let's review the science on their relationship, and then answer this question:

In research discussed previously from Sweden's Uppsala University (Uddenfeldt *et al.* 2010), it was found that among 8,150 people, contracting GERD more than doubled the incidence of adult onset asthma. Furthermore, obesity and GERD significantly increased the risk of asthma among the middle aged and the elderly.

University of Washington researchers (Debley *et al.* 2006) studied GERD symptoms and asthma among adolescents who had asthma. They studied 2,397 students from six Seattle middle schools. They found GERD in 19% of current asthmatic children, and among only 2.5% of the whole student population. GERD symptoms were also more severe among the asthmatic children compared to non-asthmatic children with GERD. Asthmatic children required urgent medical treatment five times more than did the non-asthmatic children with GERD. Asthmatic children with GERD required more asthma medication than asthmatics without GERD. Asthmatic children with GERD also had more severe asthma episodes.

Researchers from Barcelona's Hospital de la Santa Creu i Sant Pau (Plaza *et al.* 2006) found that among 56 patients with persistent coughing, 21% had gastroesophageal reflux. More than one in five, in other words.

Researchers from Columbia University's College of Physicians and Surgeons (DiMango *et al.* 2009) studied 304 asthmatics and found that 38% also had reflux. While they found little difference in lung function and bronchial medication use, they did find that the GERD sufferers had significantly more severe asthma symptoms, had to use more oral steroids (typically reserved for retracted asthma). GERD asthmatics also had poorer quality of life scores than the asthmatics without GERD.

Researchers from the Korea's Inha University College of Medicine (Kang *et al.* 2010) studied 85 young children with recurrent wheezing. They found that 48% had serious gastrointestinal reflux. They also found that 12% of the GERD patients were allergic to eggs or milk, while 20% of the non-GERD patients were allergic to eggs or milk. They concluded that while GERD predisposed asthma, GERD did not predispose food allergies, as had been previously assumed.

Researchers from the University of Utah Health Sciences Center (Peterson *et al.* 2009) studied the relationships between exercise-induced asthma and gastroesophageal reflux. They studied 31 volunteers, 20 of which had asthma. They found that 73% of the asthmatic subjects had abnormal pH (pH levels associated with GERD) during treadmill tests. They commented that people may be misdiagnosed with asthma when they simply have respiratory symptoms related to exercise and GERD.

GERD Prevalence Among Western Society

Before we can better understand the relationship between asthma and GERD, we should probably look at the science on GERD itself.

Studies have shown that GERD incidence is higher among more developed countries—and significantly greater in those countries whose populations eat primarily a 'western' diet.

This is illustrated dramatically by comparing GERD rates between China and the U.S.

Researchers from the University of Hong Kong (Wong *et al.* 2003) conducted a study of GERD among Chinese populations. In total, 2,209 adult volunteers participated in the study. The research discovered that 2.5% of the population experienced some heartburn weekly, 9% experienced heartburn monthly, and nearly 30% experienced some heartburn at least once in the past year.

In comparison, about a third of the U.S. population experiences heartburn at least monthly, and about 10% experience heartburn daily (Friedman *et al.* 2008). About 18-20% of Americans experience heartburn weekly (Locke *et al.* 1997).

In other words, Americans experience heartburn about 7.6 times more frequently than do the Chinese (18-20% versus 2.5%). That means that Americans have 760% more weekly heartburn than the Chinese. Furthermore, slightly more Americans experience daily heartburn than the number of Chinese who experience heartburn monthly. This could be translated to Americans having over thirty times more severe heartburn. However it is calculated, Americans have dramatically more GERD than the Chinese.

In addition to diet, we can also include air pollution and stress as possible GERD factors. However, we should note that cities in China are significantly more crowded, with more pollutants—especially in the way of soot and heavy metals—than U.S. cities. So the difference seems to relate primarily to diet.

GERD-Related Asthma and Acid Suppressing Medications

Furthermore, acid-suppression medication does not quell asthmatic hypersensitivity, as has been assumed. Physicians have assumed that the relationship between asthma and GERD was based on stomach acid leaking into the esophagus and bronchial passages, where it theoretically irritates the airways. Unfortunately, this theory has not panned out well in the research:

Researchers from Brazil's University of São Paulo Medical School (Araujo *et al.* 2008) studied the relationship between acid infusion and GERD-associated asthma. They monitored the esophageal pH and bronchial responsiveness among 20 GERD-asthma patients. They found that acid-infusion did not increase bronchial hyperresponsiveness among the GERD-related asthmatics. They concluded: *"These findings strongly question the significance of acid infusion as a model to study the pathogenesis of GERD-induced asthma."*

In other words, the leaking of acids into the esophagus is not the primary cause for GERD-related asthma.

Further illustrating this, researchers from Norway's Østfold County Hospital (Størdal *et al.* 2005) studied 38 children who presented with asthma and gastroesophageal reflux. They were given acid suppression medication omeprazole or placebo for 12 weeks, while undergoing monitoring for esophageal pH control.

Repeated pH monitoring confirmed that the acid suppression medication indeed inhibited acid secretion in the children. However, the total symptom scores were not significantly different between the omeprazole group and the placebo group. Lung function and asthma medication use were also comparable between the two groups. The researchers concluded: *"Omeprazole treatment did not improve asthma symptoms or lung function in children with asthma and GERD."*

Researchers from Italy's University of Verona (Ferrari *et al.* 2007) studied 29 asthmatic patients, 17 of which had acid reflux. They tested the patients with pH monitoring and challenges with methacholine and capsaicin (both irritating coughs), followed by the acid-blocking medication omeprazole. They found that inhibiting gastric acids does not halt bronchial hyperresponsiveness. However, they did find that blocking acid may somehow block the cough stimulus *("tussive sensitivity")*.

This is not a verdict on acid-suppressor medication for GERD-related asthma. And to be fair, some evidence, such as (González Morales *et al.* 1998), that indicates that acid-suppressor medications may help some GERD-asthma symptoms in some cases. The point being made here is that the research indicates that asthma with GERD is more complicated than simply gastric acids irritating the airways.

Furthermore, it appears that acid-suppressing medication may actually trigger asthma. Harvard Medical School researchers (Dehlink *et al.* 2009) studied 29,490 children diagnosed with allergy or prescriptions for allergy medications. They found that 5,645 of the children were also exposed to acid suppression medications via their pregnant mothers. The research found that acid-suppressive medication during pregnancy increased the rate of the children developing asthma by more than 50%. The researchers concluded: *"These data provide first evidence of a significant association between in utero exposure to acid-suppressive drugs and the risk of developing childhood asthma."*

GERD-Related Asthma and Drooling

Here is another piece to the puzzle to consider: Research has shown that early drooling, if it is not corrected, can lead to an asthmatic condition.

Medical researchers from Italy's University of Catania (Serra *et al.* 2007) found that 90-95% of children who drool also have gastroesophageal reflux. In most children, this will resolve by itself by 12-15 months of age. But in 5-10% of children, GERD continues. They observed that this will often accompany eventual asthma symptoms as well as inflammatory diseases of the middle ear.

Why is this? What does continued drooling have to do with asthma, while temporary drooling does not? Let's continue with the science before we make any conclusions.

Cause or Result?

We might consider the perspective and research of Drs. V. Singh and N.K. Jain, who treated five patients who were having nocturnal asthma attacks that concurred with gastroesophageal reflux symptoms. They gave asthmatic patients ephedrine or a placebo. Throughout the trial, the patients kept a diary of their asthma and GERD symptoms. They found that the asthma treatment alone improved both their asthma and GERD symptoms. The researchers titled their research paper: *"Asthma as a Cause For, Rather than a Result of, Gastroesophageal Reflux."* (Singh and Jain 1983)

We do not subscribe to this limited notion. Rather, as this thesis clearly indicates, asthma and GERD are connected by a common thread: The health of the mucosal membranes.

The Mucosal Conclusion

Since we know from the research that the acids rising into the esophagus do not directly cause or exacerbate the symptoms of asthma, we have to consider the commonalities between the two conditions. While asthma causing GERD—as was proposed by

Singh and Jain—does not seem likely, there must be a common cause for both conditions.

The answer lies in the mechanics of both conditions. GERD takes place because there are two conditions within the stomach. The first is the thinning of the mucosal membrane that lines the stomach. This membrane protects the stomach from the acids presented by the gastric cells and acidic foods. The gastric acids, meant to destroy microorganisms in our foods and help break down the nutrients, do not irritate the stomach of healthy persons. A healthy person produces sufficient alkaline mucous in the stomach to protect the cells from the acid.

The second situation that occurs in GERD is the weakening of the sphincter muscle at the entry of the stomach from the esophagus. This muscle controls the valve that keeps stomach acids and foods from backing up into the esophagus. Most medical experts propose that this is the result of overeating and/or going to bed after a big meal.

However, the problem here is that many people overeat and go to bed full and do not experience heartburn. Surely these people also have a backup of food and acids from the stomach, yet they do not experience heartburn. Holiday meals are a good example. After a gigantic holiday meal, people will roll around for the next few hours with part of their esophagi full of food, as it gradually is admitted into the stomach.

Do all of these people experience heartburn? No. Only a small percentage of these people who regularly overeat will experience GERD. Therefore, we can conclude that overeating and the subsequent sphincter weakening is also not the sole cause of GERD.

We also know that for many, GERD follows the use of certain medications. These include, beta-blockers, NSAIDs, COX-inhibitors, sedatives, antidepressants, calcium channel blockers, progestin and others.

What is the connection? Now we have several associations: asthma, GERD, certain medication use, and heartburn from stomach acids and foods.

There can only be one issue that truly links all of these: The health of the mucosal membranes. The stomach, esophagus and the airways are each coated with protective mucosal membranes.

The stomach is coated with a protective gastric mucosal membrane. The esophagus and airways are also coated with protective mucosal membranes. Special mucosal glands within the cell matrix of all three epithelial regions secrete a combination of protective mucopolysaccharides, glycoproteins and ionic fluids. These are further complexed by probiotics and immune cells, which protect their epithelial cells from infection and toxins.

Certain medications, such as the ones mentioned above, will interrupt the cyclooxygenase enzyme pathway. One of the cyclooxygenase enzyme pathways stimulates the secretion of mucosal glands around the body. In addition, the nutrient deficiency, dehydration, toxin overload and/or stress can change the content and the volume of these all-important mucosal secretions: Again not just in the stomach, but among all mucosal secretions. This is why the same acid-blocker and anti-inflammatory medications that halt mucosal secretions can also cause dry mouth.

Now should the mucosal secretions be halted from nutrient deficiencies, dehydration, nervous issues, toxin overload and/or stress, the mucosal glands will not lack the ability to produce enough of the protective coating over those epithelial regions. Regardless of the cause, this leaves the epithelia cells in these regions exposed to stomach acids in the case of GERD, and toxins or other asthma triggers in the case of asthma.

The fact is, deficiencies and toxins among the body's mucosal membranes typically occur together. This is the reason GERD also accompanies asthma: There is a deficiency in the body's ability to produce and maintain healthy mucosal membranes while there is an overload of toxins.

Furthermore, GERD is not the only indication that mucosal membrane problems result in asthmatic hypersensitivity.

For example, isn't it interesting that doctors have noticed that when there is a sinus infection, the typical cortisone medications do not seem to work for their asthma patients? Once the sinus infection is gone, the cortisone oral medications and nebulizers work just fine. But not during a severe sinusitis infection. What is the cause for this predicament?

The reason is that *asthma is an expression of inflammation combined with a deficiency among the airway mucosal membranes.* During sinusitis, the mucous membranes are super-inflamed and swollen. A thick layer of mucous has been secreted within the sinus cavities: This is called *mucous hypersecretion.* This mucous hypersecretion interrupts the normal anti-inflammatory abilities of cortisone or cortisol. Cortisol and cortisone inhibit the inflammatory process by blocking interleukin cytokines. An ongoing infection and/or toxemia within the mucosal membranes blocks the ability of these chemicals to adequately block the inflammatory process.

Another piece of evidence that connects asthma with the health of the mucosal membranes comes from a study by researchers at Brigham and Women's Hospital in Boston (Cohen *et al.* 2010). The researchers studied the effects of smoke inhalation on corticosteroid medications among 1,041 asthmatic children who were five to twelve years old. They found that those children who were exposed to cigarette smoke at home had significantly less response to cortisone treatment. In other words, like sinusitis, the smoke exposure stimulated mucosal hypersecretions that interfered with the cortisone medications. The hypersecretion of the mucosal membranes is blocking the ability of cortisol or cortisone to inhibit inflammatory mediators.

The bottom line is that defective mucosal membranes interrupt our body's natural healing capacity. Thickened mucous membranes slow down the body's natural processes of inflammation and resolution. Furthermore, thinned, defective membranes open our epithelial tissues to exposure to toxins and other harmful agents, putting additional stress upon our tissues and organs..

Chapter Four
Our Mucosal Police

Practically all of our body's mucosal membranes are populated with probiotic and controlled pathogenic bacteria in a healthy body. Our probiotic bacteria police our mucosal membranes. They—along with our body's own immune cells—protect our epithelial layers from infections and invasions of toxins. This protection comes in the form of producing various antibiotics and enzymes that break down toxins.

Here we'll discuss the various probiotics and other microorganisms that inhabit our mucosal membranes, and cover some studies that illustrate the importance of these mucosal probiotics have upon our mucosal health.

First let's review the major probiotics that inhabit the mucosal membranes of our oral and nasal cavities, our intestines, airways, skin and other regions:

The Bad and Not So Bad Microorganisms

Here are some of the microorganisms that have been shown to colonize within the mucosal membranes of the skin, mouth, upper respiratory tract, intestines and other regions. While some of these may be considered pathogenic in larger colonies, they may also be part of the biotic balance that exists within the body, and are therefore necessary to maintain health.

Actinomyces sp.

These bacteria will live within the mouth and the pharynx. They are tiny bacteria, and are prevalent in soils, plants, and animals. They are known to be cooperative with various other bacteria, both probiotic and pathogenic. Working in combination with *Streptomyces*, for example, *Actinomyces* sp. can produce antibiotics such as actinomycin.

Clostridium sp.

These bacteria will typically inhabit the lower intestines and colon, although they may also inhabit the mouth and pharynx. Some of the more common species include *Clostridium difficile, Clostridium tetani,* and *Clostridium perfringens*. They are often implicated in various intestinal disorders.

Corynebacterium sp.

These bacteria are quite hardy and will inhabit the skin surfaces, the mouth, the nasal cavity, the pharynx, the conjunctiva of the eyes, the lower intestines and the vagina. Some species have been implicated in acne. *Corynebacterium diphtheriae* is quite common in the intestines, even to the point of being considered part of our healthy flora. When their populations become too large, however, they can cause a number of disease conditions, including diphtheria.

Escherichia coli and other *Enterobacteriaceae*

Enterobacteriaceae such as *E. coli* and *Proteus* sp. may dwell and thrive in the mouth, the nasal cavity, the pharynx, the eye conjunctiva, skin surfaces, the intestinal tract, the vagina and the urethra. *E. coli* are normal residents of most humans, but are still the source of disease when their populations grow. They have been known to be lethal in large populations. This illustrates the important role probiotics play in keeping populations of *E. coli* and other bacteria in control.

Enterococcus faecalis (formerly *Streptococcus faecalis*)

These mostly pathogenic bacteria are normal residents of even healthy intestines. They can also dwell within the mouth, pharynx, urethra and vagina. They balance and strengthen our probiotics when in reasonable numbers. In larger numbers, however, they can be the cause for a number of diseases. Like other bacteria, several strains of *Enterococcus faecalis* have become antibiotic-resistant in recent years.

Haemophilus influenzae

H. influenzae is often the cause of a number of respiratory tract infections, especially among children. They are found in the nasal cavity, the mouth, the lungs, the pharynx, the eye conjunctiva and the colon and lower intestines. Many strains of *Haemophilus influenzae* are now also resistant to a number of antibiotics.

Mycoplasmas

These microorganisms are known by their absence of a cell wall. They will commonly dwell in the lower intestines, the vagina, the mouth, the pharynx, and the urethra. One of the more pathogenic species is *Mycoplasma pneumoniae,* which are known to cause a disease referred to as walking pneumonia.

Neisseria meningitides

Neisseria meningitides bacteria inhabit primarily the pharynx, but will also live in the nasal cavity, the mouth and the vagina. These bacteria are the central cause for meningitis, which can be lethal. A combination of probiotics and an active immune system may readily control these bacteria, preventing serious infection while creating immunity to them.

Pseudomonas aeruginosa

These bacteria typically dwell on the skin, in the mouth, in the pharynx, in the walls of the urethra and within the colon. *P. aeruginosa* is hardy, and can live in oxygen and low-oxygen environments. *Pseudomonas aeruginosa* can infect wounds and enter through skin openings. They can cause lung infections, urinary tract infections and kidney infections. *Pseudomonas* has also been known to cause joint infections in a condition called septic arthritis.

Spirochetes

These corkscrew-shaped bacteria of different species can live without oxygen and will embed themselves into skin, nerves, root canals, organs and various other places. Spirochetes can infect the mouth, the pharynx and the lower intestines. One of the more vigorous types is the *Borrelia burgdorferi,* the bacteria implicated in lyme disease. *Treponema pallidum* is another aggressive spirochete, known for their involvement in syphilis.

Staphylococcus aureus

Most of us house these bacteria as normal residents. When controlled, they present little or no danger. They can live on skin surfaces, in the nose, in the mouth, in the vagina, in the pharynx and within the intestines. They are not probiotic. However, as they compete with probiotics for territory, they will strengthen the body's probiotics. Many strains of *Staphylococcus aureus* are extremely pathogenic, however, especially antibiotic-resistant strains such as MRSA. Aggressive *S. aureus* can also become flesh eating, should it be allowed to grow out of control on tissue surfaces. *S. aureus* can be one of the most aggressive and dangerous bacteria within an immunosuppressed body with depleted probiotic colonies.

Staphylococcus epidermidis

These hardy probiotic or eubiotic organisms live on most of the body's epithelial surfaces. They thrive in the nasal cavity, in the pharynx, on the skin, in the conjunctiva of the eyes, in the lower urethra, in the vagina and in the colon and lower intestines. In the right colony numbers, *Staphylococcus epidermidis* can aggressively protect our skin and other membranes. *Staphylococcus epidermidis* will also adapt to varying temperatures and moisture content. They will also produce unique territorial acids that provide a protective layer for our skin and membrane surfaces. This protective acidic layer repels toxins, other bacteria, fungi and viruses.

Streptococcus mitis

These bacteria live primarily within the oral cavity and the pharynx. *Streptococcus mitis* are fairly normal residents of a healthy human body and help balance probiotic colonies. However, they can become pathogenic should they be allowed to outgrow our probiotic populations.

Streptococcus pyrogenes
These bacteria dwell primarily within the oral cavity, the pharynx, the vagina, the conjunctiva of the eyes, and on the surface of the skin. They may also inhabit the intestines, but to a lesser degree. These bacteria are the central cause for strep throat and tonsillitis. *Streptococcus pyrogenes* can also cause pneumonia, rheumatic diseases, nephritis, and heart disease. They also stimulate inflammation, causing the swelling of tissues.

Streptococcus pneumoniae
These are fairly normal inhabitants of the respiratory tract. They also can live within the mouth, the vagina, the pharynx, and the nasal cavity. *Streptococcus pneumoniae* are the central cause for most cases of pneumonia. About 50% of the human population is thought to have *S. pneumoniae* inhabitants within the upper respiratory tract. This means that for those who have not contracted pneumonia, these populations are likely under control. This is the case for numerous organisms. While we have been taught to avoid them at all costs, in reality many of us host all or many of them. In a healthy body, colonies of territorial probiotics, with the help of the immune system, keep them managed.

Streptococcus mutans
S. mutans thrive primarily in the oral cavity and pharynx. These bacteria are the central cause for plaque formation around the teeth, and the main cause for dental caries and periodontal disease. *S. mutans* secrete acids that break down the enamel of our teeth, which causes cavities. They also thrive off simple starches and sugars. This is the reason that refined sugars and simple carbohydrates are known to cause cavities.

The Good Micros
While the previous list contains probiotics in certain colony sizes, there are also clear probiotics, even in larger colony sizes. These all inhabit our mucosal membranes and protect our bodies. Here we also list some of the research associated with the supplementation of these probiotics—illustrating their importance to our mucosal membranes.

Streptococci
Bacteria from the genus Streptococcus play an important role in both disease and disease prevention. This is because when some species of *Streptococcus* become dominant, they will cause disease. In this scenario, some species of streptococci are quite aggressive and can cause lethal infections. A number of strains have also become antibiotic-resistant. Streptococci of different species and strains will inhabit the oral, nasal and pharyngeal cavities, as well as the intestines and other regions. They also produce a vari-

ety of bacteriocins that act as antibiotics to repel and kill other microorganisms. Here we will focus primarily upon the two dominant and related species, *Streptococcus salivarius* and *Streptococcus thermophilus.*

Streptococcus salivarius

Streptococcus salivarius are vigorous probiotic bacteria that station themselves throughout the upper respiratory tract, but primarily inhabit the oral cavity and pharynx. *S. salivarius* are the primary and most aggressive of our oral cavity probiotic bacteria. They are extremely territorial, and produce a number of antibiotics, including salivaricin A and salivaricin B, along with a host of other antibiotic substances.

They are also permanent residents in the human body. Our resident strains are inherited from mom. Mama transfers her resident strains through a combination of birthing, breast milk and kissing; although kissing and breast milk are likely the primary means. *Streptococcus salivarius* are extremely aggressive and will be the dominant species in a healthy mouth. This means that *Streptococcus salivarius* are organizers. To do this, they produce a number of enzymes and acids that manage the growth of other bacteria. One might conclude that *Streptococcus salivarius* are one of the most important bacteria to maintaining the health of the body, because they are the principal gatekeepers when it comes to preventing the entry and survival of infective microorganisms. As mentioned above, one of the mechanisms *S. Salivarius* utilize is the production of salivaricin. Salivaricin is recognized as one of the most potent group of antibiotics. While salivaricin A and salivaricin B have been isolated, it is certain that *S. salivarius* are constantly adjusting their antibiotic biochemistry to match new infective agents and their respective weaknesses.

Human clinical research has shown that *S. salivarius* can:
- Reduce dental plaque
- Reduce dental caries
- Inhibit gingivitis
- Inhibit *Streptococcus pyrogenes* (and strep throat)
- Prevent mastitis among breast-feeding mothers
- Reduce ulcerative colitis

Streptococcus thermophilus

Streptococcus thermophilus are considered subspecies of *S. salivarius.* Not surprisingly, *Streptococcus thermophilus* have been known to benefit the immune system in a number of ways. *Streptococcus thermophilus* are also commonly used in yogurt making. They are also used in cheese making, and are even sometimes found in pasteurized milk. They will colonize at higher temperatures, from 104-113 degrees F. This is significant because this bacterium readily produces lactase, which breaks down lactose. These are the only known streptococci that do this. Like other supplemented probiotics, *S. thermophilus* are temporary microorganisms in the human body. Their colonies will typically inhabit the system for a week or two before exiting. During that time, however, they will help set up a healthy environment to support resident colony growth. Like other probiotics, *S. thermophilus* also produce a number of different antibiotic substances and acids that deter the growth of pathogenic microorganisms.

Human clinical research has shown that *S. thermophilus* can:
- Reduce acute diarrhea (rotavirus and non-rotavirus)
- Reduce intestinal permeability
- Inhibit *H. pylori*
- Help manage AIDS symptoms
- Increase lymphocytes among low-WBC patients
- Increase IL-1beta
- Decrease IL-10
- Increase tumor necrosis factor-alpha (TNF-a)
- Increase absorption of dairy
- Decrease symptoms of IBS
- Inhibit *Clostridium difficile*
- Increase immune function among the elderly
- Restore infant microflora similar to breast-fed infants
- Increase CD8+
- Increase IFN-gamma
- Reduce acute gastroenteritis (diarrhea)
- Reduce baby colic
- Reduce symptoms of atopic dermatitis
- Reduce nasal cavity infections
- Increase HDL-cholesterol
- Increase growth in preterm infants
- Reduce intestinal bacteria
- Reduce upper respiratory tract infections from *Staphylococcus aureus*, *Streptococcus pneumoniae*, beta-hemolytic streptococci, and *Haemophilus influenzae*
- Increase HDL cholesterol
- Reduce urine oxalates (kidney stones)
- Reduce *S. mutans* in the mouth
- Reduce flare-ups of chronic pouchitis
- Reduce LDL-cholesterol in overweight subjects
- Reduce ulcerative colitis

The Lactobacilli

Lactis means "milk" in Latin. Lactobacilli are primarily found in the small intestines, although they will also inhabit the oral cavity, the nasal cavity, and the pharynx. Lactobacilli lower the pH of their environment by converting long-chain saccharides (complex sugars) such as lactose to lactic acid. This conversion process effectively inhibits pathogen growth and creates the appropriate acidic environment for other probiotics to colonize.

Lactobacillus salivarius

Lactobacillus salivarius are typical residents of most humans—although supplemented versions will still be transients. They are also found in the intestines of other animals. *L. salivarius* will dwell in the mouth, the nasal cavity, the pharynx, the small intestines, the colon, and the vagina. They are hardy bacteria that can live in both oxygen and oxygen-free environments. *L. salivarius* is one of the few bacteria species that can also thrive in salty environments. They can also survive many medications.

L. salivarius produce prolific amounts of lactic acid, which makes them hardy defenders of the teeth and gums. They also produce a number of antibiotics, and are speedy colonizers. Upon ingestion, they quickly combat pathogenic bacteria and defend their territory. Because of their hardiness, they will readily take out massive numbers of pathogens immediately. *L. salivarius* are also known to be able to break apart complex proteins.

Human clinical research has shown that *Lactobacillus salivarius* can:
- Inhibit *S. mutans* in the mouth
- Reduce dental carries
- Reduce gingivitis and periodontal disease
- Reduce mastitis
- Reduce risk of strep throat caused by *S. pyogenes*
- Reduce ulcerative colitis and IBS
- Inhibit *E. coli*
- Inhibit *Salmonella* spp.
- Inhibit *Candida albicans*

Lactobacillus reuteri

L. reuteri is a species found residing permanently in humans. As a result, most supplemented strains attach to mucosal membranes, though temporarily, and stimulate the colony growth of resident *L. reuteri* strains. *L. reuteri* will colonize in the oral cavity, the nasal cavity, and the pharynx, stomach, duodenum and ileum regions. *L. reuteri* will also significantly modulate the immune response of the gastrointestinal mucosal membranes. This means that *L. reuteri* are effective for many of the same digestive ailments that *L. acidophilus* are used for. *L. reuteri* also have several other effects, including the restoration of our oral cavity bacteria. They also produce a significant amount of antibiotics.

Human clinical research has shown that *L. reuteri* can:
- Inhibit gingivitis

- ❖ Reduce pro-inflammatory cytokines
- ❖ Help re-establish the pH of the vagina
- ❖ Stimulate growth and feeding among preterm infants
- ❖ Inhibit and suppress *H. pylori*
- ❖ Decrease dyspepsia
- ❖ Increase CD3+ in HIV patients
- ❖ Reduce nausea
- ❖ Reduce flatulence
- ❖ Reduce diarrhea (rotavirus and non-rotavirus)
- ❖ Reduce TGF-beta2 in breast-feeding mothers (reduced risk of eczema)
- ❖ Reduce *Streptococcus mutans*
- ❖ Stimulate the immune system
- ❖ Reduce plaque on teeth
- ❖ Inhibit vaginal candidiasis
- ❖ Decrease symptoms of IBS
- ❖ Increase CD4+ and CD25 T-cells in IBS
- ❖ Decrease TNF-alpha in IBS patients
- ❖ Decrease IL-12 in IBS
- ❖ Reduce IgE eczema in infancy
- ❖ Reduce infant colic
- ❖ Restore vagina pH
- ❖ Reduce colds and influenza
- ❖ Stabilize intestinal barrier function (reducing intestinal permeability)
- ❖ Decrease atopic dermatitis

Lactobacillus acidophilus

Lactobacillus acidophilus are by far the most familiar probiotic bacteria to most of us, and are also by far the most-studied to date. They are one of the main residents of the human gut, although supplemented strains will still be transient. They are also found in the mouth and vagina. *L. acidophilus* grow best in warm (85-100 degrees F) and moist environments. Many are facultative anaerobic, meaning they can grow in oxygen-rich or oxygen-poor environments. *L. acidophilus* bacteria were first discovered by Ilya Metchnikoff in the first decade of the twentieth century. Within a few years, *L. acidophilus* remedies were found in many venues, but they were poorly handled because many did not understand how easily probiotics would die outside of the intestines. Then in the late 1940s, scientists from the University of Nebraska began focused studies on *Lactobacillus acidophilus* to determine how to produce them, maintain them, and supply them as medicines.

Probably the most important benefit of *L. acidophilus* is their ability to inhibit the growth of pathogenic microorganisms, not only in the gut, but also throughout the body. *L. acidophilus* significantly control and rid the body of *Candida albicans* overgrowth, which can invade various tissues of the body if unchecked. They also inhibit *Escherichia coli*, which can be fatal in large enough populations. They can also inhibit the growth of *Helicobacter pylori*—implicated in ulcers; *Salmonella*—a genus of deadly infectious bacteria; and *Shigella* and *Staphylococcus*—both potentially lethal infectious bacteria. It should be noted that *L. acidophilus'* ability to block these infectious agents will depend upon the size of the pathobiotic colonization and the size of the *L. acidophilus* colonies. *L. acidophilus* produces a variety of antibiotic substances, including acidolin, acidophillin, lactobacillin, lactocidin and others.

L. acidophilus lessen pharmaceutical antibiotic side effects; aid lactose absorption; help the absorption of various nutrients; help maintain the mucosa; help balance the pH of the upper intestinal tract; create a hostile environment for invading yeasts; and inhibit urinary tract and vaginal infections.

L. acidophilus also produce several digestive enzymes, including lactase, lipase and protease. Lactase is an enzyme that breaks down lactose. Several studies have shown that milk- or lactose-intolerant people are able to handle milk once they have established colonies of *L. acidophilus*. Lipase helps break down fatty foods, and protease helps break down protein foods.

Human clinical research indicates that *L. acidophilus* can:
- Lower LDL and total cholesterol
- Help digest milk
- Increase growth rates
- Reduce stress-induced GI problems
- Inhibit *E. coli*
- Reduce infection from rotavirus
- Reduce necrotizing enterocolitis
- Reduce intestinal permeability
- Control *H. pylori*
- Modulate PGE2 and IgA
- Reduce dyspepsia
- Modulate IgG
- Relieve and inhibit IBS and colitis
- Inhibit keratoconjunctivitis (in eye drops)
- Inhibit and control *Clostridium* spp.
- Inhibit *Bacteroides* spp.
- Inhibit and resolve acute diarrhea
- Reduce vaginosis and vaginitis
- Decrease triglycerides
- Increase appetite
- Increase growth in preterm infants
- Inhibit *Candida* spp. overgrowths

- Produce B vitamins and other nutrients
- Reduce anemia
- Increase vaccine efficiency
- Produce virus-specific antibodies
- Reduce allergic response
- Reduce urinary oxalate levels
- Inhibit antibiotic-related diarrhea
- Decrease allergic symptoms
- Inhibit upper respiratory infections
- Increase (good) HDL-cholesterol
- Inhibit tonsillitis
- Reduce blood pressure
- Inhibit viruses
- Increase leukocytes
- Increase calcium absorption

Lactobacillus helveticus

L. helveticus is a probiotic species made popular in Switzerland. Latin *Helvetia* refers to the country of Switzerland. *L. helveticus* is used in cheese making. *L. helveticus* is used as starter bacteria for Swiss cheese and several other cheeses. *L. helveticus* will also inhabit the oral cavity temporarily as these cheeses are eaten. *L. helveticus* grow optimally between 102 and 122 degrees F. One of the reasons *L. helveticus* are favored cheese starters is because they produce primarily lactic acid and fewer metabolites, which can make the cheese taste bitter or sour.

Human clinical research has shown that *L. helveticus* can:
- Reduce blood pressure among hypertensive patients
- Produce ACE-inhibitor molecules
- Increase sleep quality and duration
- Increase general health perception
- Increase serum levels of calcium
- Decrease PTH (parathyroid hormone—marker for bone loss)
- Normalize gut colonization similar to breast-fed infants among formula-fed infants

Lactobacillus casei

L. casei are typically transient bacteria that will inhabit the mouth, pharynx, nasal cavity and intestines. They are commonly used in a number of food applications and industrial applications. These include culturing cheese and other milk products, and fermenting green olives. *L. casei* is found naturally in raw milk and in colostrum—meaning they are typical residents of cows. *L. casei* have been reported to reduce allergy symptoms and increase immune response. This seems to be accomplished by regulating the immune system's CHS, CD8 and T-cell responsiveness. However, this immune stimulation seems to be evident primarily among immunosuppressed patients (Guerin-Danan *et al.* 1998). This of course is an indication that probiotics can somehow uniquely respond to the host's particular condition. Some strains of *L. casei* are also very aggressive, and within a mixed probiotic supplement or food, they can dominate and even remove other bacteria.

Human clinical research has shown that *L. casei* can:
- Inhibit pathogenic bacterial infections
- Reduce occurrence, risk and symptoms of IBS
- Inhibit severe systemic inflammatory response syndrome
- Decrease C-reactive protein (CRP)
- Inhibit pneumonia
- Inhibit respiratory tract infections
- Inhibit bronchitis
- Maintain remission of diverticular disease
- Inhibit *H. pylori* (and ulcers)
- Reduce allergy symptoms
- Inhibit *Pseudomonas aeruginosa*
- Decrease milk intolerance
- Increase CD3+ and CD4+
- Increase phagocytic activity
- Support liver function
- Decrease risk of cirrhosis
- Decrease cytokine TNF-alpha
- Stimulate the immune system
- Inhibit and reduce diarrhea episodes
- Produce vitamins B1 and B2
- Prevent recurrence of bladder cancer
- Stimulate cytokine interleukin-1beta (IL-1b)
- Stimulate interferon-gamma
- Inhibit *Clostridium difficile*
- Reduce asthma symptoms
- Reduce constipation
- Decrease beta-glucuronidase (associated with colon cancer)
- Stimulate natural killer cell activity (NK-cells)
- Increase IgA levels
- Increase lymphocytes
- Decrease IL-6 (pro-inflammatory)
- Increase IL-12 (stimulates NK-cells)
- Reduce lower respiratory infections
- Inhibit *Candida* overgrowth
- Inhibit vaginosis
- Prevent colorectal tumor growth
- Restore NK-cell activity in smokers

- ❖ Stimulate the immune system among the elderly
- ❖ Increase oxygen burst activity of monocytes
- ❖ Increase CD56 lymphocytes
- ❖ Decrease rotavirus infections
- ❖ Decrease colds and influenza
- ❖ Reduce risk of bladder cancer
- ❖ Increase (good) HDL-cholesterol
- ❖ Decrease triglycerides
- ❖ Decrease blood pressure
- ❖ Inhibit viral infections
- ❖ Inhibit malignant pleural effusions secondary to lung cancer
- ❖ Reduce cervix tumors when used in combination radiation therapy
- ❖ Inhibit tumor growth of carcinomatous peritonitis/stomach cancer
- ❖ Break down nutrients for bioavailability

Lactobacillus rhamnosus

This species was previously thought to be a subspecies of *L. casei*. *L. rhamnosus* is a common ingredient in many yogurts and other commercial probiotic foods. *L. rhamnosus* have also been extensively studied over the years. Much of this research has focused upon a particular strain, *L. rhamnosus* GG. *L. rhamnosus* GG have been shown in numerous studies to significantly stimulate the immune system and inhibit a variety of infections. *L. rhamnosus* will also dwell in the mouth, pharynx and nasal cavity on a transient basis, but not for very long. This strain also has shown to have good intestinal wall adhesion properties. This is not to say, however, that non-GG strains will not perform similarly. In fact, studies with *L. rhamnosus* GR-1, *L. rhamnosus* 573/L, and *L. rhamnosus* LC705 strains have also shown positive results. The GG strain (LGG is trademarked by the Valio Ltd. Company in Finland) was patented in 1985 by two scientists, Dr. Sherwood Gorbach and Dr. Barry Goldin (hence the Gs). This patent and trademark, of course, gives these companies the incentive to fund expensive research to show the properties of this strain. Thanks to them, we have found that *Lactobacillus rhamnosus* (or the GG strain specifically) has a number of the health-promoting properties.

Human clinical research has shown that *L. rhamnosus* can:
- ❖ Inhibit a number of pathogenic bacterial infections
- ❖ Improve glucose control
- ❖ Reduce risk of ear infections
- ❖ Reduce risk of respiratory infections
- ❖ Decrease beta-glucosidase
- ❖ Inhibit vaginosis
- ❖ Reduce eczema
- ❖ Reduce colds and influenza

- Stimulate the immune system
- Increase IgA levels in mouth mucosa
- Increase IgA levels in mothers breast milk
- Inhibit *Pseudomonas aeruginosa* infections in respiratory tract
- Inhibit *Clostridium difficile*
- Increase immune response in HIV/AIDS patients
- Decrease symptoms of HIV/AIDS
- Inhibit rotavirus
- Inhibit enterobacteria
- Reduce IBS symptoms
- Decrease IL-12, IL-2+ and CD69+ T-cells in IBS
- Reduce constipation
- Inhibit vancomycin-resistant enterococci (antibiotic-resistant)
- Reduce the risk of colon cancer
- Modulate skin IgE sensitization
- Inhibit *H. pylori* (ulcer-causing)
- Reduce atopic dermatitis in children
- Increase Hib IgG levels in allergy-prone infants
- Reduce colic
- Stimulate infant growth
- Stimulate IgM, IgA and IgG levels
- Stabilize intestinal barrier function (decreased permeability)
- Increase IFN-gamma
- Modulate IL-4
- Help prevent atopic eczema
- Reduce *Streptococcus mutans*
- Stimulate tumor killing activity among NK-cells
- Modulate IL-10 (anti-inflammatory)
- Reduce inflammation
- Reduce LDL-cholesterol levels

Lactobacillus plantarum

L. plantarum has been part of the human diet for thousands of years, and will live in the mouth and the pharynx transiently, and the intestines on a longer-term basis. They are active in cultures of sauerkraut, gherkin and olive brines. They are used to make sourdough bread, Nigerian ogi and fufu, kocha from Ethiopia, and sour mifen noodles from China, Korean kim chi and other traditional foods. *L. plantarum* are also found in dairy and cow dung, so it is a common resident of cow intestines, which is one reason why cow dung is considered in India as being antiseptic.

L. plantarum is a hardy strain. The bacteria have been shown to survive all the way through the intestinal tract and into the feces. Temperature for optimal growth is 86-95 degrees F. *L. plantarum* are not permanent residents, however. When supplemented, they vigorously attack pathogenic bacteria, and create an environment hospitable for incubated resident strains to expand. *L. plantarum* also produce lysine, and a number of antibiotics including lactolin.

Human clinical research has shown that *L. plantarum* can:
- Reduce burn infections (topical)
- Increase burn healing
- Strengthen the immune system
- Help restore healthy liver enzymes (in mild alcohol-induced liver injury)
- Reduce frequency and severity of respiratory diseases during the cold and flu season
- Reduce intestinal permeability
- Inhibit various intestinal pathobiotics (such as *Clostridium difficile*)
- Reduce Th2 (inflammatory) levels and increase Th1/Th2 ratio
- Reduce inflammatory responses
- Reduce symptoms and aid healing of multiple traumas among injured patients
- Reduce fungal infections
- Reduce IBS symptoms
- Reduce pancreatic sepsis (infection)
- Reduce systolic blood pressure
- Reduce leptin levels (good for weight loss)
- Reduce interleukin-6 (IL-6) levels
- Reduce adhesion of vein endothelial cells by monocytes (risk of atherosclerosis)
- Reduce postoperative infection
- Reduce risk of pneumonia
- Reduce kidney oxalate levels
- Decrease flatulence
- Stimulate immunity in HIV children

Lactobacillus bulgaricus

We owe the *bulgaricus* name to Ilya Mechnikov, who named it after the Bulgarians—who used *L. bulgaricus* to make the fermented milks that appeared to be related to their extreme longevity. In the 1960s and 1970s, Russian researcher Dr. Ivan Bogdanov focused on the secretions of *L. bulgaricus* and later on fragmented cell walls of the bacteria. Early studies indicated antitumor effects. As the research progressed into clinical research and commercialization, it became obvious that *L. bulgaricus* cell fragments have a host of immune system stimulating benefits.

L. bulgaricus bacteria are transients that assist *bifidobacteria* colony growth. *L. bulgaricus* stimulate the immune system and have antitumor effects. They also produce antibiotic and antiviral substances such as bulgarican and others. *L. bulgaricus* bacteria have been reported to have anti-herpes effects as well. *L. bulgaricus* require more heat to colonize than many probiotics—at 104-109 degrees F.

Human clinical research has shown that *L. bulgaricus* can:
- ❖ Reduce intestinal permeability
- ❖ Decrease IBS symptoms
- ❖ Help manage HIV symptoms
- ❖ Stimulate TNF-alpha
- ❖ Stimulate IL-1beta
- ❖ Decrease diarrhea (rotavirus and non-rotavirus)
- ❖ Decrease nausea
- ❖ Increase phagocytic activity
- ❖ Increase leukocyte levels
- ❖ Increase immune response
- ❖ Increase CD8+ levels
- ❖ Lower CD4+/CD8+ ratio (lower CD4+—associated with inflammation)
- ❖ Increase IFN-gamma
- ❖ Lower total cholesterol
- ❖ Lower LDL levels
- ❖ Lower triglycerides
- ❖ Inhibit viruses
- ❖ Reduce *S. mutans* in the mouth
- ❖ Increase absorption of dairy (lactose)
- ❖ Increase white blood cell counts after chemotherapy
- ❖ Increase IgA specific to rotavirus (increased immunity against rotavirus)
- ❖ Reduce intestinal bacteria

Lactobacillus brevis

L. brevis are natural residents of cow intestines. They are therefore found in raw milk, colostrum, and cheese. For those who consume these frequently, *L. brevis* will temporarily inhabit the oral cavity and pharynx. They are transient in humans, but there is also the possibility that they can reside longer-term or permanently within the human intestines.

Human clinical research has shown that *L. brevis* can:
- ❖ Reduce periodontal disease
- ❖ Reduce PGE2 levels
- ❖ Reduce IFN-gamma levels
- ❖ Reduce mouth ulcers
- ❖ Reduce urinary oxalate levels (kidney stones)
- ❖ Decrease *H. pylori* colonization

Gum Disease and Dental Cavities

The gums and teeth are coated with legions of different bacteria—some probiotic and some pathogenic. Typical oral bacteria include *Streptococcus mutans, Streptococcus salivarius*, *Lactobacillus salivarius*, *E. coli*, *Streptococcus pyogenes*, *Porphyromonas gingivalis*, *Tannerella forsynthensis* and *Prevotella intermedia*. With a diet containing too many simple sugars and poor dental hygiene, the pathogenic bacteria can overwhelm the probiotics, causing infected gums and teeth. As pathogenic populations of *S. mutans, S. pyogenes, P. gingivalis, T. forsynthensis* and *P. intermedia* come into greater numbers, serious infections can occur. These conditions are often symptomized by gingivitis, teeth root infection, jawbone infections and general periodontal disease.

Streptococcus mutans was first isolated in 1924, but it was not linked to dental caries until the early 1960s. *S. mutans* and other cavity-forming bacteria consume sugars and carbohydrates from our foods, and produce destructive acids. These acids interact with the calcium in our tooth enamel, forming plaque. It is this interaction and plaque-formation that create cavities. There is now reason to believe that, like probiotics, *S. mutans* can be passed on from mother to infant.

This leads us to wonder whether *Streptococcus mutans* might actually be a eubiotic: a probiotic at controlled colony sizes. Like some other eubiotic yeasts and bacteria, perhaps it is a natural resident of the mouth that simply has grown beyond its healthy populations because of our eating and lifestyle imbalances.

All of the bacteria mentioned above and others can reside in both healthy and infected mouths. The strategy promoted by the modern medical and dental industries is to try to kill virtually all bacteria with various antiseptic mouthwashes and toothpastes. As we can see from continuing statistics on gingivitis and dental caries, these strategies are not working very well. A better strategy may be to use nature's probiotic populations to create a balance between the healthy bacteria and the disease-promoting bacteria. If probiotic populations are maximized, they will deplete and manage the pathogenic bacteria populations.

Let's see how this is supported by the research:

Researchers from the Istanbul's Yeditepe University Dental School (Caglar *et al.* 2008) gave oral lozenges of *Lactobacillus reuteri* or placebo to 20 healthy young women. After sucking on one lozenge a day for 10 days, salivary *Streptococcus mutans* levels were significantly reduced among the probiotic group, compared to the placebo group and before treatment.

Scientists from Yeditepe University (Caglar *et al.* 2007) gave placebo or *Lactobacillus reuteri* probiotic chewing gum to 80 healthy young adults for three weeks. The *L. reuteri* gum significantly reduced levels of salivary *Streptococcus mutans* compared to placebo and before treatment.

Scientists from Italy's University of L'Aquila, Department of Experimental Medicine (Riccia *et al.* 2007) gave 8 healthy volunteers and 21 chronic periodontitis patients *Lactobacillus brevis* lozenges. The probiotic treatment led to the total disappearance of all clinical symptoms among all patients. They also had a significant decrease in inflammatory markers nitrite/nitrate, PGE2, matrix metalloproteinase, and saliva IFN-gamma levels.

In another dental school study, *Lactobacillus reuteri* ATCC 55730 or placebo was given to 120 young adults through straw or lozenge daily for 3 weeks. *Streptococcus mutans* were significantly reduced in both probiotic groups as compared to the placebo group and before treatment (Caglar *et al.* 2006).

Researchers at Japan's Tohoku University Graduate School of Dentistry (Shimauchi *et al.* 2008) treated 66 human volunteers with freeze-dried *Lactobacillus salivarius* WB21 lozenge tablets or a placebo for 8 weeks. Periodontal testing confirmed that the probiotic group had significantly greater improvements in plaque index and probing pocket depth compared to the placebo group and before treatment.

Researchers from Turkey's Yeditepe University dental school (Caglar *et al.* 2008) gave 24 healthy young adult volunteers ice-cream containing *Bifidobacterium lactis* Bb-12 or a placebo ice cream for 40 days. Salivary *Streptococcus mutans* counts were significantly reduced in the probiotic ice cream group compared to the placebo group and before treatment.

Scientists from the University of Copenhagen (Twetman *et al.* 2009) gave three groups either chewing gum with placebo or two strains of *Lactobacillus reuteri* for 10 minutes a day for two weeks. Their gums were examined and given immunoassays for gingivitis inflammation. Bleeding on probing was significantly less among the probiotic subjects. TNF-alpha and IL-8 significantly decreased among the probiotic group. IL-1beta also decreased during the chewing period. The researchers concluded that, *"The reduction of pro-inflammatory cytokines in GCF may be proof of principle for the probiotic approach combating inflammation in the oral cavity."*

Researchers from the Institute of Dentistry at the University of Helsinki (Näse *et al.* 2001) investigated the effect of *Lactobacillus rhamnosus* GG on dental caries. Milk with or without *Lactobacillus rhamnosus* GG was given to 594 children ages 1 to 6 years old. The probiotic group had significantly less dental caries and significantly lower mutans streptococcus counts by the end of the study—especially among the 3- to 4-year-olds.

Scientists from the Universidad Nacional Autónoma de Mexico (Bayona *et al.* 1990) gave 245 seven-year-old children chewable tablets of either pyridoxine (vitamin B6) with heat-killed probiotics (streptococci and lactobacilli) or tablets with pyridoxine once a week for 16 weeks. Four evaluations were made over a two-year period from the beginning of the study. There was a 42% reduction of dental caries among the probiotic group compared to the placebo group.

Scientists from Sweden's Malmö University (Krasse *et al.* 2006) gave *Lactobacillus reuteri* or placebo to 59 patients with moderate to severe gingivitis. After 2 weeks of treatment, the gingival index and plaque index were established from measurements of two teeth surfaces and from saliva. The average gingival index and plaque index was significantly lower in the *L. reuteri* probiotic groups. The researchers concluded that, "*Lactobacillus reuteri* was efficacious in reducing both gingivitis and plaque in patients with moderate to severe gingivitis."

Finnish researchers from the University of Helsinki (Ahola *et al.* 2002) found that the long-term consumption of milk containing *Lactobacillus rhamnosus* GG significantly reduced dental caries. They found this same effect from probiotic cheese ingestion. To illustrate this later effect, the researchers gave 74 young adults a placebo or 60 grams of probiotic cheese per day for three weeks. There were significantly lower salivary *Streptococcus mutans* counts among the probiotic cheese group.

Italian scientists (Petti *et al.* 2001) gave healthy volunteers either yogurt with *Streptococcus thermophilus* and *Lactobacillus bulgaricus* or non-probiotic ice cream for 8 weeks. The probiotic group had lower levels of salivary *Streptococcus mutans* than the control group. However, *L. bulgaricus* was only transiently detected in the oral cavity, indicating that it did not colonize well within the mouth [in contrast with observations of other species such as *L. reuteri*].

Irritable Bowel Syndrome and Crohn's Disease

IBS is one of those diseases that physicians like to qualify as an autoimmune disease. As we've discussed earlier, the concept that the body's immune system is attacking itself for no reason is not logical. There are reasons the immune system might target cells from within the body. These can range from the cells being damaged by environmental toxins, endotoxins, oxidative (free) radicals, viruses, to the immune system itself being damaged. How do probiotics intermix within these possibilities?

The research illustrates that probiotics directly attack foreign invaders like bacteria, viruses and fungi, often before they can damage the cells of the intestinal walls. Probiotics can also bind to oxidative radicals formed by many types of toxins. Probiotics will also line the intestinal cells, creating a barrier for toxins to enter the blood. They secrete lactic acid and other biochemicals that prevent endotoxic microorganisms from flourishing. Probiotics will also signal the immune system with the identities of pathogens, and then assist in their eradication.

Deficiencies of probiotics in the intestines usually result in overgrowths of pathogenic microorganisms like *Clostridia* spp., *E. coli*, *H. pylori* and *Candida* spp. These damage the cells of the intestinal wall and produce endotoxins that poison intestinal cells. In addition, a lack of probiotics means that food will not be properly broken down, as probiotics help break down many large food molecules into bioavailable nutrients. This means the intestinal cells will become under-nourished too.

Toxins from our foods will also more easily reach the intestinal wall cells without the protective agency that probiotics provide. For this reason, the intestinal cells have more exposure to various toxic chemicals from our foods and environment, including pesticides, herbicides and preservatives. These can damage intestinal cells to the point where they do not function normally. They can also mutate through adaptation to toxin exposure. Toxin exposure and subsequent genetic alteration can cause the immune system to launch an inflammatory attack on intestinal cells, in an effort to rid them from the body. This can result in the inflammation and pain associated with Crohn's and IBS.

Here is some research supporting these conclusions:

Researchers from the Medical University of Warsaw (Gawrońska *et al.* 2007) investigated 104 children who had functional dyspepsia, irritable bowel syndrome, or functional abdominal pain. They gave the children either placebo or *Lactobacillus rhamnosus* GG. for 4 weeks. The probiotic group had overall treatment success (25% versus 9.6%) compared to the placebo group. The IBS probiotic group had even more treatment success compared to the placebo IBS group (33% versus 5%). The probiotic group also had significantly reduced pain frequency.

French researchers (Drouault-Holowacz *et al.* 2008) gave probiotics or a placebo to 100 patients with irritable bowel syndrome. Between the first and fourth weeks of treatment, the probiotic group had significantly less abdominal pain (42% versus 24%) than the placebo group.

Researchers from Poland's Curie Regional Hospital (Niedzielin *et al.* 2001) gave *Lactobacillus plantarum* 299V or placebo to 40 IBS patients. IBS symptoms significantly improved for 95% of the probiotic patients versus just 15% of the placebo group.

Forty IBS patients took *Lactobacillus acidophilus* SDC 2012, 2013 or a placebo for four weeks in research at the Samsung Medical Center and Korea's Sungkyunkwan University School of Medicine (Sinn *et al.* 2008). The probiotic group had a 23% reduction in pain and discomfort while the placebo group showed no improvement.

Scientists from Italy's University of Parma (Fanigliulo *et al.* 2006) gave *Bifidobacterium longum* W11 or rifaximin (an IBS medication) to 70 IBS patients for two months. The probiotic patients reported fewer symptoms and greater improvement than the rifaxmin patients. The researchers commented: "The abnormalities observed in the colonic flora of IBS suggest, in fact, that a probiotic approach will ultimately be justified."

Researchers from the University of Helsinki (Kajander *et al.* 2008) treated 86 patients with IBS with either a placebo or a combination of *Lactobacillus rhamnosus* GG, *L. rhamnosus* Lc705, *Propionibacterium freudenreichii* subsp. *Shermanii* JS and *Bifidobacterium animalis* subsp. *lactis.* After 5 months, the probiotic group had a significant reduction of IBS symptoms, especially with respect to distension and abdominal pain. The researchers concluded that, "this multi-species probiotic seems to be an effective and safe option to alleviate symptoms of irritable bowel syndrome, and to stabilize the intestinal microbiota."

Scientists from the Canadian Research and Development Centre for Probiotics and The Lawson Health Research Institute in Ontario (Lorea Baroja *et al.* 2007) studied 20 IBS patients, 15 Crohn's patients, 5 ulcerative colitis patients, and 20 healthy volunteers. All subjects were given a yogurt supplemented with *Lactobacillus rhamnosus* GR-1 and *L. reuteri* RC-14 for 30 days. IBS inflammatory markers were tested in the bloodstream. CD4(+) CD25(+) T-cells increased significantly among the probiotic IBS group. Tumor necrosis factor (TNF)-alpha(+)/interleukin (IL)-12(+) monocytes decreased for all the groups except the IBS probiotic group. Myeloid DC decreased among most probiotic groups, but was also stimulated in IBS patients. Serum IL-12, IL-2(+) and CD69(+) T-cells also decreased in probiotic IBS patients. The researchers also concluded that, "Probiotic yogurt intake was associated with significant anti-inflammatory effects…"

Researchers from the General Hospital of Celle (Plein and Hotz 1993) gave *Saccharomyces boulardii* or placebo to 20 Crohn's disease patients with diarrhea flare-ups. After ten weeks, the probiotic group had a significant reduction in bowel movement frequency compared with the control group. The control group's bowel movement frequency rose in the tenth week and then subsided to initial frequency levels—consistent with flare-ups.

In another study from Finland (Kajander *et al.* 2005), a placebo or combination of *Lactobacillus rhamnosus* GG, *L. rhamnosus* LC705, *Bifidobacterium breve* Bb99 and *Propionibacterium freudenreichii* subsp. *shermanii* JS was given to of 103 patients with IBS. The total symptom score (abdominal pain + distension + flatulence + borborygmi) was 7.7 points lower among the probiotic group. This represented a 42% reduction in the symptoms of the probiotic group compared with a 6% reduction of symptoms among the placebo group.

In a study from Yonsei University College of Medicine in Korea (Kim *et al.* 2006), 40 irritable bowel syndrome patients were given either a placebo or a combination of *Bacillus subtilis* and *Streptococcus faecium* for four weeks. The severity and frequency of abdominal pain decreased significantly in the probiotic group.

Researchers from Sweden's Lund University Hospital (Nobaek *et al.* 2000) gave 60 patients with irritable bowel syndrome either a placebo or daily rose-hip drink with *Lactobacillus plantarum* for four weeks. Enterococci levels increased among the placebo group were unchanged in the test group. Flatulence was significantly reduced among the probiotic group compared with the placebo group. At a 12-month follow-up, the probiotic group maintained significantly better overall GI symptoms and function than the placebo group.

New York scientists (Hun 2009) gave 44 IBS patients either a placebo or *Bacillus coagulans* GBI-30 for 8 weeks. The probiotic group experienced significant improvements in abdominal pain and bloating symptoms versus the placebo group.

Scientists at Ireland's University College in Cork (O'Mahony *et al.* 2005) studied 77 irritable bowel syndrome patients with abnormal IL-10/IL-12 ratios—indicating a proinflammatory, Th1 status. The patients were given a placebo, *Lactobacillus salivarius* UCC4331 or *Bifidobacterium infantis* 35624 for eight weeks. IBS symptoms were logged daily and assessed weekly. Tests included quality of life, stool microbiology, and blood samples to test peripheral blood mononuclear cell release of inflammatory cytokines interleukin (IL)-10 and IL-12. Patients who took *B. infantis* 35624 had a significantly greater reduction in abdominal pain and discomfort, bloating and distention, and bowel movement difficulty, compared to the other groups. IL-10/IL-12 ratios—indicative of Th1 proinflammatory metabolism—were also normalized in the probiotic *B. infantis* group.

Researchers from the Umberto Hospital in Venice in Italy (Saggioro 2004) studied probiotics on seventy adults with irritable bowel syndrome. They were given 1) a placebo; 2) a combination of *Lactobacillus plantarum* and *Bifidobacterium breve*; or 3) a combination of *Lactobacillus plantarum* and *Lactobacillus acidophilus* for four weeks. After 28 days of treatment, pain scores measuring different abdominal regions decreased among the probiotic groups by 45% and 49% respectively, versus 29% for the placebo group. The IBS symptom severity scores decreased among the probiotic groups after 28 days by 56% and 55.6% respectively, versus 14% among the placebo group.

Sixty-eight patients with irritable bowel syndrome were treated at the TMC Hospital in Shizuoka, Japan (Tsuchiya *et al.* 2004) with either placebo or a combination of *Lactobacillus acidophilus*, *Lactobacillus helveticus* and *Bifidobacteria* for twelve weeks. The probiotic treatment was either "effective" or "very effective" in more than 80% of the IBS patients. In addition, less than 5% of the probiotic group reported the treatment as "not effective," while more than 40% of the placebo patients reported their placebo treatment as "not effective." The probiotic group also reported significant improvement of bowel habits.

Researchers from Britain's University of Manchester School of Medicine (Whorwell *et al.* 2007) gave a placebo or *Bifidobacterium infantis* 35624 to 362 primary care women with irritable bowel syndrome in a large-scale, multicenter study. After four weeks of treatment, *B. infantis* was significantly more effective than the placebo in reducing bloating, bowel dysfunction, incomplete evacuation, straining, and the passing of gas.

Scientists from Denmark's Hvidovre Hospital and the University Hospital of Copenhagen (Wildt *et al.* 2006) gave 29 colitis-IBS patients either *Lactobacillus acidophilus* LA-5 and *Bifidobacterium animalis* subsp. *lactis* BB-12, or a placebo for twelve weeks. The probiotic treatment group had a decrease in bowel frequency from 32 per week to 23 per week. Furthermore, the probiotic group had an average reduction in the frequency of liquid stools from 6 days per week to 1 day per week.

Scientists at Poland's Jagiellonian University Medical College (Zwolińska-Wcisło *et al.* 2006) tested 293 ulcer patients, 60 patients with ulcerative colitis, 12 patients with irritable bowel syndrome and 72 patients with other gastrointestinal issues. Compared to placebo, *Lactobacillus acidophilus* supplementation resulted in a lessening of symptoms, a reduction of fungal colonization, and increased levels of immune system cytokines TNF-alpha and IL-1 beta.

Medical researchers from Finland's University of Helsinki (Kajander *et al.* 2007) sought to understand the mechanism of probiotics' proven ability to reduce IBS symptoms. They gave either a placebo or a combination of *Lactobacillus rhamnosus* GG, *Lactobacillus rhamnosus* Lc705, *Propionibacterium freudenreichii* subsp. *shermanii* JS and *Bifidobacterium breve* Bb99 to 55 irritable bowel syndrome patients. After six months of treatment, composition of feces and intestinal microorganism content illustrated a significant drop in glucuronidase levels in the probiotic group compared to the placebo group. The researchers concluded that there was a complexity of different factors, and so far unknown mechanisms explaining "the alleviation of irritable bowel syndrome symptoms by the multispecies probiotic."

Digestive Conditions

Chronic digestive problems, which include bloating, indigestion, and cramping are often symptoms of IBS, Crohn's disease or colitis. These diseases (IBS, etc.) are also typically accompanied by chronic pain and intestinal inflammation, however. Occasional indigestion, bloating and cramping is often associated with a developing case of dysbiosis caused by antibiotic use, poor diet, or an overgrowth of specific pathogenic microorganisms. Enzyme deficiency can be caused by probiotic deficiencies. Probiotics produce a number of enzymes, including protease and lipase—necessary for the break down of proteins and fats. Poor digestion is often the result of a lack of these and other enzymes. Gastrointestinal difficulties in general are often caused by dysbiosis. This can include an overgrowth of yeasts, pathogenic bacteria or both. Here are a few of the many studies showing that digestion can improve with probiotic use:

French researchers (Guyonnet *et al.* 2009) gave *Bifidobacterium lactis* DN-173010 with yogurt strains to 371 adults reporting digestive discomfort for 2 weeks. 82.5% of the probiotic group reported improved digestive symptoms compared to 2.9% of the control group.

Another group of French scientists (Diop *et al.* 2008) gave 64 volunteers with high levels of stress and incidental gastrointestinal symptoms either a placebo or *Lactobacillus acidophilus* Rosell-52 and *Bifidobacterium longum* for three weeks. At the end of the three weeks, the stress-related gastrointestinal symptoms of abdominal pain, nausea and vomiting decreased by 49% among the probiotic group.

Allergies and Eczema

Allergies have been increasing over the past few decades. Modern medical research is puzzled with this progression. Why are suddenly more people becoming allergic to the plants and pollens that have surrounded humans for thousands of years? This is a huge topic, but we do know from the research that the lack of healthy probiotic colonies is at least a contributing factor.

Probiotics mechanisms have been increasingly connected to inflammatory and allergic responses. They play a critical role in maintaining the epithelial barrier function of the intestinal tract. Allergies appear to increase with intestinal permeability. Without an adequate intestinal barrier, larger food molecules, endotoxins and microorganisms can enter the bloodstream more easily. These increase the body's total toxin burden, making it more sensitive to environmental inputs such as pollen.

Research from Sweden's Linköping University (Böttcher *et al.* 2008) gave *Lactobacillus reuteri* or a placebo to 99 pregnant women from gestational week 36 until infant delivery. The babies were followed for two years after birth, and analyzed for eczema and allergen sensitization and immunity markers. Probiotic supplementation lowered TGF-beta2 levels in mother's milk and babies' feces and slightly increased IL-10 levels in mothers' colostrum. Lower levels of TGF-beta2 are associated with lower sensitization and lower risk of IgE-associated eczema.

German researchers (Grönlund *et al.* 2007) tested 61 infants and mother pairs for allergic status and bifidobacteria levels from 30-35 weeks of gestation and from one-month old. Every mother's breast milk contained some type of bifidobacteria, with *Bifidobacterium longum* found most frequently. However, only the infants of allergic, atopic mothers had colonization with *B. adolescentis*. Allergic mothers also had significantly less bifidobacteria in their breast-milk versus non-allergic mothers. Infants of allergic mothers also had less bifidobacteria in the feces than did infants from non-allergic mothers.

Japanese scientists (Xiao *et al.* 2006) gave 44 patients with Japanese cedar pollen allergies *Bifidobacterium longum* BB536 for 13 weeks. The probiotic group had significantly decreased symptoms of rhinorrhea (runny nose) and nasal blockage versus the placebo group. The probiotic group also had decreased activity among plasma T-helper type 2 (Th2) cells and increased activity among Japanese cedar pollen-specific IgE. The researchers concluded that the results, "suggest the efficacy of BB536 in relieving allergic symptoms, probably through the modulation of Th2-skewed immune response."

Researchers from the Wellington School of Medicine and Health Sciences at New Zealand's University of Otago (Wickens *et al.* 2008) studied the association between probiotics and eczema in 474 children. Pregnant women took either a placebo, *Lactobacillus rhamnosus* HN001, or *Bifidobacterium animalis* subsp *lactis* strain HN019 starting from 35 weeks gestation, and their babies received the same treatment from birth to 2 years old. The probiotic infants given *L. rhamnosus* had significantly lower incidence of eczema compared with infants taking the placebo. There was no significant difference between the *B. animalis* group and the placebo group, however.

Researchers from Japan's Kansai Medical University Kouri Hospital (Hattori *et al.* 2003) gave 15 children with atopic dermatitis either *Bifidobacterium breve* M-16V or a placebo. After one month, the probiotic group had a significant improvement of allergic symptoms.

Japanese scientists (Ishida *et al.* 2003) gave a drink with *Lactobacillus acidophilus* strain L-92 or a placebo to 49 patients with perennial allergic rhinitis for eight weeks. The probiotic group showed significant improvement in runny nose and watery eyes symptoms, along with decreased nasal mucosa swelling and redness compared to the placebo group. These results were also duplicated in a follow-up study (2005) of 23 allergy sufferers by some of the same researchers.

Researchers from Tokyo's Juntendo University School of Medicine (Fujii *et al.* 2006) gave 19 preterm infants placebo or *Bifidobacterium breve* supplementation for three weeks after birth. Anti-inflammatory serum TGF-beta1 levels in the probiotic group were elevated on day 14 and remained elevated through day 28. Messenger RNA expression was enhanced for the probiotic group on day 28 compared with the placebo group. The researchers concluded that, "These results demonstrated that the administration of *B. breve* to preterm infants can up-regulate TGF-beta1 signaling and may possibly be beneficial in attenuating inflammatory and allergic reactions in these infants."

Scientists from Britain's Institute of Food Research (Ivory *et al.* 2008) gave *Lactobacillus casei* Shirota (LcS) to 10 patients with seasonal allergic rhinitis. The researchers compared immune status with daily ingestion of a milk drink with or without live *Lactobacillus casei* over a period of 5 months. Blood samples were tested for plasma IgE and grass pollen-specific IgG by an enzyme immunoassay. Patients treated with *Lactobacillus casei* milk showed significantly reduced levels of antigen-induced IL-5, IL-6 and IFN-gamma production compared with the placebo group. Levels of specific IgG also increased and IgE decreased in the probiotic group. The researchers concluded that, "These data show that probiotic supplementation modulates immune responses in allergic rhinitis and may have the potential to alleviate the severity of symptoms."

Researchers from the Skin and Allergy Hospital at the University of Helsinki (Kukkonen *et al.* 2007) studied the role of probiotics and allergies with 1,223 pregnant women carrying children with a high-risk of allergies. A placebo or lactobacilli and bifidobacteria combination with GOS was given to the pregnant women for 2 to 4 weeks before delivery, and their babies continued the treatment after birth. At two years of age, the infants in the probiotic group had 25% less chance of eczema and 34% less chance of contracting atopic eczema.

The same researchers from the Skin and Allergy Hospital and Helsinki University Central Hospital (Kukkonen *et al.* 2009) studied the immune effects of feeding probiotics to pregnant mothers. 925 pregnant mothers were given a placebo or a combination of *Lactobacillus rhamnosus* GG and LC705, *Bifidobacterium breve* Bb99, and *Propionibacterium freudenreichii* ssp. *shermanii* for four weeks prior to delivery. Their infants were given the same formula together with prebiotics, or a placebo for 6 months after birth. During the infants' six-month treatment period, antibiotics were prescribed less often among the probiotic group by 23%. In addition, respiratory infections occurred less frequently among the probiotic group through the two-year follow-up period (even after treatment had stopped) compared to the placebo group (an average of 3.7 infections versus 4.2 infections).

Finnish scientists (Kirjavainen *et al.* 2002) gave 21 infants with early onset atopic eczema a placebo or *Bifidobacterium lactis* Bb-12. Serum IgE concentration correlated directly to *Escherichia coli* and bacteroides counts, indicating the association between these bacteria with atopic sensitization. The probiotic group had a decrease in the numbers of *Escherichia coli* and bacteroides.

Sonicated *Streptococcus thermophilus* cream was applied to the forearms of 11 patients with atopic dermatitis for two weeks. This led to a significant increase of skin ceramide levels, and a significant improvement of their clinical signs and symptoms—including erythema, scaling and pruritus (Di Marzio *et al.* 2003).

Japanese researchers (Odamaki *et al.* 2007) gave yogurt with *Bifidobacterium longum* BB536 or plain yogurt to 40 patients with Japanese cedar pollinosis for 14 weeks. *Bacteroides fragilis* significantly changed with pollen dispersion. The ratio of *B. fragilis* to bifidobacteria also increased significantly during pollen season among the placebo group but not in the *B. longum* group. Peripheral blood mononuclear cells from the patients indicated that *B. fragilis* microorganisms induced significantly more Th2 cell cytokines such as interleukin-6, and fewer Th1 cell cytokines such as IL-12 and interferon. The researchers concluded that, "These results suggest a relationship between fluctuation in intestinal microbiota and pollinosis allergy. Furthermore, intake of BB536 yogurt appears to exert positive influences on the formation of anti-allergic microbiota."

Scientists from the Department of Oral Microbiology at Japan's Asahi University School of Dentistry (Ogawa *et al.* 2006) studied skin allergic symptoms and blood chemistry of healthy human volunteers during the cedar pollen season in Japan. After supplementation with *Lactobacillus casei*, activity of cedar pollen-specific IgE, thymus, chemokines, eosinophils, and interferon-gamma levels all decreased among the probiotic group.

Researchers from the School of Medicine and Health Sciences in Wellington, New Zealand (Sistek *et al.* 2006) determined in a study of *Lactobacillus rhamnosus* and *Bifidobacteria lactis* on 59 children with established atopic dermatitis that food-sensitized children responded significantly better to probiotics than did other atopic dermatitis children.

French scientists (Passeron *et al.* 2006) found that atopic dermatitis children improved significantly after three months of *Lactobacillus rhamnosus* treatment, based on SCORAD levels of 39.1 before and 20.7 afterward.

Scientists from Finland's National Public Health Institute (Piirainen *et al.* 2008) gave a placebo or *Lactobacillus rhamnosus* GG to 38 patients with atopic eczema for 5.5 months—starting 2.5 months before birch pollen season. Saliva and serum samples taken before and after indicated that allergen-specific IgA levels increased significantly among the probiotic group versus the placebo group (using the enzyme-linked immunosorbent assay (ELISA)). Allergen-specific IgE levels correlated positively with stimulated IgA and IgG in saliva, while they correlated negatively in the placebo group. The researchers concluded that the research showed that *L. rhamnosus* GG displayed "immunostimulating effects on oral mucosa seen as increased allergen specific IgA levels in saliva."

Children with cow's milk allergy and IgE-associated dermatitis were given a placebo or *Lactobacillus rhamnosus* GG and a combination of four other probiotic bacteria (Pohjavuori *et al.* 2004). The IFN-gamma by PBMCs at the beginning of supplementation was significantly lower among cow's milk allergy infants. However, cow's milk allergy infants receiving *L. rhamnosus* GG had significantly increased levels of IFN-gamma, showing increased tolerance.

The British medical publication *Lancet* published a study (Kalliomäki *et al.* 2003) where 107 children with a high risk of atopic eczema were given either a placebo or *Lactobacillus rhamnosus* GG during their first two years of life. Fourteen of 53 children receiving the probiotic developed atopic eczema, while 25 of 54 of the children receiving the placebo contracted atopic eczema by the end of the study.

In a study from the University of Western Australia School of Pediatrics (Taylor *et al.* 2006), 178 children born of mothers with allergies were given either *Lactobacillus acidophilus* or a placebo for the first six months of life. Those given the probiotics showed reduced levels of IL-5 and TGF-beta in response to polyclonal stimulation (typical for allergic responses), and significantly lower IL-10 responses to vaccines as compared with the placebo group. These results illustrated that the probiotics had increased allergen resistance among the probiotic group of children.

Researchers from the Department of Otolaryngology and Sensory Organ Surgery at Osaka University School of Medicine in Japan (Tamura *et al.* 2007) studied allergic response in chronic rhinitis patients. For eight weeks, patients were given either a placebo or *Lactobacillus casei* strain Shirota. Those with moderate-to-severe nasal symptom scores at the beginning of the study given probiotics experienced significantly reduced nasal symptoms compared to the placebo group and before treatment.

Intestinal Permeability

For years, traditional practitioners described a digestive disorder termed "leaky gut syndrome." This was largely dismissed by the medical establishment as anecdotal and non-existent. In recent years, however, research on intestinal drug absorption by the pharmaceutical industry has confirmed that the lining of the small intestine is subject to alteration, dramatically affecting absorption and permeability. As this research has progressed, it has become apparent that nutrient absorption can be significantly reduced due to permeability alteration. Worse, increased intestinal permeability syndrome (IIPS) may well be implicated in many allergic and arthritic conditions.

These diseases are related to the fact that permeability allows macromolecules—larger peptides, toxins and even invading microorganisms—into the bloodstream. Once these foreigners arrive in the bloodstream, the immune system may activate a variety of inflammatory responses as a defense measure. For example, the invasion of pathogenic microorganisms through the intestinal wall can result in bacterial translocation throughout the body—stimulating inflammatory responses (Baik 2004; Yasuda *et al.* 2006). Illustrating this mechanism, Blastocystis hominis—pathogenic bacteria typically found in the intestines—have been found within synovial (joint) membranes of arthritic patients (Kruger et al. 1994).

The intestinal brush barrier is a complex mucosal layer of enzymes, probiotics and ionic fluid. It forms a protective surface medium over the intestinal epithelium. It also provides an active nutrient transport mechanism. This mucosal layer is stabilized by the grooves of the intestinal microvilli. It contains glycoproteins and other ionic transporters, which attach to nutrient molecules, carrying them across intestinal membranes. Meanwhile the transport medium requires a delicately pH-balanced mix of ionic chemistry able to facilitate this transport of amino acids, minerals, vitamins, glucose and fatty acids. The mucosal layer is policed by billions of probiotic colonies, which help process incoming food molecules, excrete various nutrients, and control pathogens. In the proper mucosal environment, probiotics will produce several B vitamins and potent antibiotics (DeWill and Kudsk 1999).

The brush barrier is a triple-filter that screens for molecule size, ionic nature and nutrition quality. Much of this is performed via four mechanisms existing between the intestinal microvilli: tight junctions, adherens junctions, desmosomes, and of course probiotics. The tight functions form a bilayer interface between cells, controlling permeability. Desmosomes are points of interface between the tight junctions, and adherens junctions keep the cell membranes adhesive enough to stabilize the junctions. These junction mechanisms together regulate permeability at the intestinal wall.

This mucosal brush barrier creates the boundary between intestinal contents and our bloodstream. Should the mucosal layer chemistry become altered, its protective and ionic transport mechanisms become weakened, allowing toxic or larger molecules to be presented to the microvilli junctions. This contact can irritate the microvilli, causing a subsequent inflammatory response. This is now considered a contributing cause of IBS.

This situation also weakens the microvilli junctions, allowing the larger molecules immediate access to the bloodstream.

Intestinal permeability is caused by a number of factors. Alcohol is one of the most irritating substances to the mucosal lining and junctions. In addition, many pharmaceutical drugs, notably NSAIDs, have been identified as damaging to the mucosal chemistry and intestinal junction strength. Foods with high arachidonic fatty acid capability (such as trans-fats and animal meats); low-fiber, high-glucose foods; and high nitrite-forming foods have been suspected for their ability to compromise the intestinal lining. Toxic substances such as plasticizers, pesticides, herbicides, chlorinated water and food dyes are also suspected. Substances that increase PGE-2 response also negatively affect permeability (Martin-Venegas *et al.* 2006).

In addition, the overuse of antibiotics can cause a die-off of the all-important resident probiotic colonies. When intestinal probiotic colonies are decreased, pathogenic bacteria and yeasts can outgrow probiotic colonies. Pathogenic bacteria growth invades the brush barrier, introducing an influx of endotoxins (the waste matter of these microorganisms) into the bloodstream together with some of the microorganisms themselves.

Holistic doctors have attributed the influx of macromolecules into the bloodstream as a major cause for the increasing occurrence of food allergies in western society. Typically, intestinal barriers let only smaller molecules access to the liver and bloodstream—usually beneficial nutrients. Should larger, undigested food molecules enter the bloodstream—even if from a food consumed for decades—the body's immune system will not recognize them. This can lead to IgA and/or IgE responses, stimulating heightened histamine levels. This in turn can cause skin and/or sinus inflammatory responses.

This scenario is happening more frequently in western society. A food that has been a source of nutrition for many years begins to be identified by the immune system as toxic. This unfortunate circumstance results not only in the possibility of allergic response to some foods: Nutritional deficiencies can also result. Research is finally confirming these mechanisms (Laitinen and Isolauri 2005; Fasano and Shea-Donohue 2005).

Inflammatory responses resulting from IIPS are thus associated with sinusitis, allergies, psoriasis, asthma, arthritis and other inflammatory disorders. Overgrowth of *Candida albicans,* a typical fungal inhabitant of the digestive system at controlled populations, has also been attributed to IIPS. Systemic Candida infections have a route of translocation via IIPS.

The research has supported the link between IIPS and liver damage (Bode and Bode 2003). Alcohol consumption has also been associated with IIPS (Ferrier *et al.* 2006). Alcohol also damages probiotic populations (Bongaerts and Severijnen 2005).

In a study by scientists from China's Qilu Hospital and Shandong University (Zeng *et al.* 2008), 30 irritable bowel syndrome patients with intestinal wall permeability were given either a placebo or a fermented milk beverage with *Streptococcus thermophilus, Lactobacillus bulgaricus, Lactobacillus acidophilus* and *Bifidobacterium longum.* After four weeks, intestinal permeability reduced significantly among the probiotic group.

Researchers from Greece's Alexandra Regional General Hospital (Stratiki *et al.* 2007) gave 41 preterm infants of 27-36 weeks gestation a formula supplemented with *Bifidobacterium lactis* or a placebo. After 7 days, bifidobacteria counts were significantly higher, head growth was greater, and the lactulose/mannitol ratio (a marker for intestinal permeability) was significantly lower after 30 days in the probiotic group as compared to the placebo group. The researchers concluded that, "bifidobacteria supplemented infant formula decreases intestinal permeability of preterm infants and leads to increased head growth."

Granada medical researchers (Lara-Villoslada *et al.* 2007) gave *Lactobacillus coryniformis* CECT5711 and *Lactobacillus gasseri* CECT5714 or a placebo to 30 healthy children after having received conventional yogurt containing *Lactobacillus bulgaricus* and *Streptococcus thermophilus* for three weeks. The supplemented yogurt significantly inhibited *Salmonella cholerasuis* adhesion to intestinal mucins compared to before probiotic supplementation. The probiotic supplementation also increased IgA concentration in feces and saliva.

German scientists (Rosenfeldt *et al.* 2004) gave *Lactobacillus rhamnosus* 19070-2 and *L. reuteri* DSM 12246 or a placebo to 41 children. After six weeks of treatment, the frequency of GI symptoms were significantly lower (10% versus 39%) among the probiotic group as compared to the placebo group. In addition, the lactulose-to-mannitol ratio was lower in the probiotic group, indicating to the researchers that, "probiotic supplementation may stabilize the intestinal barrier function and decrease gastrointestinal symptoms in children with atopic dermatitis."

Researchers from the People's Hospital and the Jiao Tong University in Shangha (Qin *et al.* 2008) gave *Lactobacillus plantarum* or placebo to 76 patients with acute pancreatitis. Intestinal permeability was determined using the lactulose/rhamnose ratio. Organ failure, septic complications and death were also monitored. After 7 days of treatment, microbial infections averaged 38.9% in the probiotic group and 73.7% in the placebo group. 30.6% of the probiotic group colonized potentially pathogenic organisms, as compared to 50% of patients in the control group. The probiotic group also had significantly better clinical outcomes compared to the control group. The researchers concluded that *Lactobacillus plantarum* "can attenuate disease severity, improve the intestinal permeability and clinical outcomes."

Polyps, Diverticulosis and Diverticulitis

Polyps, diverticulosis and diverticulitis are abnormalities within the intestines or colon. They have been associated with Crohn's, IBS and ulcerative colitis, as well as intestinal cancer. They also have been seen forming seemingly without other disease pathologies. Diverticulosis is the bulging of sections of the intestines. When a bulging area weakens and bursts, that is called diverticulitis. A polyp, on the other hand, is a growth on the inside of the intestinal wall. These may be either benign, or cancerous. All of these conditions are associated with intestinal probiotics, because healthy probiotic colonies are essential to the health of the intestinal wall. We can see the evidence from the research:

Scientists from Sweden and Ireland (Rafter *et al.* 2007) gave placebo or *Lactobacillus rhamnosus* GG and *Bifidobacterium lactis* Bb12 to 43 polyp patients (who also had surgery for their removal) for 12 weeks. The probiotics significantly reduced colorectal proliferation and improved epithelial barrier function (reducing intestinal permeability) among the polyp patients. Testing also showed decreased exposure to intestinal genotoxins among the probiotic polyp patient group.

Researchers from The Netherlands' University Hospital Maastricht (Goossens *et al.* 2006) gave *Lactobacillus plantarum* 299v or a placebo to 29 polyp patients twice a day for two weeks. Fecal sample examinations and biopsies were collected during colonoscopy. *L. plantarum* 299v significantly increased probiotic bacteria levels from fecal tests and from rectal biopsies. Ascending colon populations were not significantly greater, however.

Researchers from the Digestive Endoscopy Unit at Italy's Lorenzo Bonomo Hospital (Tursi *et al.* 2008) treated 75 patients with symptomatic diverticulosis. Mesalazine and/or *Lactobacillus casei* DG were given for 10 days each month. Of the 71 patients that completed the study, 66 (88%) were symptom-free after 24 months. The researchers concluded that mesalazine and/or *Lactobacillus casei* were effective in maintaining diverticulosis remission for an extended period, assuming continued treatment.

Ulcers

Just a couple of decades ago, medical scientists and physicians were certain that ulcers were caused by too much acid in the stomach and the eating of spicy foods. This assumption has been debunked over the past two decades as researchers have confirmed that at least 80% of all ulcers are associated with *Helicobacter pylori* infections.

While acidic foods and gastrin produced by the stomach wall are also implicated with symptoms of heartburn and acid reflux, we know that a healthy stomach has a functional barrier that should prevent these normal food and gastric substances from harming the cells of the stomach wall. This barrier is called the mucosal membrane. This stomach's mucosal membrane contains a number of mucopolysaccharides and phospholipids that, together with secretions from intestinal and oral probiotics, protect the stomach cells from acids, toxins and bacteria invasions.

As doctors and researchers work to eradicate *H. pylori*, which infects billions of people worldwide, they are finding that *H. pylori* is becoming increasingly resistant to many of the antibiotics used in prescriptive treatment. Research from Poland's Center of Gastrology (Ziemniak 2006) investigated antibiotic use on *Helicobacter pylori* infections: 641 *H. pylori* patients were given various antibiotics typically applied to *H. pylori*. The results indicated that *H. pylori* had developed a 22% resistance to clarithromycin and 47% resistance to metronidazole. Worse, a 66% secondary resistance to clarithromycin and metronidazole was found, indicating *H. pylori*'s increasing resistance to antibiotics.

H. pylori bacteria do not always cause ulcers. In fact, only a small percentage of *H. pylori* infections actually become ulcerative. Meanwhile, there is some evidence that *H. pylori*—like *E. coli* and *Candida albicans*—may be a normal resident in a healthy intestinal tract, assuming it is properly balanced and managed by strong legions of probiotics.

Here are some research data that confirms the ability probiotics have in controlling and managing *H. pylori* overgrowths. Here we will also see probiotics' ability to arrest ulcerative colitis and even mouth ulcers:

Researchers from the Academic Hospital at Vrije University in The Netherlands (Cats *et al.* 2003) gave either a placebo or *Lactobacillus casei* Shirota to 14 *H. pylori*-infected patients for three weeks. Six additional *H. pylori*-infected subjects were used as controls. The researchers determined that *L. casei* significantly inhibits *H. pylori* growth. This effect was more pronounced for *L. casei* grown in milk solution than in the DeMan-Rogosa-Sharpe medium (a probiotic broth developed by researchers in 1960).

Mexican hospital researchers (Sahagún-Flores *et al.* 2007) gave 64 *Helicobacter pylori*-infected patients antibiotic treatment with or without *Lactobacillus casei* Shirota. *Lactobacillus casei* Shirota plus antibiotic treatment was 94% effective and antibiotic treatment alone was 76% effective.

Researchers from the Department of Internal Medicine and Gastroenterology at Italy's University of Bologna (Gionchetti *et al.* 2000) gave 40 ulcerative colitis patients either a placebo or a combination of four strains of lactobacilli, three strains of bifidobacteria, and one strain of *Streptococcus salivarius* subsp. *thermophilus* for nine months. The patients were tested monthly. Three patients (15%) in the probiotic group suffered relapses within the nine months, versus 20 (100%) in the placebo group.

Italian scientists from the University of Bologna (Venturi *et al.* 1999) also gave 20 patients with ulcerative colitis a combination of three bifidobacteria strains, four lactobacilli strains and *Streptococcus salivarius* subsp. *thermophilus* for 12 months. Fecal samples were obtained at the beginning, after 10 days, 20 days, 40 days, 60 days, 75 days, 90 days, 12 months and 15 days after the (12 months) end of the treatment period. Fifteen of the 20 treated patients achieved and maintained remission from ulcerative colitis during the study period.

British researchers from the University of Dundee and Ninewells Hospital Medical School (Furrie *et al.* 2005) gave 18 patients with active ulcerative colitis either *B. longum* or a placebo for one month. Clinical examination and rectal biopsies indicated that sigmoidoscopy scores were reduced in the probiotic group. In addition, mRNA levels for human beta defensins 2, 3, and 4 (higher in active ulcerative colitis) were significantly reduced among the probiotic group. Inflammatory cytokines tumor necrosis factor alpha and interleukin-1alpha were also significantly lower in the probiotic group. Biopsies showed reduced inflammation and the regeneration of epithelial tissue within the intestines among the probiotic group.

Scientists from Italy's Raffaele University Hospital (Guslandi *et al.* 2003) gave *Saccharomyces boulardii* or placebo to 25 patients with ulcerative colitis unsuitable for steroid therapy, for 4 weeks. Of the 24 patients completing the study, 17 attained clinical remission—confirmed endoscopically.

Researchers from Switzerland's University Hospital in Lausanne (Felley *et al.* 2001) gave fifty-three patients with ulcerative *H. pylori* infection milk with *L. johnsonii* or placebo for three weeks. Those given the probiotic drink had a significant *H. pylori* density decrease, reduced inflammation and less gastritis activity from *H. pylori*.

Lactobacillus reuteri ATCC 55730 or a placebo was given to 40 *H. pylori*-infected patients for 4 weeks by researchers from Italy's Università degli Studi di Bari (Francavilla *et al.* 2008). *L. reuteri* effectively suppressed *H. pylori* infection, decreased gastrointestinal pain, and reduced other dyspeptic symptoms.

Scientists from the Department of Internal Medicine at the Catholic University of Rome (Canducci *et al.* 2000) tested 120 patients with ulcerative *H. pylori* infections. Sixty patients received a combination of antibiotics rabeprazole, clarithromycin and amoxicillin. The other sixty patients received the same therapy together with a freeze-dried, inactivated culture of *Lactobacillus acidophilus*. The probiotic group had an 88% eradication of *H. pylori* while the antibiotic-only group had a 72% eradication of *H. pylori*.

Scientists from the University of Chile (Gotteland *et al.* 2005) gave 182 children with *H. pylori* infections placebo, antibiotics or probiotics. *H. pylori* were completely eradicated in 12% of those who took *Saccharomyces boulardii*, and in 6.5% of those given *L. acidophilus*. The placebo group had no *H. pylori* eradication.

Researchers from Japan's Kyorin University School of Medicine (Imase *et al.* 2007) gave *Lactobacillus reuteri* strain SD2112 in tablets or a placebo to 33 *H. pylori*-infected patients. After 4 and 8 weeks, *L. reuteri* significantly decreased and suppressed *H. pylori* in the probiotic group.

In a study of 347 patients with active *H. pylori* infections (ulcerous), half the group was given antibiotics and the other half was given antibiotics with yogurt (*Lactobacillus acidophilus* HY2177, *Lactobacillus casei* HY2743, *Bifidobacterium longum* HY8001, and *Streptococcus thermophilus* B-1). The yogurt plus antibiotics group had significantly more eradication of the *H. pylori* bacteria, and significantly less side effects than the antibiotics group (Kim, *et al.* 2008).

Lactobacillus brevis (CD2) or placebo was given to 22 *H. pylori*-positive dyspeptic patients for three weeks before a colonoscopy by Italian medical researchers (Linsalata *et al.* 2004). A reduction in the UBT delta values and subsequent bacterial load ensued. *L. brevis* CD2 stimulated a decrease in gastric ornithine decarboxylase activity and polyamine. The researchers concluded: "Our data support the hypothesis that *L. brevis* CD2 treatment decreases *H. pylori* colonization, thus reducing polyamine biosynthesis."

Thirty *H. pylori*-infected patients were given either probiotics *Lactobacillus acidophilus* and *Bifidobacterium bifidum* or placebo for one and two weeks following antibiotic treatment by British researchers (Madden *et al.* 2005). Those taking the probiotics had a recovery of normal intestinal microflora, damaged during antibiotic treatment. The researchers also observed that those taking the probiotics throughout the two weeks showed more normal and stable microflora than did those groups taking the probiotics for only one out of the two weeks.

Researchers at the Nippon Medical School in Tokyo (Fujimori *et al.* 2009) gave 120 outpatients with ulcerative colitis either a placebo; *Bifidobacterium longum;* psyllium (a prebiotic); or a combination of *B. longum* and psyllium (synbiotics) for four weeks. C-reactive protein (pro-inflammatory) decreased significantly only with the synbiotic group, from 0.59 to 0.14 mg/dL. In addition, the synbiotic therapy experienced significantly better scores on symptom and quality-of-life assessment.

Scientists from the Department of Medicine at Lausanne, Switzerland's University Hospital (Michetti *et al.* 1999) tested 20 human adults with ulcerative *H. pylori* infection with *L. acidophilus johnsonii*. The probiotic was taken with the antibiotic omeprazole in half the group and alone (with placebo) in the other group. The patients were tested at the start, after two weeks of treatment, and four weeks after treatment. Both groups showed significantly reduced *H. pylori* levels during and just following treatment. However, the probiotic-only group tested better than the antibiotic group during the fourth week after the treatment completion.

Medical scientists from the Kaohsiung Municipal United Hospital in Taiwan (Wang *et al.* 2004) studied 59 volunteer patients infected with *H. pylori*. They were given either probiotics (*Lactobacillus* and *Bifidobacterium* strains) or placebo after meals for six weeks. After the six-week treatment period, the probiotic group "effectively suppressed *H. pylori*," according to the researchers.

In the Polish study mentioned earlier (Ziemniak 2006), 641 *H. pylori* patients were given either antibiotics alone or probiotics with antibiotics. The two antibiotic-only treatment groups had 71% and 86% eradication of *H. pylori*, while the antibiotic-probiotic treatment group had 94% eradication.

Researchers from the Cerrahpasa Medical Faculty at Istanbul University (Tasli *et al.* 2006) gave 25 patients with Behçet's syndrome (chronic mouth ulcers) six *Lactobacillus brevis* CD2 lozenges per day at intervals of 2-3 hours. After one and two weeks, the number of ulcers significantly decreased.

Vaginosis and Vaginitis

The vagina is lined with probiotic bacteria just as the mouth is. These bacteria protect the woman's internal tissues and organs from being overwhelmed by pathogenic bacteria, yeasts and other pathogens. Without a balance of probiotic bacteria, overgrowths can take place easily. Normal colonies within a healthy vagina include lactobacilli, *Gardenella vaginalis*, *Candida albicans* and other microorganisms—all existing in balance.

Vaginosis is the alteration of the normal microbiological ecology. Vaginitis is an overgrowth of pathogenic bacteria, and their resulting infection. Two common infective microorganisms within the vagina are *Candida albicans* and *Trichomonas vaginalis*. The use of antibiotics, antiseptics and chemical toxins can stress probiotic populations, allowing overgrowths to take place.

Vaginitis can easily lead to urinary tract infections as pathogenic bacteria colonies expand. Vagina microbial infection is often symptomized by stinging sensations and a fishy odor from the vagina. As we'll discuss later and as indicated in the research, internal supplementation (through the mouth) and external application (into the vagina) both have been shown to help replenish the probiotic populations within the vagina.

Estrogen production can also be a factor. Researchers from Israel's HaEmek Medical Center (Colodner *et al.* 2003) determined from research that, "The lack of lactobacilli in the vagina of postmenopausal women due to estrogen deficiency plays an important role in the development of bacteriuria."

Researchers from the School of Medicine at Italy's Università degli Studi di Siena (Delia *et al.* 2006) treated 60 healthy women with vaginosis with either a vaginal suppository containing *Lactobacillus acidophilus* or a suppository containing *Lactobacillus acidophilus* and *Lactobacillus paracasei* F19. At the end of three months of treatment—and again three months afterward—both groups showed significant improvement in vaginosis, a significant reduction in vaginal pH, and significant decrease in vagina odor.

In a study from the University of Milan (Drago *et al.* 2007), forty women with vaginosis took a douche with *Lactobacillus acidophilus* for six days. After treatment, only 7.5% of the women still had the vaginosis. The odor typical in vaginosis discontinued in all the women, and the pH went to normal levels of 4.5 in 34 of the 40 women.

Scientists from the University of Western Ontario (Reid *et al.* 2001) gave 42 women oral encapsulated *Lactobacillus rhamnosus* GR-1 plus *Lactobacillus fermentum* RC-14 probiotics, or *L. rhamnosus* GG orally for 28 days. Vaginal flora—normal in only 40% of the cases—resolved to healthy flora in 90% of the women in the GR-1 group, and the 7 of 11 women with microbial vaginosis at the beginning of the study were resolved within a month. *L. rhamnosus* GG did not have an effect.

In a similar study (Reid *et al.* 2003), 64 women were given placebo or *Lactobacillus rhamnosus* GR-1 and *Lactobacillus fermentum* RC-14 daily for 60 days. The treatment resulted in the restoration from microbial vaginosis microflora to normal lactobacilli-colonized microflora in 37% of the women treated with the probiotic, versus only 13% among the placebo group.

Researchers from Israel's Central Emek Hospital (Shalev *et al.* 1996) gave 46 microbial vaginosis patients either yogurt with live *L. acidophilus* or a placebo for several months. The probiotic group had significantly less vaginosis than the control group.

Researchers from Sweden's Uppsala University Hospital (Hallén *et al.* 1992) gave 60 women infected with microbial vaginosis either a placebo or *Lactobacillus acidophilus*. At the end of the study, 16 of the 28 women treated with lactobacilli had normal vaginal wet smear results while no improvement occurred among the 29 women treated with the placebo. Infective vagina bacteroides were eliminated from 12 of 16 women in the probiotic group.

Italian scientists (Cianci *et al.* 2008) investigated the use of *Lactobacillus rhamnosus* GR-1 and *Lactobacillus reuteri* for the treatment and prevention of vaginosis and microbial vaginitis. Fifty women with diagnosed microbial vaginosis and vaginitis took either a placebo or an oral combination of *Lactobacillus rhamnosus* GR-1 and *Lactobacillus reuteri* RC-14 following antibiotic therapy. The researchers found that 92% of the patients significantly benefited from the probiotic treatment.

Scientists from Brazil's Universidade de Sao Paulo (Martinez *et al.* 2009) gave 64 women with microbial vaginosis tinidazole with placebo or with a combination of oral *Lactobacillus rhamnosus* GR-1 and *Lactobacillus reuteri* RC-14 daily for four weeks. The probiotic group experienced a cure rate of 87%, while the placebo group experienced a 50% cure rate. Normal vagina flora resumed in 75% of the probiotic group and in only 34% of the placebo group. This research team (2009) found similar results in another study on 55 women with vulvovaginal candidiasis.

Researchers from the Department of Obstetrics and Fetomaternal Medicine at Austria's Medical University of Vienna (Petricevic and Witt 2008) tested 190 women with microbial vaginosis. They were given either placebo or topical plus oral *Lactobacillus rhamnosus* after antibiotic treatment for 7 days. Sixty-nine of 83 (or 83%) in the probiotic group significantly improved, versus 31 of the 88 women (35%) in the placebo group.

Another study done by researchers from the Medical University of Vienna (Petricevic *et al.* 2008) gave *Lactobacillus rhamnosus* GR-1 and *Lactobacillus reuteri* RC-14 or placebo to 72 postmenopausal women with vaginosis for seven days. Both the placebo group and the probiotic group had received antibiotic treatment for seven days prior. Four weeks after treatment concluded, 60% (21 of 35) of the probiotic group demonstrated a significant improvement, while only 6 of the 37 non-probiotic subjects (16%) showed the same level of improvement.

Candida Infections

Candida albicans is a normal inhabitant of the intestinal tract and several other locations throughout the body. Complications arise when *Candida* populations have been allowed to grow beyond their normal levels. Lower probiotic populations allow these fungi to easily grow beyond their healthy levels, infecting the intestines, vagina and many other parts of the body. The consumption of probiotics can help return *Candida* back to its normal population levels, as probiotics manage and control their colonies by secreting chemicals that limit their growth.

Researchers from Long Island Jewish Medical Center's Division of Infectious Diseases (Hilton, *et al.* 1992) studied thirty-three patients with vulvovaginal candida infections. Infection rates decreased by a third among patients consuming an eight-ounce yogurt (orally) with *Lactobacillus acidophilus* for six months. The infection rate was 2.54 per six months in the control group versus 0.38 in the yogurt group, while *Candida* spp. colonization rates were 3.23 in the control group versus only 0.84 in the yogurt group—through the six-month testing period.

Ear Infections

Most of us would laugh at the prospect that probiotics would help or prevent ear infections. Think again.

Scientists from Sweden's University of Gothenburg (Skovbjerg *et al.* 2009) studied the effect of probiotic treatment on secretory otitis media—an ear infection with fluid in the middle ear cavity. Sixty children suffering from chronic secretory otitis media who were scheduled for tympanostomy tube insertion were given a nasal spray of placebo, *Streptococcus sanguinis* or *Lactobacillus rhamnosus* for 10 days prior to surgery. "Complete or significant clinical recovery" occurred in 7 of 19 patients treated with *S. sanguinis;* in 3 of 18 patients treated with *L. rhamnosus;* and in 1 of 17 of the placebo patients.

Respiratory Infections

There is sufficient evidence that pathogenic bacteria such as *Staphylococcus aureus, Streptococcus pneumoniae* and *Heomonphilus influenzae* can infect the lungs. Little research seems to have been done to confirm whether or not the lungs also harbor probiotic bacteria, however. Research has confirmed that probiotic bacteria inhabit the nasal cavity, the mouth and the throat. Research has also confirmed that both ingested probiotics and probiotic sprays reduce lung infections. Probiotics in the lungs does not seem so radical: Certainly not as radical as the evidence showing probiotics from the intestinal tract can somehow inhibit bacteria in the lungs and nasal cavity.

In a study also mentioned earlier, scientists from the Swiss National Accident Insurance Institute (Glück and Gebbers 2003) gave 209 human volunteers either a conventional yogurt or a combination of *Lactobacillus* GG (ATCC 53103), *Bifidobacterium* sp. B420, *Lactobacillus acidophilus* 145, and *Streptococcus thermophilus* every day for 3 weeks. Nasal microbial flora was measured at the beginning, at day 21 and at day 28 (a week after). Significant pathogenic bacteria were found in most of the volunteers' nasal cavities at the beginning of the study. The consumption of the probiotic-enhanced milk led to a 19% reduction of pathogenic bacteria in the nasal cavity. The researchers concluded that, "The results indicate a [possible] linkage of the lymphoid tissue between the gut and the upper respiratory tract."

Scientists from Barcelona (Cobo Sanz *et al.* 2006) gave 251 children aged 3 to 12 years milk either with or without *Lactobacillus casei* for 20 weeks. The probiotic group of children experienced significantly less low respiratory tract infections, bronchitis and/or pneumonia (32% vs. 49%). The probiotic children also had a reduction in the duration of fatigue (3% vs. 13%). There was also a difference in the duration of sicknesses among the probiotic children compared to the placebo group.

French scientists (Forestier *et al.* 2008) assessed whether ventilator-associated pneumonia in intensive care units could be prevented or lessened by the use of probiotics.

The 17-bed intensive care unit at the Clermont-Ferrand Teaching Hospital was used to test 208 patients with an intensive care unit stay of more than 48 hours. Patients were fed a placebo or *Lactobacillus rhamnosus* through a nasogastric feeding twice daily from their third day in the unit until discharge. Infective *Pseudomonas aeruginosa* cultures were measured at admission, once a week, and upon discharge. Bacteriological tests of the respiratory tract also were done to determine patient infections. The study results indicated that *P. aeruginosa* respiratory colonization and/or infection was significantly reduced among the probiotic group. Ventilator-associated pneumonia by *P. aeruginosa* in the probiotic group was reduced by more than 50% compared to the placebo group.

Researchers from the University of Arkansas' Medical School (Wheeler *et al.* 1997) studied 15 asthmatic adults in two 1-month crossover periods with placebo or yogurt containing *L. acidophilus*. The probiotic consumption increased immune system interferon gamma and decreased eosinophilia levels.

Greek scientists from the Faculty of Medicine of the University of Thessaloniki (Kotzampassi *et al.* 2006) gave a placebo or probiotic combination to 65 elderly critically ill, mechanically ventilated, multiple trauma patients for 15 days. The combination consisted of *Pediococcus pentosaceus* 5-33:3, *Leuconostoc mesenteroides* 32-77:1, *L. paracasei* subsp. *paracasei* 19; and *L. plantarum* 2,362; and inulin, oat bran, pectin and resistant starch as prebiotics. The probiotic patients had significantly lower levels of infection, sepsis and death than did the placebo group. Number of days in the ICU and number of days under ventilation were significantly reduced compared to the placebo group. The researchers concluded that: "The administration of this synbiotic formula in critically ill, mechanically ventilated, multiple trauma patients seems to exert beneficial effects in respect to infection and sepsis rates and to improve the patient's response, thus reducing the duration of ventilatory support and intensive care treatment."

Scientists from the University of Buenos Aires (Río *et al.* 2002) studied the incidence and severity of respiratory tract infections by giving 58 normal or undernourished children from 6 to 24 months old either a placebo or a combination of live *Lactobacillus acidophilus* and *Lactobacillus casei* probiotics. Their respiratory episodes were classified as pneumonia, bronchitis, recurrent obstructive bronchitis or upper respiratory tract infections. Total episodes in the probiotic group were 34; and 69 episodes occurred among the placebo group. The probiotic combination significantly suppressed pneumonia and bronchitis in both the normal and undernourished probiotic groups.

Chapter Five
What Harms Our Mucosal Membranes?

Synthetic Toxins

The mucosal membranes of different parts of our bodies are damaged by a number of toxins, microorganisms and other elements. There are a variety of mechanisms that produce this damage to our membranes. The most common is the oxidation of lipids, also called lipid peroxidation. Many substances are toxic because they are unstable. When they come into contact with the body's mucosal membranes, or epithelia, they can oxidize the lipids. The cell membranes are made of lipids, and the mucosal membranes contain numerous glycolipids.

These lipids are broken down by toxins. This effectively thins or damages the mucosal membranes. This damage effectively allows other exposures to penetrate the mucosal membrane region and irritate or damage the epithelia. This damage then produces the symptoms of inflammation that we see around the body in the form of the mucosal conditions we discussed earlier, including GERD, asthma, COPD, eczema, allergies and so on.

Let's discuss some of the common elements that harm practically any mucosal membrane they come into contact with. Typically, exposure will be persistent and acute, however. This is because our mucosal membranes are quite hardy. A healthy person will typically be able to resist the occasional exposure to one or a few of these toxins. A unhealthy person, or one with weakened probiotic colonies or otherwise immunosuppression may not be so lucky.

Clinical research by Professor John G Ionescu, Ph.D. (2009) concluded that environmental pollution is clearly associated with the development of mucosal membrane-related hypersensitivities. Dr. Ionescu's research indicated that environmental noxious agents, including many chemicals, contribute to the total immune burden, producing increased susceptibility for intolerances due to inflammation.

According to Dr. Ionescu, toxic inputs such as formaldehyde, smog, industrial waste, wood preservatives, microbial toxins, alcohol, pesticides, processed foods, nicotine, solvents and amalgam-heavy metals have been observed to be mediating toxins that produce the physical susceptibilities for toxin sensitization and subsequent inflammation.

This is also consistent with findings of other scientists—that chemicals overload the immune system and damage our mucosal membranes.

Chemical toxins such as DDT, PBDEs, dioxin, formaldehyde, benzene, butane and chlorinated chemicals are fat-soluble. Thus they can build up within the mucosal membranes and systemically ruin their structure and protective abilities.

Other compounds, such as phthalate plasticizers and parabens also damage our membranes, but they typically do not accomplish this through lipid peroxidation. Still, they produce free radicals that damage our membranes and epithelia.

Furthermore, as the immune system gears up to overdrive due to the overloading of multiple toxins, it becomes weaker and hypersensitive. This can cause a host of issues, including allergies, irritable bowel syndrome and many others.

In conjunction with a mandate to lower toxin levels among the state's residents, in 2010 the Minnesota Department of Health compiled and released a list of the most toxic chemicals used in consumer products, building materials, pesticides, hair dyes, detergents, aerosols, cosmetics, furniture polish, herbicides, paints, cleaning solutions and many other common sources. The list also referenced research connecting the toxins to disease conditions.

The list contained 1,755 chemicals.

For each of these toxins, the liver and immune system must launch a variety of macrophages, T-cells and B-cells to break them apart and escort them out of the body. This means that each toxin represents an additional load the immune system must carry.

We might compare this to moving dirt. A small handful of dirt can be carried around easily, and dispersed without much effort. However, a truckload of dirt is another matter completely. What can we do with a truckload of dirt? If we dumped a truckload of dirt on our lawn, we'd have a hill of dirt that would bury the access to our front door and annihilate our lawn and/or garden.

This is a useful comparison because while our bodies can handle a small amount of toxins quite easily, modern society is increasingly dumping toxic 'dirt' into our atmosphere, water and foods, effectively inundating our bodies 'by the truckload.'

With this increased burden, the research shows that the body's defenses are lowered and our mucosal membranes are weakened.

Plasticizers and Parabens

Today, plasticizers and parabens are common amongst many of our medications, toys, foods packaged in plastic and other consumer items. Phthalates are also found in many household items. While phthalates have shorter half-lives than some toxins, they have been implicated in systemic inflammatory issues, hormone disruption, cancers and other conditions. Many cosmetics and antiperspirants contain parabens. These can thin or damage our mucosal membranes, and are thus readily absorbed into the skin where they can provoke inflammatory responses (Crinnion 2010).

Foods and Beverages

The foods and beverages that deplete our mucosal membranes, not surprisingly, are some of the same ones that increase the risk of asthma in the research. These also increase systemic inflammation because they contribute free radicals and other toxins, stimulating inflammation.

These include:
- Alcohol
- Foods/beverages high in refined sugars
- Highly processed foods/beverages
- Foods/beverages high in refined salt
- Foods high in saturated fats
- Fried foods and fast foods
- Foods that are burnt or overcooked
- Foods containing chemical additives

These foods and beverages serve to irritate the mucous membranes. This is because they either directly contribute free radicals to the body, or the oxidation occurs as they make contact with the mucosal membranes and body cells.

Lifestyle Factors

A number of activities also reduce our mucosal health. These include:
- Stress
- Anxiety
- Anger
- Lack of sunshine

As for anger and stress, when our body is stressed, our body switches to fight-or-flight metabolic mechanisms that pull energy away from the processes of the sub-mucosal glands and gastric glands—which produce our mucosal membrane fluids. This is why a person who is nervous or anxious will also often have dry mouth and an upset stomach. They are not producing enough mucosal secretions to protect those epithelial cells.

The others on the list are either toxins that directly alter the pH of our mucosal membranes, or simply infect them.

A lack of sunshine robs the body of vitamin D and key pineal/pituitary master hormones. As for hydration, we'll discuss this again shortly.

Most pharmaceuticals are toxic to the mucosal membranes. This is why a significant side effect of most medications is dry mouth and an upset stomach. These chemicals can deplete our mucosal membranes and/or block mucosal secretions by virtue of inhibiting the COX-2 process. This also goes for other drugs, chemicals, pollutants, and so on.

Heavy Metals

Heavy metals are metal elements that exist naturally in trace quantities within our soils, waters and foods. However, extraordinary levels of heavy metals such as cadmium, lead and mercury are produced by humanity's industrial complex in the manufacturing of various consumer items.

We can cite many studies that have associated heavy metal exposure to immunosuppression. Mercury is one of these.

For example, in multicenter research from the Department of Medicine from the Lavoro Medical Center in Bari, Italy (Soleo *et al.* 2002), researchers studied the effects of low levels of inorganic mercury exposure on 117 workers. They compared these with 172 general population subjects. They found no difference in the white blood cell count between the two groups. However, the worker group exposed to mercury had increased levels of CD4+ and CD8+ cytokines, and CD4+ levels were particularly high. These indicated a state of systemic inflammation. In addition, significantly lower levels of interleukin (IL-8) occurred among the exposed workers—indicating immunosuppression.

This research concluded that even low levels of environmental exposure to mercury and other heavy metals (beyond the trace levels normally found in nature) suppresses the immune system and stimulates mucosal membrane defects.

Cadmium is another heavy metal bombarding us. Among consumer products, cadmium is used in a number of metal coatings, batteries and colorings. Most cigarettes also contain cadmium.

Asenic, tungsten, nickel, copper and others are considered heavy metals when their levels are out of balance with others. There are at least 70 trace minerals that our bodies utilize—mostly for enzymatic reactions. Practically every heavy metal is used in the body's mucosal membranes at very minute levels, including the ones mentioned above. This means that levels of these in our diets and water should be in trace amounts, as might be contained in natural rock salt.

When levels of any heavy metal become more than minute, then they throw off our body's enzyme activity, creating imbalances within our metabolism and mucosal membrane health. While imbalances can usually be tolerated for a short duration as the body seeks to correct itself, a continuous intake of heavy metals can lead to serious illness

Water Pollutants

Our industrial society has been dumping massive amounts of synthetic chemistry into our waters for many decades, and we are paying the price. Water contamination comes from manufacturing, wastewater streams from houses, air pollution, ship and boat waste streams and pollutants, run-off from farms and the gutters and streets. All of these to one degree or another end up in our drinking water supplies.

While municipalities have extensive chlorination systems in place to clear microbiological content, removal systems for chemical pollutants are still in various stages of development. As a result, our drinking water supplies have numerous contaminants.

Even some of the cleaning agents used in some municipal water supplies are toxic. This includes trichloroethylene. Trichloroethylene is a chlorinated hydrocarbon used to separate oil from water. The solvent was popularized in the dry cleaning business, and is a common cleansing agent in many local water municipalities.

Pharmaceutical medicines in our water supplies make for a perfect example. In 2007, researchers from Finland's Abo Akademi University (Vieno *et al.*) released a study showing that pharmaceutical beta-blockers, antiepileptic drugs, lipid regulators, anti-inflammatory drugs and fluoroquinolone drugs were all found in river waters. The concentrations of these were well above drinking water limits. The researchers also found that water treatment only eliminated an average of 13% of the concentration of these pharmaceuticals. This means that 87% of these pharmaceutical medicines remained in the drinking water, ready to dose each and every person drinking that water with prescription medication.

Other pollutants that are commonly found in our drinking water supplies include PCBs, and other biphenol compounds, dioxin, chlorine metabolites, pesticides, herbicides, petroleum byproducts, nitrates, and many others.

Agricultural runoff is a huge source of drinking water contamination. In addition, nitrogen-rich fertilizers choke rivers and oceans with extra nitrogen, causing abnormal blooms of algae. These massive algal blooms cut off oxygen supplies and lead to the die-offs of many species of marine life. *Dead zones* have been reportedly growing in many of the world's waterways, as we will discuss shortly. The cause is the massive use of nitrogen-based synthetic fertilizers.

The use of pesticides on agricultural land, playgrounds, parks, home lawns, and gardens throughout the United States is staggering, and it is growing. In 1964, approximately 233 million pounds of pesticides were applied in the U.S. By 1982, this amount tripled to 612 million pounds. In 1999, the U.S. Environmental Protection Agency reported that some five *billion* pounds of these chemicals were applied per year throughout America's crops, forests, parks, and lawns.

One of the more increasingly popular pesticides is imidacloprid, a neonicotinoid. Introduced by Bayer in 1994, imidacloprid is used against aphids and similar insects on over 140 different crops. Touted as a chemical with a fairly short half-life of thirty days in water and twenty-seven days in anaerobic soil, imidacloprid's half-life is about 997 days in aerobic soil. While it has a lower immediate toxicity compared with hazards like DDT, imidacloprid's use is now widespread. It is rated by the EPA and WHO as *"moderately toxic"* in small doses. Larger doses can disrupt liver and thyroid function. While this pesticide does well at killing off increasingly resistant pests, it has also been shown to decimate bee populations.

Cleaning agents are used with or rinsed by water. They will thus immediately enter our greywater systems. According to the U.S. Poison Control Centers, about ten percent of all toxin exposure is caused by cleaning products, with almost two-thirds involving children under six years old. While we might be shocked to find a child toying with a bottle of drain cleaner containing sulfuric acid, hydrochloric acid and lye, we do not think twice about feeding this same product into our waterways. We wear gloves to protect our skin from the harmful affects of ammonia and bleach while we do our cleaning but assume they disappear once poured down the sink.

An example of this is 1,4-dioxane, a common ingredient in many shampoos and other cleaning products. The California EPA documented that 1,4-dioxane is a carcinogen that can also damage kidneys, nerves and lungs. It biodegrades very slowly and is becoming a threat to drinking water supplies. This is but one of many.

In a 2002 U.S. Geological Survey report on stream water contaminants, 69% of stream samples revealed non-biodegradable detergents, and 66% of the samples contained disinfectant chemicals. Phosphates—central ingredients in many commercial laundry soaps—have been banned for dumping in over eleven states in the U.S. because of their dangerous effects upon the environment. Yet many people still use these soaps without any consideration of their effects upon our waters.

Biphenyls are considered *xenoestrogens,* or endocrine system disruptors. Long-term effects as their residues build up in the tissues of aquatic species, and bio-accumulate up the ladder to our cells, organs and tissue systems. Research has found that biphenyls have produced sexual re-orientation of fish in some water supplies.

Our waters are filling up with plastic particles. As plastics break down into smaller particles, they are absorbed by filtering marine plants and aquatics and passed up the food chain. Research led by Captain Charles Moore of the *Algalita Marine Research Foundation* (2001; 2002; 2008) found an astounding six-to-one ratio of plastic particles-to-plankton in some areas. This means that for every pound of algae—the key nutrient for nearly all marine life—there are six pounds of plastic in the oceans. This also means that our marine life is eating plastic particles with their meals: and so are humans who eat fish.

Captain Moore was first alerted to the plastic problem in 1997 when he sailed through a region of the Pacific Ocean between Hawaii and California called the *North Pacific Gyre*. He came upon a large area of floating garbage, consisting primarily of plastic debris. The *Great Pacific Garbage Patch* is now documented from a number of studies, the earliest from a 1988 National Oceanic and Atmospheric Administration paper.

Requiring some 500 years to breakdown, plastics are known to disrupt hormones and accumulate hydrocarbons as mentioned earlier. It is estimated that about twenty percent of the plastic polluting our waters comes from discarded plastic pellets used to make plastic by manufacturers. These pellets are being swept or blown into the water from careless manufacturers and transport companies. The other eighty percent of the ocean's plastics is estimated to come from daily consumer use and the careless littering of waterways and runoffs.

These combined factors are increasingly problematic to a human population seeking to sustain life on the planet. Research by Slovenian researchers Tatjana Tisler and Jana Zagorc-Koncan (2003) has shown that we are drastically underestimating the effects of toxic industrial waste. Our typical method for toxicity research has been to study each individual chemical and its possible toxicity. What we are missing with this type of research is the combined effects of the thousands of chemicals we are putting into our waters. As these chemicals mix, they create a toxic soup of new chemical combinations. Some of these are combinations are exponentially more toxic than the individual chemicals.

Toxic Microorganisms

Microorganisms and their endotoxins are collectively called *biological pollutants*. These microorganisms include bacteria, viruses, fungi and mold.

Bacteria can come from rotting food, plants, people and pets. Dander also can carry these creatures. Viruses can lodge within our mucosal membranes initially, eventually infecting our cells as they penetrate. Viruses damage DNA within the cells, and reproduce through the body via the DNA damage.

Microorganisms can grow on anything wet—especially mold. Almost any type of sitting water or dampness will grow mold, especially those in dark areas (as many fungi abhor sunlight).

Research has confirmed that infective microorganisms from viruses, bacteria and fungi can stimulate serious mucosal membrane defects. As we'll discuss later, microorganism infection requires a responsive living immune system—as we'll discuss in the next chapter. While a periodic super-cleanse might be helpful to clear microorganism toxins, a vibrant living immune system will consistently protect the body against infection. Let's talk about the possible microorganism infections we can face.

Bacteria were first discovered in 1673 by Dutch scientist Antony van Leeuwenhoek. Leeuwenhoek began writing letters to the Royal Society of London about the images he was seeing in his newly invented microscope. In 1674, Leeuwenhoek described his microscopic creatures as "wound serpent-wise and orderly arranged, after the manner of the copper or tin worms." He described "many very little living animalcules."

There are a variety of different

Types of Microbes

Fungi	Yeasts, molds and others; over 100,000 species; live in earth, air, water and damp, moist environments; can infect the body via food, water, air, and skin
Bacteria	Single-celled organisms; live in water, earth, air, on and inside other living organisms; can infect via food, water, air, and skin
Viruses	Non-living; genetic mutation triggers; exist in water, earth, air and skin; infect by altering cellular DNA, and spreading through ongoing cell division and mutation
Mycoplasmas	Ancient slow-moving bacteria; live primarily on earth and water; infect mostly via food, water and touch
Parasites	Tiny organisms that infect and live within another living organism. Includes worms, protozoa and amoeba
Thermophiles	Opportunistic bacteria that can live in very hot environments, such as deserts, boiling water or even in ovens
Psychophiles	Opportunistic bacteria that can live in the very cold, such as the artic or in freezers
Nanobacteria	Extremely small bacteria that typically have a hard calcium shell. Are thought to cause some diseases considered autoimmune.

Bacterial Infections

Today we are dealing with a multitude of infections from all of these types of microorganisms. Growing infectious diseases from this list include lyme disease (*Borrelia burgdorferi*), pneumonia, staphylococcus, streptococcus, salmonella, *E. coli*, cholera, listeria, salmonella, Shigella, dengue fever, yellow fever, tuberculosis, cryptosporidiosis, hepatitis, rabies and others. Many of these microorganisms are growing despite our antibiotic and antiviral medications. Some are growing because of unsafe sex, unclean water or changes in land use. Many are growing because of new opportunities arising from our destruction of nature. Many are becoming resistant to our antibiotics. These are often referred to as *superbugs*.

One of the more dangerous of these superbugs is methicillin-resistant *Staphylococcus aureus* (MRSA). MRSA rates are on the rise, and nearly every hospital—the crown jewels of our antimicrobial kingdom—is infected with MRSA. In a 2007 survey of 1200 U.S. hospitals, 46 of every 1,000 hospital inpatients are colonized or infected with MRSA, with 75% of those becoming infected. Among the general population, the incidence of MRSA has skyrocketed from 24 cases per 100,000 people in 2000 to 164 cases per 100,000 people in 2005 (Hota *et al.* 2007). This means that MRSA is infecting nearly seven times the number of people it did in 2000.

The virulence of *Staphylococcus aureus* was first realized in 1929 by Alexander Fleming, a microbiologist who cultured a combination of *Staphylococcus aureus* in the vicinity of a growing mold. He noticed that the penicillin mold would kill some bacteria and not others. Fleming soon realized that *Staphylococcus aureus* adapted quickly to the penicillin. It became resistant. Even to this day, *Staphylococcus aureus* is still one of the most antibiotic-resistant bacteria.

Staphylococcus aureus is also one of the most lethal bacteria known to man. It secretes three cell-killing toxins: alpha toxin, beta toxin and leukocidin. Together these poisons bind to and dissolve cell membranes, allowing cytoplasm and cell contents to leak out. This, of course, immediately kills the cell. The immune system also has difficulty attacking and removing *Staphylococcus aureus* because it secretes enzymes that neutralize the immune system's attack strategies. *Staphylococcus aureus* adapts very quickly, so the more we throw at it, the stronger it becomes.

Multiple pathogenic microorganisms can grow and prosper within the mouth, teeth and gums. These include *Streptococcus mutans, Streptococcus pyogenes, Porphyromonas gingivalis, Tannerella forsynthensis* and *Prevotella*. Additional microbes can grow within root canals. Root canals provide protected spaces for bacterial growth. Bacteria infecting root canals can include a variety of steptococci, staphylococci, and even dangerous spirochetes such as *Borrelia burgdorferi* among many others. Just about any bacteria that can infect the body internally can hibernate inside root canals. Because root canals are enclosed and the tissues around them die, the immune system cannot reach these areas to remove bacteria. As a result, a growing number of diseases are now being associated with root canal-harbored bacteria.

As these microbial populations grow, they not only can infect teeth and gums with gingivitis: They can also infect various other parts of the body. Infected gums have been implicated in a variety of fatal disorders, including heart disease, lung disease, liver disease, kidney disease, septic arthritis and others. A recent report from the Jos University Teaching Hospital in Nigeria (Adoga *et al.* 2009) reported that, "Most often the cause of cervical necrotizing fascitis is of dental origin." Necrotizing fascitis is a growing lethal infection of multiple bacteria that rapidly destroy tissues around the body, causing death very quickly.

Bacterial infections can cause an overload on the immune system because they produce endotoxins that form radicals in the body.

Lipopolysaccharides are common bacteria endotoxins. Lipopolysaccharides make up the cell membranes of gram negative bacteria, and they make up a significant part of their waste stream. Lipopolysaccharides also have shown in research to produce inflammation and damage our mucosal membranes.

For example, *Helicobacter pylori, Clostridium* spp. and *E. coli* are known to exert damage to the mucosal membranes of our stomach, intestines and colon. This causes ulcers, irritable bowel syndrome and other intestinal disorders.

Viral Infections

Viruses that infect the lower respiratory tract or digestive tract can produce significant inflammatory conditions. These include pneumonia, viral dysentery, influenza and so many others.

An example of a serious virus is the respiratory syncytial virus (RSV). RSV is fairly common among premature children. As a result, doctors often give premature children anti-viral medications during infancy to help prevent an RSV infection. RSV has specifically been shown to cause wheezing in children, and other conditions later on.

Another virus is the human metapneumovirus (hMPV). This virus also can infect the lower respiratory airways. In a study from Iran's Shiraz University of Medical Sciences (Moattari *et al.* 2010) of 120 children found that 17% of the children were infected with hMPV.

Researchers from the City University of New York (Dowd *et al.* 2009) explored the association of various viral infections among U.S. families of different socioeconomic means. Using the Third National Health and Nutrition Examination Survey (NHANES III), they found that infections of herpes simplex virus-1 (HSV-1), cytomegalovirus, hepatitis A and B related to higher levels of illness among U.S. children over the age of six. They also found that non-white children with lower family income, and parents with lower levels of education, had greater incidences of these infections.

Certainly, while infections relate to exposure, they relate more to a weakened or compromised immune system. As to family income and education, these also likely relate to a weakened and compromised immune system due to a lack of wholesome foods. Other research has shown that Americans of lower income status tend to consume more processed and inexpensive mass market foods containing more fried foods, additives and refined sugars.

Surprisingly, the human rhinovirus (HRV), which will cause the common cold in most people, can also infect the lower respiratory airways. Indeed, the association between HRV during infancy and a weakened immune system later in life is stronger with HRV than with other viruses (Jackson and Lemanske 2010).

This study confirms what other studies have indicated: An early serious viral lung infection seriously penetrates and weakens our mucosal membranes. This opens the body to these infective agents.

Yeast, Molds and other Fungi

Yeast and mold are members of the fungi family. While many fungi such as mushrooms are protective to the immune system, an overburdened immune system can become sensitive to microorganism yeasts and molds. Yeasts can become infective and can directly overload the immune system. Mold and their airborne spores can also overload the immune system. This makes these fungi can contribute to an already-overloaded system.

Mold spores reproduce and float through both the outdoor and indoor air. Once they land, they can begin multiplying into larger cultures. While there are several species of mold, almost all require moisture to grow and populate. A concentration of spores riding the indoor air currents can cause various sensitivities, allergies, and sickness (Sahakian *et al.* 2008).

Mold spores also produce a number of substances called mycotoxins, which can create health concerns if inhaled. Homeowners and renters should be aware of this, and make sure the houses they live in have no water entry into the basement. Moist appliances like air conditioners, bathtubs, bathroom carpets, and air ducts can also grow mold.

For these reasons, we might want to frequently check the various corners and dark places in our houses and workplaces for moisture, because the fungal or bacterial populations growing on these surfaces will only get bigger with time—disbursing toxins into the air as they grow. Once found, the area should be dried, the mold or bacteria should be cleaned up (water with a few drops of rubbing alcohol, vinegar or chlorine will kill most mold or bacteria) thoroughly. If a mold growth is over several feet, a mold specialist may need to be called in to eliminate the mold.

This was confirmed by researchers from the National University of Singapore (Tham *et al.* 2007), who found that home dampness and indoor mold is linked to an increase in asthma and allergy symptoms among children. They studied 4,759 children from 120 daycare centers. After eliminating other possible effects, home humidity was significantly associated with increased rates of allergic rhinoconjunctivitis. As discussed earlier, allergic rhinoconjunctivitis is the inflammation of the conjunctiva and sinuses as a result of histamine release following an allergic immune response. As mold infects our mucosal membranes, the body can respond with inflammation and hypersensitivity.

Overgrowths of yeasts like *Candida albicans* can also contribute to or overload the immune system. While Candida is a typical resident of the immune system, when it is unchallenged by our probiotic system it can grow to incredible colony sizes. Like most other organisms, it is typically not the Candida organism that overloads the immune system: it is the endotoxins that these microscopic living beings produce.

Candida albicans can grow conjunctively with *Staphylococcus aureus,* resulting in the accelerated growth of both microorganisms. This can result in a tremendous burden for the immune and probiotic systems as they try to defend against the incursion of combined yeast and bacteria infections.

The Superbugs

Normally, healthy mucosal membranes, with their enhanced probiotic colonies, will resist and protect us from most infective microorganisms. That is, unless those probiotics are themselves taken out or weakened by antibiotics.

The use of antibiotics has soared over the past few decades. Today, over 3,000,000 pounds of pure antibiotics are taken by humans annually in the United States. This is complemented by the approximately 25,000,000 pounds of antibiotics given to animals each year.

Meanwhile, many of these antibiotics either are given in vain or are ineffectual. The example is respiratory infections, which are typically viral infections. The Centers for Disease Control states that, *"Almost half of patients with upper respiratory tract infections in the U.S. still receive antibiotics from their doctor."* This said, the CDC also warns that *"90% of upper respiratory infections, including children's ear infections, are viral, and antibiotics don't treat viral infection. More than 40% of about 50 million prescriptions for antibiotics each year in physicians' offices were inappropriate."*

Indeed, the growing use of antibiotics has also created a Pandora's Box of superbugs. As bacteria are repeatedly hit with the same antibiotic, they learn to adapt. Just as any living organism does (yes, bacteria are alive), bacteria learn to counter and resist repeatedly utilized antibiotics. As a result, many bacteria today are resistant to a variety of antibiotics. This is because bacteria tend to adjust to their surroundings. If they are attacked enough times with a certain challenge, they are likely to figure out how to avoid it and thrive despite it.

This has been the case for a number of other new antibiotic-resistant strains of bacteria. They have simply evolved to become stronger and more able to counteract these antibiotic measures.

This phenomenon has created *multi-drug resistant organisms.* Some of the more dangerous MDROs include species of *Enterococcus, Staphylococcus, Salmonella, Campylobacter, Escherichia coli,* and others. Superbugs such as MRSA are only the tip of the bacterial iceberg.

Another growing infectious bacterium is *Clostridium difficile.* This bacterium will infect the intestines of people of any age. Among children, this is one of the world's biggest killers—causing acute, watery diarrhea. It is also a growing infection among adults. Every year *C. difficile* infects tens of thousands of people in the U.S. according to the Mayo Clinic. Worse, *C. difficile* are increasingly becoming resistant to antibiotics and infections from clostridia are growing in incidence each year.

Pharmaceutical Toxins

As we discussed in the last chapter, pharmaceuticals can harm the mucosal membranes, causing inflammatory responses.

Practically any and every synthetic pharmaceutical can add to our body's total toxin burden. This is because the body must eventually break down any synthetic chemical in order to purge it from the body. The isolated or active chemical within the pharmaceutical may have its biological effect upon the body, but it must be broken down at some point. The body rarely if ever utilizes these chemicals as nutrients, in other words. They are foreigners to the body. Thus, enzymes such as glutathione must break down these chemical molecules into forms that can be excreted in urine, sweat, exhalation or stool.

This breakdown and disposal process requires work by the body's detoxification systems. This means that they further burden or stress a system that must remove many other toxins within the body, including other environmental toxins, microorganisms and their endotoxins, inflammatory mediators, broken-down cells and other toxins the body must get rid of. In other words, pharmaceuticals can contribute to, and even become another straw that breaks the camel's back.

Illustrating this, researchers from Britain's Imperial College (Shaheen *et al.* 2008) studied the association between acetaminophen use and asthma incidence among 1,028 asthmatics and healthy matched controls. They found that the weekly use of acetaminophen was significantly related to a diagnosis of asthma. The researchers concluded that: *"These data add to the increasing and consistent epidemiological evidence implicating frequent paracetamol [acetaminophen] use in asthma in diverse populations."*

Researchers from Norway's Oslo University Hospital (Bakkeheim *et al.* 2011) studied 1,016 mothers and their children from birth until six months old, and then followed up with the children at 10 years old. They found that acetaminophen use by the mother during the first trimester significantly increased incidence of allergic rhinitis at age ten. Furthermore, girls given acetaminophen had more than double the asthma incidence at age ten.

While these pharmaceuticals may be of concern specifically, we should look at any pharmaceutical as having the potential to increase the body's total toxic burden and raise the risk of mucosal membrane defects.

We can add to this discussion particular drugs and drug types that have been shown to be particularly toxic to our mucosal membranes due to their mechanisms of shutting down the healthy secretion of our mucosal membranes:

COX Inhibitors

NSAIDs provide pain relief and reduced inflammation by interrupting the enzyme cyclooxygenase. Cyclooxygenase or COX oxidizes certain fatty acids to initiate a chain reaction that produces prostaglandins and thromboxane. These are key components involved in the process of healing wound sites and removing pathogens. The COX process also stimulates the secretion of the mucins around the body that make up the bulk of our mucosal membranes.

The three main COX enzymes are COX-1, COX-2 and COX-3. NSAIDs will inhibit the activity of both COX-1 and COX-2. The problem with inhibiting the COX-1 enzyme is that this blocks the metabolic process that produces protective secretions among the mucosal membranes of our esophagus, stomach and duodenum. Without this protective lining, our stomach can be damaged by our food and the gastric acids our stomach cells produce. This blocking of our protective mucus is what causes the ulcer and GI pain characteristic of NSAID use.

When these secretions are halted, various conditions begin to pop up, including heartburn, ulcers, gastric bleeding, intestinal problems and others. The common issue relates to the mucosal membranes in these regions.

This is the reason there are so many different COX-inhibiting drugs: They each cause a number of sometimes lethal side effects.

Let's review a few of these:

Acetylsalicylic acid (ASA) or aspirin (Aspirin, Ecotrin®, many others; over the counter) is a synthetic molecule designed to mimic the effects of willow bark and meadowsweet herb. For thousands of years, herbalists and ancient healers used both willow bark and meadowsweet for the relief of pain. In 1828, salicin was isolated from the bark of the willow tree by Joseph Buchner. Two years later, salicin was isolated from the flower of the meadowsweet plant by Johann Pagenstecher. In 1838, a method of isolating salicylic acid from willow extract was discovered by the Italian Raffaele Piria. Meanwhile, German chemist Karl Jacob Lowig isolated the same salicylic acid from meadowsweet extract. In 1874, salicylic acid began to be produced for commercial use. Twenty-three years later, in 1897, Charles Garhardt, a chemist at the Friedrich Bayer & Company, synthesized a similar derivative by adding an acetyl group (OCOOH), to produce the more stable acetylsalicylic acid. The Bayer company proceeded to call it *aspirin* and began large-scale production shortly thereafter.

Aspirin's mechanism of action in the body continued to be mysterious, however. Finally, in 1971, Sir John Vane determined that aspirin's active constituent, acetylsalicylic acid, inhibited prostaglandin synthetase (later identified as cyclooxygenase) causing its anti-inflammatory and anti-thrombosis effects. Sir John Vane received the Nobel Prize for Medicine in 1982 for this hypothesis.

Like willow and meadowsweet, aspirin has an immediate effect of reducing pain. Aspirin binds to cylooxygenase-2 within the cells. This allows it to block the pain and inflammatory process. Cylooxygenase-2 produces prostaglandins that in turn send messages to the brain that a particular part of the body is injured. When cylooxygenase-2 is blocked, the process of converting arachidonic acid to prostaglandins is halted.

Cylooxygenase-2 also stimulates the production of thromboxanes. These stimulate the process of blood clotting within the platelets—called platelet aggregation. This is again part of the healing process, because if a blood vessel were to be pierced, our blood would leak out, causing immediate death unless the vessel was sealed somehow. In other words, thromboxanes stimulate clotting, preventing our bodies from bleeding to death when injured.

Adverse Side Effects: This also produces the side effect that aspirin is also known for—as a blood thinner. Because many heart attacks, strokes and other cardiovascular problems are caused by blood clots, low-dose aspirin is used to keep the blood thinner than normal. This also creates another problem, however: The tendency to bleed slows down wound healing. And because it takes increasing amounts of aspirin to provide the same pain relief when used continuously, this adverse effect can become more dangerous.

The problem with ASA, like other isolated chemicals, is that its positive effects come with a price of several adverse effects. Aspirin is notorious for damaging the lining of the stomach, and causing a variety of digestive issues, including acid reflux, ulcers, nausea and gastritis. Aspirin has also been known to cause liver toxicity, Reye's syndrome (especially in children), and tinnitus—ringing of the ears. Aspirin's blood-thinning effects can create internal bleeding from a variety of internal injuries. The dangerous part of this is that the person may be bleeding internally without knowing it.

Acetaminophen or paracetamol: (many brands; over the counter) Acetaminophen, on the other hand, can in some ways be more dangerous than aspirin. A number of studies have confirmed that acetaminophen causes acute liver damage and kidney failure. Some research has indicated that more than a third of Americans take acetaminophen at least once per month. The ubiquitous advertising by the many drug manufacturers that include acetaminophen as an active ingredient have removed much if not all consumer concern for the dangers of acetaminophen. Instead of seeing it as a potentially harmful drug, consumers have grown accustomed to acetaminophen on the bathroom shelf, ready to take at the first sign of a headache or body ache.

Current theory holds that acetaminophen works by blocking the oxidized COX enzyme, thereby blocking prostaglandin production but not thromboxane synthesis. Apparently, for this reason, acetaminophen does not produce the same level of blood thinning. Some believe the COX-3 enzyme is also blocked, but COX-3 is not connected to inflammation, so this theory is disputed.

In addition to acetaminophen, there are several other ingredients in many of the popular NSAID brands. These can include chlorpheniramine, dextromethophan, diphenhydramine, guaifenesin, pamabrom, pseudoephedrine and doxylamine. These provide antihistamine (blocking histamine production), anticholinergic (blocking the neurotransmitter acetylcholine), decongestant and diuretic properties.

Adverse Side Effects: One of the basic problems with acetaminophen is that it will cause acute liver failure. In a 2009 study done at the University of Maryland's School of Medicine (Mindikoglu *et al.* 2009), 661 acute liver failure patients that were forced to undergo a liver transplant to survive were analyzed. The study concluded that 40% of all the liver failures were as a result of acetaminophen use. As for the other larger drug categories, 8% of the liver failures resulted from antituberculosis drugs, 7% from antiepileptic drugs, and 6% from antibiotics. In comparison with the other drugs, the acetaminophen-caused liver failure patients also required more dialysis.

Acetaminophen can also cause stomach bleeding and gastric upset. A recent study (Beasley *et al.* 2008) has also showed acetaminophen can increase asthma, eczema and conjunctivitis in young children.

Adverse effects of some ancillary drug ingredients included in many acetaminophen-containing OTC drugs include liver damage, nausea, vomiting, fluid loss, hypertension, anxiety and tachycardia.

Ibuprofen: (prescription and over the counter) is a fast-acting drug that provides anti-inflammatory effects and pain relief for a few hours. Brand names Advil®, Nuprin® and Motrin® use ibuprofen as the central active agent. Ibuprofen is an NSAID that inhibits both COX-1 and COX-2. This has the combined effect of reducing inflammation, reducing fever associated with inflammation, and relaxing tense muscles. Because the inflammatory process is inhibited by the blocking of the COX-2 conversion process, there is a reduction of pain associated with the inflammation.

Adverse Side Effects: As mentioned, one of the most concerning side effects of ibuprofen is its blocking of critical COX-1 enzymes, robbing the digestive tract of its healthy mucosal linings. Problems that result from constant ibuprofen use include GI bleeding, ulcers, acid reflux and indigestion. These can in turn cause nausea, vomiting, diarrhea and ulcers in the esophagus.

Side effects from ibuprofen also include a thinning of the blood, which increases the risk of bleeding. Liver enzymes are often significantly raised during ibuprofen use. This indicates possible liver damage over time. Other side effects have included dizziness, headaches, high blood pressure and loss of sexual potency. Other side effects that have been seen include heart problems, kidney damage, and lung damage. Some heart attacks have occurred with higher dosages. Ibuprofen also sometimes causes photosensitivity.

Naproxen and naproxen sodium: (OTC and prescription) Also anti-inflammatory, pain-relieving agents. Naproxen is the active constituent in Anaprox®, Midol Extended Relief® and others. The U.S. is one of the few countries in the world that allows the sale of naproxen over the counter. Canada and Australia are one of the few others that do.

Adverse Side Effects: Naproxen has many of the same side effects that other NSAIDs have. It has a history of causing GI bleeding, ulcers, and complete perforations of the stomach. Naproxen has also caused circulation problems, breathing problems, liver damage, problems with blood clotting and others. Naproxen has also been implicated in heart attacks and strokes.

A 2006 study (ADAPT) of 2528 human subjects showed that naproxen has a significant risk of cardiovascular-related deaths, heart attacks and strokes. Out of 713 patients on naproxen, 8.25% suffered a heart attack, a stroke, or heart failure, while only 5.68% of the placebo group suffered any of these events.

Meloxicam: (Mobic®; prescription only) This is a COX inhibitor, but this drug requires less dosing per day because it takes longer for the body to break down. This, however, is also a possible cause for concern, as it may further burden the liver and/or kidneys.

Adverse Side Effects: As with other COX-1 and COX-2 inhibitors, meloxicam causes gastrointestinal bleeding, ulcers, perforation and other intestinal difficulties. Headaches and tinnitus have also been reported.

Etodolac: (Lodine®; prescription only) This is another COX enzyme conversion inhibitor, with medium dosing required.

Adverse Side Effects: The research has shown that etodolac can cause headaches, nausea, diarrhea, constipation, dizziness, drowsiness, kidney impairment, rashes, constipation, abdominal pain and ringing in the ears. Like the other COX inhibitors, etodolac also causes GI bleeding and ulcer issues. Anyone with a history of heart disease or asthma is warned against the product by the manufacturer.

Nabumetone: (Relafen®; prescription only) is another NSAID that is prescribed to relieve pain associated with rheumatoid arthritis and osteoarthritis.

Adverse Side Effects: Like the other COX inhibitors, nabumentone causes GI bleeding, ulcers and other intestinal issues. Studies have also shown that nabumentone also can cause nausea, liver toxicity, dizziness, abdominal pain, and the inability for the blood to clot effectively.

Research has shown that etodolac can cause headaches, nausea, diarrhea, constipation, dizziness, drowsiness, kidney impairment, rashes, constipation, abdominal pain, lightheadedness, and ringing in the ears. Anyone with a history of heart disease or asthma is warned against the product by the manufacturer.

Sulindac: (Clinoril®; prescription only) Another nonspecific COX inhibitor.
Adverse Side Effects: Like other COX inhibitors, GI bleeding and ulcerous effects in the stomach and small intestines are common side effects. Also, rashes, kidney impairment, lightheadedness, ringing in the ears, weakness, internal bleeding, liver toxicity and an exacerbating of asthma and hives have been reported.

Choline magnesium salicylate: (Trilasate®; prescription only) is a salicylate, like aspirin. It thus acts the same, by blocking COX enzyme conversion. However, the risk of Reye's syndrome, compared to aspirin, is apparently slightly reduced with this drug.
Adverse Side Effects: Gastrointestinal bleeding and ulcers in the stomach and small intestines are side effects of all isolated salicylates. Liver toxicity, internal bleeding, and tinnitus have also been seen among users of this form of salicylate.

Ketoprofen: (prescription only, Orudis®, Oruvail®) is another NSAID that blocks the COX enzyme conversion process. This reduces pain and inflammation.
Adverse Side Effects: Ketoprofen has similar side effects as many of the other NSAIDs in that it can cause GI bleeding, intestinal cramping, ulcerations, nausea, vomiting, and diarrhea. In addition, there are a number of other side effects with ketoprofen. These include headaches, fainting, persistent sore throats, stiff necks, rashes, itching, yellowing eyes and dark urine—indicating liver issues.

Diclofenac; (Cataflam®, Voltaren®, Arthrotec®; prescription only) **oxaprozin;** (Daypro®) **diflusinal;** (Dolobid®) **piroxicam;** (Feldene®) and **indomethicin** (Indocin®) are all COX inhibitor NSAIDs. Thus, they all block the inflammatory cascade that helps the body protect and heal itself and the production of mucosal membrane lining of the stomach and other mucosal surfaces.
Adverse side effects: Very similar to the other NSAIDs. They all can cause gastrointestinal problems. They can all cause ulcers because they block the body's secretion of protective mucosal lining in the stomach and small intestine. They also can cause cardiovascular problems and potentially bleeding issues, and to varying degrees, headaches and nausea.

Chemical Food Additives

This is a large topic, because so many processed foods are chock full of many different artificial additives. These include hundreds of artificial food colors, preservatives, stabilizers, flavorings and a variety of food processing aids. A number of these additives have been found to cause sensitivities in some people.

Illustrating the effects that food additives can have, Australian researchers (Dengate and Ruben 2002) studied 27 children with irritability, restlessness, inattention and sleep difficulties. The researchers saw many of these symptoms subside after putting the children on the Royal Prince Alfred Hospital Diet, which is absent of food additives, natural salicylates, amines and glutamates.

Using preservative challenges, the researchers were also able to determine that the preservatives significantly affected the children's behavior and physiology adversely.

Researchers from Britain's University of Southampton (Bateman *et al.* 2004) screened 1,873 three-year old children for hyperactivity and the consumption of artificial food colors and preservatives. They gave the children 20 mg daily of artificial colors and 45 mg daily of sodium benzoate, or a placebo mixture. The additive group showed significantly higher levels of hyperactivity than the group that did not consume the artificial colors and preservative.

While these studies are not proof that these food additives are allergens, we can say that with confidence that they can cause food intolerances, as hyperactivity is considered a reaction to eating these "foods."

Once an additive has caused intolerance symptoms such as those from the research above, there is always the possibility that the immune system may begin to become sensitive to some of the foods these additives are associated with. This likelihood increases should the immune system become continually exposed to the foods together with the additives over a considerable period of time.

Sulfites

Sulfites provide a classic case. The sulfite ion will aggressively preserve a food. Sulfites can also produce wheezing, tightness of the throat and other symptoms almost immediately after eating foods preserved with them. However, the effects of sulfites may not be as significant as often portrayed. It may well be that many sulfite-sensitivities seen among wine drinkers are actually the product of the alcohol rather than the sulfites.

Illustrating this, researchers from Australia's Centre for Asthma (Vally *et al.* 2007) tested eight wine-sensitive subjects with sulfite wine and non-sulfite wine. The researchers found that the wine sensitivities were unlikely caused by the sulfites in the wine.

Today, sulfites are used to preserve many wines, dehydrated potatoes and numerous dried fruits. Sulfites include potassium bisulfite, sulfur dioxide, potassium matabisulfite and others. Often labels do not disclose the use of sulfites, because the preservative may have been used early in the processing of the raw ingredients instead of added into the finished product. In addition, under current U.S. labeling laws, if an ingredient such as sulfite is less than 10 parts per million, there is no requirement for putting the ingredient on the panel.

Sulfite sensitivity may be the result of B12 deficiency. In a study presented to the American Academy of Allergy and Immunology, 18 sulfite-sensitive persons were given sublingual B12. The B12 effectively blocked adverse reactions to sulfites in 17 of the 18 (Werbach 1996).

Monosodium Glutamate

Monosodium glutamate also gets a lot of attention for producing sensitivity symptoms. This has also been echoed among a number of studies.

To better understand this, Harvard researchers (Geha *et al.* 2000) set out to study the effects of MSG sensitivities in a multi-center study. They found that of 130 human volunteers who thought they were sensitive to MSG, 38% physically responded to MSG with allergic symptoms. However, 13% also responded to a placebo (they thought contained MSG). Subsequent retesting continued to show inconsistent responses among some of those who thought they were MSG-sensitive.

This led the researchers to conclude that people who believe they are sensitive tend to react more strongly to MSG, but their responses were not always consistent. This of course may be the result of differing levels of tolerance and periods of sensitivity—again depending upon immunity.

This research still confirms that MSG can cause sensitivity responses. Possibly MSG may be overhyped somewhat, but like so many other food additives, there is no doubt that it is not a natural part of our food supply.

Microparticles

Some researchers have suggested that substances with microparticles can lead to increased intestinal permeability and food sensitivities (Korzenik 2005).

Microparticles are particles smaller than 100 μm, but larger than 0.1 μm. (Smaller molecules, in the nanometer range, are called nanoparticles.) Products that are produced with microparticles include toothpaste and mouthwashes. Food products that contain microparticles include powdered sugars and some refined flours.

We might better classify microparticles in the same category as overly processed foods. The bottom line is that the body can become sensitive to unnaturally-processed constituents should they be exposed to intestinal tissues and bloodstream—and not be recognized by the immune system.

Artificial Sweeteners

A number of artificial sweeteners should be considered toxic. One is aspartame. Aspartame is a chemical combination of the amino acids phenylalanine and aspartic acid, bonded by methyl ester—a wood alcohol. Once inside the body, the wood alcohol and formaldehyde are released.

Another artificial sweetener sucralose. This is sweet yet not readily absorbed according to manufacturers. Yet studies have found that 11-27% is absorbed, and 20-30% of that absorbed quantity can be metabolized by the body. This requires the liver and kidneys to break it down and excrete it.

While this is a huge topic in itself, other questionable sweeteners that may provide toxicity once within the body include saccharin, acesulfame potassium and cyclamates. Stevia, mannitol and xylitol are plant-derived sweeteners that are considered by most to be relatively safe and non-toxic.

Air Pollutants

Clean air contains about 78% nitrogen, 21% oxygen, 0.9% argon, 0.03% carbon dioxide and a host of trace elements. Depending upon the location and source, outdoor air pollution can contain carbon monoxide, nitrogen dioxide, sulphur dioxide, excess carbon dioxide, ammonia, various particulates, chlorofluorocarbons (CFCs), radon daughters, and a variety of toxic metals and volatile organic compounds (VOCs).

There are several types of air pollution, and most of them can overload the body with toxins. The first is *air particle* pollution—when particulate size ranges from .1 micron to 10 microns. This type of pollution is from soot, typical of automobile exhaust, industrial smoke stack exhaust, fireplace smoke, and smoke from forest fires, barbeques and other combustion. Soot is also called *black carbon* pollution, because the excess carbon burn off from burning fossil fuels is the primary component.

Noxious gases are another type of pollution category. These include gasses such as carbon monoxide, chlorine gas, nitrogen oxide, sulphur dioxide and various other chemical gases and vapors. CFCs are a type of noxious gas.

While these two pollution types are distinct, they are often tough to differentiate. Many pollutants are actually vaporized liquids. Molecules become suspended in vapor, appearing like gases or liquid vapors. They are airborne elements derived from synthetic solid and liquid compounds.

We should also specify a difference between *indoor* and *outdoor* air pollution. There are a number of pollutants specifically pervading building ventilation systems and indoor facilities. To this, we can add outdoor pollution entering the house. Examples of indoor pollutants include formaldehyde emitted by foam, treated wood plastics, and chlorine gas emitted in indoor swimming pools.

According to a 2007 *American Lung Association State of the Air* report, 46% or about 136 million Americans live within a county having *"unhealthful"* levels of either ozone or particle-based outdoor pollution. Over 38 million Americans live in a county with *"un-*

healthful" levels of both ozone and particle pollution. A third of Americans live in *"unhealthful"* ozone level counties.

Interestingly, this is substantially better than a 2006 report indicating that almost half of Americans live in ozone-rich areas. It is unlikely that the source of ozone pollution—carbon emissions—went down this much in a year. Most likely—just as the ozone hole has been fluctuating with atmospheric rhythms—there are complicated relationships between weather systems, temperature, pressure and so on.

Meanwhile, more than ninety-three million Americans—about one in three—live in areas seasonally high in short-term particle pollution and about one in five Americans lives in an area of high year-round particle pollution. Unlike the fluctuating ozone levels, the number of high particle pollution areas has steadily increased over the past few years.

Smog

Research has illustrated that increased exposure to the particulates within smog, as well as the toxic burden presented by mercury, arsenic, sulfur dioxide, nitrogen dioxide and others, can contribute to mucosal membrane damage.

Illustrating this, researchers from Australia's University of Queensland (Barnett *et al.* 2005) studied respiratory hospital admissions among children of different ages in five Australian cities and two New Zealand cities. They found that increased rates of hospital admissions for asthma correlated with increased levels of particulate matter smaller than 2.5 micrometer and less than 10 micrometer (PM10-2.5), along with increased nitrogen and sulfur levels. A 6% hike in asthma admissions for children between five and fourteen years old related to a five parts per billion increase in nitrogen levels.

Ozone

Smog is primarily made up of ozone. There are two forms of ozone: The ozone that naturally makes up part of the stratosphere, often referred to as the ozone hole; and the ozone within the lower atmosphere, or troposphere. This latter ozone is called tropospheric ozone or ozone pollution. This form of O_3 gas is caused not by nature's interaction between radiation and the atmosphere, but through the reaction between fuel vapors from automobiles and sunlight. For this reason, smog levels tend to peak during hot weather.

Smog levels are also higher in warmer regions like Southern California and urban areas in the southern U.S., such as Atlanta. Other cities also experience greater smog levels during the summer months. Wherever higher concentrations of vehicles combine with warm sunshine, smog levels go up. The 'perfect storm' of almost constant sunshine, warm weather, and vehicle concentration makes Southern California one of the worst smog and ozone regions in the United States.

Ozone will oxidize on a cellular and internal tissue level when taken into the body. These tissues will be damaged in almost the same way other oxidized radicals damage tissues. Ozone is readily absorbed through the alveoli as a gas. From there it can enter the bloodstream and damage artery walls and tissues. Ozone is also a major mucosal membrane irritant, causing inflammation and epithelial cell damage. This can result in decreased lung capacity and/or decreased lung growth development among children.

Ozone is directly linked to the incidence and worsening of respiratory conditions such as asthma, bronchitis, and COPD. Recent research indicates that this mechanism is the oxidation of lung mucosal membrane lipids that line the cells of the lung. These oxidized lipids stimulate inflammation as the body seeks to mitigate ozone's damaging effects. The oxidation stimulates scavenger macrophages, which bind to the oxidized lipids in an effort to reverse the damage (Postlethwait 2007).

This means that ozone will release unpaired oxygen radicals, which can damage cell membranes and tissues, as we discussed earlier.

Ozone has some redeeming qualities as well. Ozone therapy is gaining recognition among the alternative medical community. Ozone is used in hot tubs as a purification measure. It is also used as an industrial cleaning and sanitizing substance. Ozone is part of our natural mix of gases in our air as well. Typical levels are between 25 and 75 parts per billion.

However, dangerous ozone levels occur with higher levels of carbon monoxide levels, sulphur dioxide, and other pollutants. Like the canary in the coalmine, high ozone levels provide a good indicator of unhealthy air. When combined with other pollutants, ozone has a worsening detrimental effect upon the body.

The EPA's Air quality index rates 85 parts per billion of ozone as unhealthy for sensitive people, and over 105 ppb as unhealthy for anyone. As ozone levels rise, it can irritate the lungs and throat, increasing the potential for inflammatory throat and lung infections. As a result, indoor ozone generating machines—which have become popular over the last decade—are discouraged by both the EPA and the FDA if they emit levels higher than 50 parts per billion.

Ironically, higher ozone levels in the air reflect its cleansing action upon other pollutants. Ozone is part of the atmosphere's normalizing systems. The very same cleaning and antibacterial effect we have begun to utilize are part of the earth's detoxification mechanisms to clean and break down particulate pollution. This doesn't mean it is healthy to breathe in ozone at these levels, however.

Particulates

Particulate pollution can produce severe toxicity. PM(10-2.5) refers to a particle size from 2.5 micron to 10 micron, and PM(2.5) refers to particle sizes below 2.5 micron. 2.5 micron or less is a *fine particulate,* while less than .1 micron is *ultra-fine.* Ultra-fine particles may also be considered noxious gas pollutants, because their molecular size is small enough to pass through the alveoli into the bloodstream.

Particles above 10 micron in size are usually trapped by the cilia and mucous membranes in the nose, throat, or mouth. As mentioned earlier, these are usually disposed through the movement of mucous or broken down by immune cells.

Fine particulates are small enough to escape this labyrinth and get into our lungs, but they are usually too large to get directly into the bloodstream. These particles can become lodged in the tissues of the lungs and bronchi and slowly break down. As they break down, their toxins become absorbed and dumped into the bloodstream. This accumulation of toxins can quickly overburden the liver and bloodstream, producing an inflammatory airway response—or damage to our mucosal membranes.

The chemical makeup of these toxins depends upon the source of the pollution. Particle pollution caused by automobile exhaust will have various fluorocarbons and nitrate particles, while coal fired power plants will emit large numbers of sulphur dioxide molecules.

Course particulate pollutants are typically caused by mining, construction, or demolition. Building demolition can rain fumes of various dangerous substances a mile or more from the demolition site.

The most blatant illustration of the demolition effect is the World Trade Center bombing of 2001. The collapse of the towers caused such a toxic fume that there are still thousands of people suffering from a slow poisoning of the lungs. Dangerous chemicals like asbestos, formaldehyde and many others were breathed by thousands of people.

This effect was not limited to rescuers and those who escaped from the twin towers. Many others who happened to be in the vicinity are now suffering. One of the more prevalent diseases has been *sarcoidosis*—a life-threatening inflammation of the lungs. As toxin deposits build up and damage the mucous membranes of the airways, scar tissue forms—making mild asthma seem like a walk in the park.

This scar tissue affects the elasticity and efficiency of the lungs, causing life-threatening lung collapse. A recent study released by nine doctors (Izbicki *et al.* 2007) who researched the delayed health effects at Ground Zero reported that firefighters and rescue workers were diagnosed with sarcoidosis at a rate of five times the incidence rate prior to 9/11.

An epidemic of respiratory disorders and lung cancer was also an unfortunate result of the Trade Center bombing. While we know asbestos is toxic to the lungs, it is still a popular building material. Many structural components of new buildings use asbestos as an ingredient. Because it is a cheap fire retardant material, buildings still go up using it. Asbestos has been linked to thyroid cancer and lung cancer in many studies, which caused a number of high profile lawsuits and residential building restrictions.

Another toxin released when buildings collapse or are demolished is benzene. Benzene has been identified as a carcinogen, and certain types of leukemia are associated with benzene exposure. Other toxins thought to be released by building collapse include mercury, lead, cadmium, dioxin, polycyclic aromatic hydrocarbons (PAHs) and polychlorinated biphenyls (PCBs). Many of these components are still used to build buildings. All of them were used in buildings a few decades ago, when many of our current skyscrapers were built.

Besides the more publicized cases of cancer and sarcoidosis, ailments associated with the WTC bombing include reactive-airways syndrome, asthma, chronic throat irritation, gastroesophageal reflux disease (GERD—also referred to as heartburn) and persistent sinusitis. Other cases thought to be associated with the WTC have included miner's lung and thyroid cancer. While many thought these disorders were temporary, new diagnoses have continually increased. This is because toxins can build up and reside in lung tissue cells, affecting future lung capacity for many years to come. Studies on firefighters involved in the rescue report an average loss of 300 milliliters of lung capacity (Senior 2003).

It is thus safe to say that exposure to these sorts of particulates may not be symptomatic for years after the exposure. This was certainly the case with those exposed to Agent Orange in Vietnam. Cases of prostate cancer, skin cancer, and chronic lymphocytic leukemia did not appear in some veterans until decades later (Beaulieu and Fessele 2003).

Particulate pollution or soot is the most dangerous form of outdoor pollution. Auto exhaust, aerosols, and chemicals from power plants and wood burning are the major sources. While the particles themselves are too small to be seen by the naked eye, they can be seen as a whole in the form of a haze in the sunlight. While the body's cilia hair and mucous membranes in the nose and throat might filter and catch some of these particles, many will make it into the lungs where they can damage the mucous membrane, producing inflammation.

Like any living organism, the earth and its atmosphere have means to cleanse toxins out of the system. The atmosphere conducts a number of self-cleaning currents, which move and break down pollutants. One such mechanism is the hydroxyl radical (OH) molecule. The immediate effect of the hydroxyl radical is to form photo-oxidants like nitric acid, which undergoes a photolysis reaction with nitrous acids. These can be highly toxic.

Humanity's intrusions into nature's course can produce other types of toxins. We might consider, for example, Owens Lake, California. For thousands of years, this beautiful lake offered respite from the heat and inhospitality of the California desert region known as Death Valley. The size of Owens lake was nearly 28,500 hectares—a huge body of water fed by the Sierra mountains. In 1900, the mountain rivers feeding the lake were diverted into the Los Angeles basin to feed a growing legion of humanity.

Within ten years, Owns Lake, which was often compared to the Aral Sea, turned into a dustbowl. Now the silt covering the water basin is coated with arsenic. Arsenic is a natural element, and in this case, it is providing resistance and restructuring for the soil at the lake bottom. This arsenic is also blowing around the region with the winds, increasing cancer rates among local residents (Raloff 2001).

Carbon Monoxide

Carbon monoxide is a substantial indoor air toxin. Carbon monoxide is released by burning gas, kerosene, or wood. It can thus arise from the use of wood stoves, fireplaces, gas stoves, generators, automobiles, kitchen stoves, and furnaces. Low concentrations of carbon monoxide in the indoor environment might cause fatigue and even chest pain.

Higher concentrations may result in headaches, confusion, dizziness, nausea, vision impairment and fever. This is due to carboxyhemoglobin formation in the bloodstream, which takes place when carbon monoxide attaches to hemoglobin instead of oxygen. This will in effect starve the body of oxygen, and higher concentrations can easily lead to death.

Acceptable carbon monoxide levels in households are about .5 to 5 parts per million. Levels near a gas stove might be 5 to 15 ppm. An improperly vented or leaking stove might cause 30 ppm or more near the stove, which becomes hazardous. The U.S. National Ambient Air Quality Standard for maximum carbon monoxide levels outside is 35 ppm for one hour and 9 ppm for eight hours. Standards for indoor carbon monoxide have not been determined.

Making sure that every appliance is vented properly is task number one in avoiding carbon monoxide poisoning. The appliance should also be checked for leaks, and those leaks should be sealed prior to use. Central heating systems should be inspected for leaks as well. Idling the car in the garage is a no-no. Open fireplaces should be avoided indoors, and wood stove doors should be kept closed. We shouldn't solely rely upon the draft up the fireplace chimney for the escape of carbon monoxide.

Nitrogen oxide

Nitrogen oxide is a gas byproduct of most engines and practically any gas-run appliance. Gas stoves, water heaters, wood stoves, gas heaters and cars are probably the biggest emitters in the home. Homes without these appliances will have very low levels of NO_2 compared to outside. Homes with these appliances may have double the levels. Nitrogen oxide can be a significant toxin if significant levels are taken in.

Researchers from Birmingham Heartlands Hospital (Tunnicliffe *et al.* 1994) tested one hour exposure to nitrogen dioxide on ten mild asthmatics with dust mite sensitivities. Forced expiratory volume (FEV1) levels were tested with non-NO_2 air, air with 100 parts per billion of NO_2, and air containing 400 ppb of nitrogen dioxide. FEV1 levels were 27%

lower between the non-NO_2 air and the 400 ppb of NO_2 air. The average FEV1 among the asthmatics was nearly three times lower in the 400 ppb NO_2 air than in the clear air. The 100 ppb NO_2 air content did not seem to make a significant difference in FEV1, however. This gives us a yardstick for determining unhealthy NO_2 levels.

Cooking and Heating

Research from the University at Albany (Kaplan 2010) has revealed that about half of the people around the world utilize biomass such as wood, agricultural residues or coal to cook by and heat their homes with.

These fuels are not completely consumed by their ignition. They leave toxic residues in the form of carbon monoxide, arsenic and others that can significantly increase the body's burden of toxins when breathed in. This in turn increases the risk of damage to our mucosal membranes.

Volatile Organic Compounds (VOCs)

Researchers from the Texas Tech University Health Sciences Center (Arif and Shah 2007) studied the effects of volatile organic compounds (VOCs). They collected data on ten VOCs and 550 adults. Aromatic compounds and chlorinated hydrocarbons were specifically categorized. Exposure to aromatic compounds increased the incidence of asthma by 63%. In addition, exposure to aromatic compounds increased wheezing incidence from the previous year by 68%, and chlorinated hydrocarbon exposure increased wheezing incidence from the previous year by 50%.

Exposures to VOCs ranged from 0.03 micrograms per cubic meter for trichloroethene up to 14 microg/m3 for toluene. In other words, the higher the level of toxic inhalation, the higher the incidence of respiratory disorders. This is because VOCs present toxins that are quickly absorbed into the bloodstream through the airways. Once in the bloodstream, the body launches an inflammatory response to remove them.

The researchers also found that as a group, Mexican-Americans experience the highest exposure levels to benzene—averaging 2.38 micrograms per cubic meter—compared with whites—who averaged 1.15 microg/m3—and blacks—who averaged 1.07 microg/m3. This relates to exposure levels that are relative to the type of work being done. In other words, this study indicates that Mexican-Americans are likely doing more work involving the use of VOCs, which in turn expose them to greater levels of benzene.

Benzene, like toluene and other VOCs, is highly disruptive to cells and tissues because of its highly reactive aromatic hydrocarbon structure. It can thus damage practically every cell and tissue system in the body, releasing numerous radicals. Not surprisingly, benzene is also known to be significantly carcinogenic.

Benzene and other VOCs can be found in many paints, glues, solvents, rubbers and many other workplace materials. Industries that use aromatic hydrocarbon solvents must provide significant ventilation and protection to avoid poisoning their workers.

First-, Second- and Third-Hand Smoke

Tobacco smoke is also an important source of indoor pollution. The American Cancer Society estimated in 2004 that 160,000 Americans die each year from lung cancer caused by smoking. Lung cancer maintains between an eleven and fifteen percent chance of survival beyond five years. It should be noted that the highest rates of global lung cancer occur for both men and women in North America and Europe (Field *et al.* 2006). Of course, these are also countries where indoor smoking rates are the highest.

Recent research has indicated that not only is second-hand smoke dangerous to non-smokers, but it has more than twice the amount of tar, nicotine and other toxins than the smoker inhales. While the smoker will inhale the smoke through the filtering mechanism provided by the packed tobacco inside the cigarette paper—and many cigarettes also have additional filters to screen out toxins—the second-hand smoker will breathe all the smoke. Second-hand smoke contains five times the amount of carbon monoxide—the lethal gas that de-oxygenates the blood—than the smoker inhales.

Second-hand smoke also contains higher levels of ammonia and cadmium. Its nitrogen dioxide levels are fifty times higher than levels considered harmful, and the concentration of hydrogen cyanide approaches toxic levels. Constant exposure to second-hand smoke increases the risk of lung disease by 25%, and increases the risk of heart disease by 10%. Second-hand smoke exposure has also been irrefutably linked to emphysema, chronic bronchitis, asthma and other ailments.

Despite significant educational programs, second-hand and third-hand smoke poisoning is still prevalent in the United States. The Centers for Disease Control's National Health and Nutrition Examination Survey from 1999-2008 (CDC 2010) revealed that between 2007 and 2008, about 88 million American nonsmokers over the age of three were consistently exposed to secondhand smoke. The good news is that the detectible blood nicotine levels among nonsmokers have declined from 52% between 1999 and 2000 to 40% between 2007 and 2008. Still, 40% is simply not acceptable. It should be noted that rates were the highest among children living in households below federal poverty levels.

Researchers from Britain's University of Southampton School of Medicine (Edgecombe *et al.* 2010) found in a study of 22 adolescents with severe asthma, that two-thirds lived with a smoker.

Researchers from the Respiratory Diseases Department of France's Hospital of Haut-Lévêque in Bordeaux (Raherison *et al.* 2008) studied 7,798 children among six cities in France. This focused on asthma and allergies among families who smoked. They found that about 20% of children were exposed to tobacco via their mother's smoking. Furthermore, they found that children born of mothers who smoked during pregnancy had significantly greater incidence of asthma.

There is now research that shows that anti-smoking laws decrease disease rates. Researchers from the Harvard School of Public Health (Dove *et al.* 2011) studied the National Health and Nutrition Examination Survey (NHANES) data—a research program run by the U.S. Centers for Disease Control and Prevention's National Center for Health Statistics (NCHS). NCHS's directive has been a continuous survey method focused on specific diseases among representative samples throughout the United States. About 5,000 persons each year are included in the data, from different counties across the nation.

The Harvard researchers used the 1999-2006 NHANES data to correlate locations that had some semblance of required smoke-free public places with asthma incidence. They found that smoke-free laws significantly reduced the odds of asthmatic symptoms among nonsmoking children and adolescents. Smoke-free laws were also linked to reduced asthma episodes ("attacks"), persistent wheeze, chronic night coughing and asthma medication use.

Synthetic Fragrances

Various scents and fragrances used in deodorizers, decorations, soaps, and furniture can be downright toxic. While a fragrance might smell like flowers or delicious foods, the typical commercial fragrance contains at least ninety-five percent synthetic chemicals. A single perfume may contain more than 500 different chemicals. Benzene derivatives, aldehydes, toluene, and petroleum-derived chemicals are just a few synthetics used in commercial fragrances. Toluene alone, for example, has been linked to respiratory disorders among previously healthy people.

For this reason, we should carefully consider any product with an ingredient called "fragrances." This includes laundry detergents, dishwashing and other soaps, shampoos and other types of hair products, disinfectants, shaving creams, fabric softeners, fragrant candles, air fresheners, and of course perfumes and colognes. Discernment also should also be given to the word "unscented," as this still may have some of the same synthetics, used instead as fragrance masking elements.

In one study (Anderson and Anderson 1997), mice were submitted to breathing with a commercial air freshener for one hour at different concentrations. A number of concentrations, including levels typically used by humans in everyday use, caused sensory and pulmonary irritation, decreased breathing velocity, and functional behavior abnormalities.

Another study, performed by the same researchers (Anderson and Anderson 1998) and published a year later, revealed that mice who were subjected to five commercial colognes or toilet water for an hour suffered various combinations of negative effects, including sensory irritation, pulmonary irritation, decreased airflow expiration, and neurotoxicity.

Skin Lotion Toxins

Many of the chemical ingredients in many sunscreens have been identified as carcinogenic. These include benzophenone-3, homosalate, 4-methyl-benzylidene camphor, octylmethoxycinnamate, and octyl-dimethyl-PABA. These five, alone or in some combination thereof, are contained in about 90% of today's commercial sunscreens. All five have showed increased cancer cell proliferation both *in vitro* and *in vivo* in a study conducted at the Institute of Pharmacology and Toxicology at the University of Zurich (Schlumpf *et al.* 2001). This study also showed negative estrogenic and endocrine effects among mice from several of these chemicals.

A study done at the University of Manitoba in Winnipeg (Sarveiya *et al.* 2004) reported that all sunscreen ingredients tested—including octymethoxycinnamate and oxybenzone—significantly penetrate the skin. The penetration of common sunscreens was found to increase the penetration of even more dangerous herbicides—a concern for agricultural workers and non-organic gardeners (Pont *et al.* 2004). Furthermore, it has been established that some organic sunscreens can cause photo-contact allergies (Maier and Korting 2005). Research from Australia's Skin and Cancer Foundation (Cook and Freeman 2001) reported 21 cases of photo-allergic contact dermatitis caused by oxybenzone, butyl methoxy dibenzoylmethane, methoxycinnamate or benzophenone. The Cook and Freeman research has led to a conclusion that these sunscreen ingredients are the leading cause of photo-allergic contact dermatitis.

Contact dermatitis is actually quite rare amongst the general population. A study at the National Institute of Dermatology in Colombia conducted a study of eighty-two patients with clinical photo-allergic contact dermatitis. Their testing showed that twenty-six of those patients—31.7%—were shown to be positive for sensitivity to one or several of the sunscreen ingredients (Rodriguez *et al.* 2006).

The widespread proliferation of these harmful sunscreen ingredients—an occurrence increasing since the 1960s sunbathing era—is a significant factor in the skin cancer epidemic. Their addition to the epidermis layer create an environment of excessive oxidative radicals, as the sun in the presence of oxygen further oxidizes these synthetic molecules without nature's balancing biomolecules. At the bare minimum, these chemicals substantially increase the toxic burden within skin cells. This burden minimizes the body's ability to neutralize the oxidizing effects of the sun's radiation—intensifying the oxidizing factor. This intensification would essentially convert the sun's rays from therapeutic to dangerous.

Prior and concurrent to the prevalent use of sunscreen, sun-worshipers have ceremoniously applied various chemical- and oil-based sun lotions onto the skin. This is done to intensify the sun's tanning effects: to obtain that rich, brown tan to look more attractive. Many chemicals are/were in these products, including various hydrocarbons, which revert to oxidized radicals when exposed to the sun. In addition to sun lotion, sunbathers also apply various other chemical-based lotions onto the skin to condition, hydrate or treat sunburn. These various moisturizing lotions also contain a variety of synthetic chemicals that can become free radicals.

Furthermore, many sunscreens available today effectively absorb UV-B rays, but let UV-A rays through. Because UV-A rays are quite dangerous out of balance with UV-B to an unhealthy body, the risk of skin cancer using these sunscreens is even higher than without any sunscreen protection. In a 2007 study from the University of California at San Diego, researchers (Gorham *et al.* 2007) reviewed 17 studies of sunscreen use and melanoma. For those studies performed in latitudes over 40 degrees from the equator where skin types are fairer, there was a more significant correlation between sunscreen use and skin cancer.

Many other skin lotions should also be considered toxic. An example is DEET, or N,N-Diethyl-meta-toluamide. DEET is an effective mosquito repellent, yes. But it also poisons us as well. Research has shown that DEET exposure causes impairments to cognition, mood issues and insomnia. Whatever we put on our skin is absorbed into the epidermal and subdermal tissues, and eventually, into the bloodstream, and in the case of DEET, into our central nervous system.

Other toxic chemicals are used for lubricants, moisturizers, exfoliants and masks. Ingredients to steer clear of include methylisothiazalone, DMDM hydantoin, octenylsuccinate (a neurotoxin), methylchloroisothiazalone and triclosan—an antibacterial ingredient that is suspected to be an endocrine disruptor. Common among most soaps and cleansers are sodium laureth sulfate and ceteareth, which can bond to carcinogen chemicals used in manufacturing, such as ethylen oxide and 1,4-dioxane.

Household Toxins

The same researchers (Anderson and Anderson 2000) found that pulmonary irritation and decreased lung capacity results from the use of synthetic mattress pads. They identified respiratory irritants such as styrene, isopropylbenzene and limonene among polyurethane mattresses. When subjecting organic cotton mattresses to the same test, the results were quite the opposite. Increased respiratory rates and tidal breathing volumes were observed with organic fiber mattresses.

Fabric softener emission is also a dangerous source of air toxicity. Several known irritants and toxins are typically found in fabric softeners, including styrene, isopropylbenzene, thymol, trimethylbenzene and phenols. In yet another study, Anderson and

Anderson subjected mice to five commercial fabric softener emissions for 90 minutes using laundry dryers. The results clearly illustrated that fabric softeners significantly irritate airways. These negative health effects were also seen resulting from emissions of clothing driers containing fabric softener pads.

The researchers (Anderson and Anderson 1999) also found that pulmonary toxicity resulted from commercial diapers, adding that a number of chemicals found in diapers were known pulmonary and sensory irritants.

Another potential indoor trigger category is propellants. Propellants are used in sprays and pump bottles to disperse fluids. While chlorofluorocarbons (CFCs) have been practically eliminated from aerosols, today's aerosols and pump sprays often involves the use of volatile organic compounds (VOCs). Noxious propellants such as isobutane, butane and propane will typically linger in the air for several minutes after spraying. They can be quite toxic.

Asbestos

Asbestos exposure has become less likely since the *Environmental Protection Agency* passed the *Asbestos Ban and Phase Out Rule* as part of the *Toxic Substances Control Act* in 1989—which was for the most part overturned in 1991 by the U.S. *Fifth Circuit Court of Appeals*. What remain are various specific bans such as those from the *Clean Air Act* and remnants of *Toxic Substances Control Act*, including some continued restrictions supported by Congressional rulings.

The CAA has stimulated various bans since 1973. The bottom line is that although paper- and cardboard-based asbestos has been banned along with certain spray-on versions, many products still contain asbestos. These include cement sheets, clothing, pipe wrap, roofing felt, floor tiles, shingles, millboard, cement pipe, and various automotive parts.

Beyond the banned items, there is no ban preventing manufacturers from using asbestos. The important thing to remember is that the EPA does not monitor manufacturers for their ingredients. In general, asbestos inclusion into today's building materials should be considered a given.

Formaldehyde

Formaldehyde has been shown to be a significant and prevalent toxin. Today so many building materials and furniture are built using formaldehyde. These include pressed wood, draperies, glues, resins, shelving, flooring, and so many other materials. The greatest source of formaldehyde appears to be those materials made using *urea-formaldehyde* resins. These include particleboard, plywood paneling, and medium density fiberboard.

Among these, medium density fiberboard—used to make drawers, cabinets and furniture tops—appears to contain the highest resin-to-wood ratio. Another sort of resin called *phenol-formaldehyde* or PF resin. PF resin apparently emits substantially less formaldehyde than the UF resins. The PF resin is easily differentiated from UF resin by its darker, red or black color. The incidental *off-gassing* of formaldehyde into the indoor environment from these resins results from sun, heat, sanding and demolition. As the formaldehyde slowly off gasses, it becomes a chemical toxin once in the body.

Other Building Material Toxins

There are many other toxins in our building materials—including many yet to be discovered. Certainly, we can safely say that any kind of building or decomposition of a modern building will likely impart various hazardous chemicals, including but not exclusively asbestos and formaldehyde.

Polybrominated diphenyl ethers or PBDEs provide one example. PBDEs is an organobromine used as a fire retardant. It is used to make automobiles, polyurethane foams, furniture, electronic goods, textiles, airplanes and of course, building materials.

This means that the air during any kind of sanding, crushing, fire or demolition should be treated with extreme caution. Using a particle or gas mask is more than a good idea under these circumstances, though it should be noted that most particle masks do not form a tight enough bond with the face to filter much at all. Best is to use a gas filter or a mask with a rubber barrier that fits tightly onto the face.

With regard to off-gassing, prior to bringing in any type of new furniture or wood into the house, it is best to off-gas the product by setting it in the sunshine for a couple of days or at least for a full day. As the sun's resonating waves connect with the material, many of its toxins are disassociated and released. Not such a good thing for the environment, but at least it will disburse outside of our immediate breathing environment. Off-gassing can help us avoid more than a potent toxin.

Fresh paint can also be toxic. This is because paint typically contains VOCs.

That 'New Car Smell'

Many other indoor pollutants exist, depending upon the structure and condition of the environment. For example, automobiles, trains, planes, or buses can provide a whole range of triggers, from carbon monoxide to lead, formaldehyde and plasticizers—which can off-gas (also called *outgassing*), especially when the weather gets warmer.

This is especially the case for new cars. That 'new car smell' is the toxic off-gassing of a mixture of plasticizers, formaldehyde and other synthetics. In the case of older cars, air vents may be clogged with a number of molds, dust and bacteria, which may spray out whenever the "air" is turned on.

It might help to periodically clean out the filters of any car—especially older ones. In the case of a newer car, we might also consider leaving the windows cracked while parking in sunny locations between drives for a few weeks, to let the various materials outgas.

Sick Buildings

Over the last thirty years, researchers have become increasingly aware that certain buildings, especially older ones with older ventilation systems, can make people sick. This effect is often termed *sick building syndrome,* or SBS. The major symptoms reported in SBS include chronic fatigue, brain fog, headaches, allergies, nausea, chronic sore throat, bronchial congestion, and others.

Toxin overload becomes apparent in the case of toxins provided by older buildings, or buildings without sufficient ventilation or cleaning policies.

For example, research from the National Center for Healthy Housing (Jacobs *et al.* 2009) found that lower-income families tend to live in older homes, where there can be poor ventilation, more water leaks, more lead paint and greater moisture and mold levels. They found that these trends also relate to increased rates of respiratory illness, obesity and lead poisoning. They saw a clear association between respiratory disorders and home ventilation, home age, and the windows of homes. In other words, higher toxin exposure.

Researchers from the Vermont Department of Health's Division of Health Surveillance (Laney *et al.* 2009) studied a 2006 respiratory disorder cluster among workers who worked in a building that had water-damage. Physicians diagnosed increased incidence of sarcoidosis and asthma among the workers, and conducted pulmonary function tests.

As the researchers investigated the data, they found that adult respiratory disorders incidence in the office workers was 3.3/1,000 person-years prior to their working in the office, and 11.5/1,000 person-years after they began working in the building. Their respiratory disorders incidence tripled, in other words.

The workers were removed from the building while it was cleaned up.

In a study of school buildings (Sahakian *et al.* 2008), 309 school employees in two older elementary schools were tested. Excess dampness produced increased incidence of respiratory irritation, wheezing and rhinitis symptoms among the employees. The older, damper school of the two also produced more illness.

SBS is indicated when multiple workers or inhabitants of a building complain of one or more of these symptoms soon after beginning to work or live in the building. Sometimes, however, SBS can develop over time, or directly after or during an extreme change in the weather. A humid summer or heavy rainfall period, for example, may stimulate a growth in mold in the ventilation system. After a smoggy summer in a city or during a fire season, the ventilation system may become clogged with soot. Workers or occupants of the building need to speak up and request from management that filters and vents be periodically cleaned and flushed. The upholstery, walls and other parts of workplaces should also be cleaned periodically.

Occupational Toxins

Scientists from the University of Texas School of Public Health (McHugh *et al.* 2010) analyzed the data from the National Health and Nutrition Examination Survey (2001-2004) to determine the relative risks of toxicity in different occupations. They found that miners, health-care workers, and teachers have significantly higher rates of respiratory disorders than other occupations, including construction workers. Miners, for example had over four times the respiratory disorders incidence than construction workers. This of course relates to their exposure to indoor air pollutants at work.

Researchers from the National Institute for Occupational Safety and Health and the Centers for Disease Control (Greskevitch *et al.* 2007) investigated respiratory disease among agricultural workers using the 1988-1998 National Centers for Health Statistics' Multiple Cause of Death Data and the 1988-1994 Third National Health and Nutrition Examination Survey data (NHANES III). They studied mortality ratios for eleven respiratory illnesses in crop farm workers, livestock workers, farm managers, landscapers, horticultural workers, forestry workers, and fishery workers. Among the different occupations, the crop farm workers and livestock farm workers suffered significantly more deaths from respiratory conditions. Pneumonia with hypersensitivity was 10 to 50 times the normal levels. Landscapers and horticultural workers suffered more deaths from lung abscesses and COPD.

Wheeze and shortness of breath were also significantly elevated among the farm workers, especially among female farm workers. Respiratory disorders were heightened among agricultural workers, especially those who also smoked.

It is notable that these occupations each present particular toxins. In the case of miners, they are exposed to coal dust and soot, together with exhaust, with minimal ventilation. In the case of agricultural workers, landscapers and horticulture workers, they are exposed to chemical pesticides and herbicides. In the cases of teachers and healthcare workers, they are exposed to the contaminants that occupy their respective buildings and ventilation systems.

Exposure to specific toxins requires extensive ventilation and filtration systems. Whether these come in the form of protective breathing gear or building HVAC systems, the toxin exposures within a workplace must be minimized. Reducing exposure is, in fact, one of the driving purposes of the U.S. Occupational Safety and Health Administration (OSHA). Toxin exposure at the workplace has reached such significant levels that OSHA has put in place many regulations, such as Material Safety Data Sheets (MSDS), in efforts to protect workers from the effects of workplace toxins.

Why such an effort to protect workers from toxins? Today there are in the neighborhood of 100,000 different synthetic chemicals available in the marketplace. The chemical industry has produced many workplace chemicals for industrial uses over the past century, and many of these chemicals have been subsequently found to be carcinogenic or otherwise toxic. Keeping track of the effects and safeguards of each of these chemical toxins is a dizzying affair. Yet it is theoretically the responsibility of any business to make efforts to protect its workers from these toxins.

Here is a small list of occupations and their toxins, and following that, a partial list of mucosal irritants:

Occupation	Exposures
Agricultural workers	Pesticides, herbicides
Plastics manufacturers	Plasticizers, VOCs, polymers
Painters	Paints/thinners (VOCs)
Drivers	Carbon, soot, formaldehyde, micro
Metal workers	Metallic dusts, heavy metals
Saw millers	Wood dust, preservatives
Janitorial and housekeepers	VOCs, cleaning chemicals
Bakers and food workers	Airborne food particles
Home builders	VOCs, formaldehyde, asbestos
Health workers	SBS, microorganisms, chemicals

And finally, here is a summary of the toxins that irritate and damage our mucosal membranes around the body:

Some Mucosal Irritants and their Sources

Source	Toxins
Air pollutants	Lead, mercury, carbon monoxide, sulfur, arsenic, nitrogen dioxide, ozone...
Carpets, rugs	Molds, dander, lice, PC-4, latex
Cigarette/Cigar/Pipe Smoke	Carbon monoxide, nicotine, aldehydes, ketones, soot, formaldehyde, others
Cosmetics	Aluminum, phosphates and chemicals
Spray cans	Propellants, other chemicals
Foods/Additives	Food colors, preservatives, trans fats, pesticides,

	arachidonic acids, acrylamide, phytanic acid, artificial flavors, refined sugars and much, much more
House	Radon, formaldehyde, pollen, dust, mold, dander, pesticides, cleaning products, asbestos, lead, paint, endotoxins
Household chemicals	Cleaners, pesticides, herbicides, paints
Insects	Endotoxins from dust mites, cockroaches and other insects
Laundry soaps	Fragrances, detergents, surfactants
Mattresses/pillows	Endotoxins, molds, formaldehyde
Mice	Various mice allergens
Microorganisms	Mold, bacteria, viruses, parasites
Paints	Lead, arsenic, VOCs, adhesives
Pets	Dander, up to 240 infectious diseases & parasites (65 from dogs/39 from cats)
Pharmaceuticals	Many-see short list on pages 112-113
Pools and spas	Chlorine byproducts such as trihalomethanes (THMs), various carbonates
Soaps and Shampoos	Fragrances, detergents, surfactants
Stoves, Fireplaces	Carbon monoxide, NO_2, arsenic, soot
Water	Chorine byproducts, pesticides, pharmaceuticals, many others
Work and school environments	SBS, practically all of the above

Chapter Six
Rebuilding Mucosal Health

Mucosal Herbs

Herbs work completely differently than do pharmaceuticals. While pharmaceuticals typically contain one or two synthesized active ingredient that can cause serious side effects, herbs typically contain hundreds of active constituents that each balance each other. As a result, many herbs will accomplish pain relief and other needs, but will also protect the health of the mucosal membranes.

The use of certain herbs for thousands of years by billions of people, and the knowledge of their use and possible misuse has been handed down through thousands of generations. We must remember too, that there has been no financial conflict of interest in the study of traditional herbs—since they grow freely. Herbal medicine has been an honorable institution of devoted individuals.

In comparison, there is a huge conflict of interest in the study of pharmaceuticals—as pharmaceutical companies can spend billions of dollars on the development of a single drug. To abandon such a drug is a proposal of mass proportions. Once a pharmaceutical company has designed a new drug, it can receive patent protection for that chemical combination, giving it up to twenty years of potential exclusivity for selling that drug—at least where patent laws exist. This means a guarantee of profits as long as doctors prescribe that drug. With a patent, there is protection from competition, guaranteeing salaries and profits for many years.

Without the doctor prescribing the medication, however, there is no continual use. Thus, market control must include both the patent and the doctor. For this reason, pharmaceutical giants focus their attention on a combination of drug research, patent protection, regulation, and marketing to both physicians and patients.

In our modern medical institutions, pathology instruction relating to diagnosis also accompanies the use of specific pharmaceutical drugs. Western medical institutions synchronize with the pharmaceutical industry because of the financial relationships between pharmaceutical companies, medical schools, medical licensure and pathology documentation. Drug research by doctors—many of whom are also medical school professors—is often funded by the pharmaceutical manufacturers. There is thus a built-in incentive for a successful outcome. As the COX anti-inflammatory drug lawsuits and investigative reporting proved over the past few years, pharmaceutical manufacturers and medical researchers can be slow to disclose information damaging to a drug's income potential.

Even if a pharmaceutical results in an improved condition for a particular ailment, there are often dangerous side effects. Some of these can be worse than the original ailment. In addition, most medications stress the liver and kidneys in one respect or another—shortening the lifespan of these critical organs. Some medications, like aminoglycoside antibiotics streptomycin, kanamycin, garamicin and others have been shown to cause kidney damage in as many as 15 percent of patients. Others, such as acetaminophen, carbamazepine, atenolol, cimetidine, phenylbutazone, acebutolol, piroxicam, mianserin, naproxen, sulindac, ranitidine, enflurane, halothane, valproic acid, phenobarbital, isoniazid and ketoconazole can cause acute dose-dependent liver damage. This is because the liver and the kidneys work together to process most chemicals out of the body. Together these organs break down and excrete the chemical byproducts of medications, resulting in their hopeful elimination from the body. During their journey out, these derivatives can damage the body's cells and tissue systems.

The P450 liver enzyme process moves chemicals through the extraction pathway in many cases. This enzyme is effective in most healthy bodies for a few chemicals at a time. Yet multiple drugs can overwhelm and deplete this pathway. With the P450 pathway overloaded by various chemicals, additional drugs can damage tissues incrementally. For this reason, a higher number of liver enzymes in a blood analysis is seen by doctors as a dangerous sign.

This means that, like most toxic chemicals, many pharmaceuticals put a burden on the liver. This is because the liver must work harder to filter and break down the chemicals—before sending them out through the kidneys, colon, lungs and/or sweat glands. This of course, directly affects mucosal membrane health.

The central issue related to the burdening of liver is the fact that synthetic chemicals are foreign to the body. Most botanicals are quite the opposite. Botanicals are highly recognized by the body, simply because humans have been consuming these and similar botanicals for thousands of years. Thus, the body processes the constituents of a botanical with a very normal pathway.

In fact, many botanical herbs provide a broad spectrum of healthy effects, which in turn increase the health of our mucosal membranes. These effects include antioxidant activity and immune stimulation. Some are also antiseptic and antibiotic as well. Some increase detoxification, stimulate the liver, increase kidney efficiency and stimulate the adrenal glands all at the same time.

While pharmaceuticals are isolated chemicals with often one central mechanism of action within the body, most botanicals have many—some even hundreds—of pharmacological constituents and complementary actions. For example, according to the research of James Duke, Ph.D. of the U.S. Department of Agriculture and Norman Farnsworth, Ph.D., a research professor at the University of Illinois, ginger contains at least 477 active constituents (Schulick 1996). While botanicals produce active biochemicals that act in a healing manner, they also produce active multiple constituents that buffer and balance each other.

Separately, one of ginger's active constituents might produce side effects along with its actions. The other constituents balance these mechanisms, however. Together the many constituents in ginger make it one of the most active and effective medicinal botanicals for many ailments. Many herbal medicine experts consider it one of the best anti-inflammatory botanicals. Like a number of other anti-inflammatory herbs, ginger has been shown to suppress the expression of both cyclooxygenase-1 and cyclooxygenase-2; yet without slowing down the production and secretion of mucosal membranes around the body. As a result, whole ginger has shown to slow leukotriene production through the blocking of the 5-lipooxygenase enzyme (Grzanna *et al.* 2005) without adverse side effects. This slows inflammation and pain without sacrificing the health of the mucosal membranes. In fact, ginger has been shown to actually stimulate mucosal membrane health.

Ginger is not alone. Research has confirmed that many other botanicals also have dozens if not hundreds of constituents.

Unlike the parade of adverse side effect-ridden COX inhibiting non-steroidal anti-inflammatory drugs introduced by the pharmaceutical industry over the past two decades, anti-inflammatory botanicals provide a level of safety and a myriad of benefits to our mucosal membranes. We might add that these pharmaceuticals—some of which have been pulled from the market because they injured hundreds of thousands of people—have required billions of dollars of taxpayer investment in regulation and oversight. The complexity of these drugs is met with a double-whammy of risk. If even a small amount of this wasted effort could be diverted to the growing and production of the anti-inflammatory botanicals discussed here, we could be saving billions of taxpayer dollars, not to speak of the damage to the environment from the dumping of toxic synthetics.

The issue modern medicine has with herbal medicine is the speed in which its therapeutic effects can be seen. This is also its benefit, however. While pharmaceuticals are fast acting, they also create imbalances within the body that require the body to work harder in other ways to detoxify the drug. Medicinal botanicals have no toxicity, but they work slower and more gradual. This forces the patient to be disciplined, and well, *patient*. It is because natural herbal medicines are complex and balanced that they tend to act more deeply. They also produce a result that is long-lasting, working with the body to strengthen its immunity and ability to resist the problem in the future.

Rather than causing negative side effects by blocking the immune system, anti-inflammatory botanicals produce *positive* side effects. While gradually reducing pain, fever and inflammation, they modulate eicanosoids and boost mucosal membrane secretions. They also stimulate detoxification; increase healthy appetite; reduce nausea; protect against ulcers; increase liver vitality; stimulate circulation; calm nerves; balance endocrine function; encourage bone healing; improve lung and gum health; and neutralize oxidative (free) radicals. Many are also antiseptic, anesthetic, and antiemetic—among so many other positive "side effects." Laboratory studies have also shown many of these to be protective against cancer as well (LaValle, 2001; Shukla and Singh 2007; Schulick 1996).

There are a number of excellent pain-relieving botanicals that physicians can consider before resorting to the array of increasingly toxic pharmaceutical analgesics. Botanicals such as white willow tree bark and meadowsweet are good examples. White willow tree bark and meadowsweet both contain a constituent called salicin. This of course is the natural version of the synthetic *acetyl-salicylic acid* we discussed in the last chapter, known by its expired patented trademark name of *aspirin*. As mentioned, acetyl-salicylic acid and its non-acetylated, isolated *salicylic acid* both come with a number of side effects, including internal bleeding and gastro-intestinal upset sometimes leading to ulceration and stomach bleeding.

Far from its natural origins, today's aspirin is usually manufactured from phenol, which can be derived from coal or isolated from other materials. The phenol is treated with sodium and then carbon dioxide under pressure, rendering salicylate. After acidification into salicylic acid, it is acetylated with acetic anhydride to yield the final product. The manufacturing facility hosting these reactions produces pollutants to yield the synthetic result. Though it successfully relieves pain, aspirin also creates adverse side effects as we have discussed.

We've discussed how NSAIDs disrupt the cyclooxygenation (COX) process, which oxidizes arachidonic acid utilizing the enzyme called cyclooxygenase. We have discussed this. By blocking COX, the production of prostaglandins and prostanoids such as thromboxane is interfered with. This also interferes with sub-mucosal gland production, and the secretion of mucosal membranes. This is the relationship between these NSAID and selective COX-inhibitors and their various GI side effects. When the stomach and intestinal mucosal membranes are not secreted, intruders and even the stomach's own acids can damage the epithelial cells of the stomach wall and the intestinal walls.

What we may not realize is that the original botanical sources of *salicylic acid*—white willow bark and meadowsweet flowers—also perform this same inhibition of COX. The difference, however, is that these botanicals also balance the actions of its salicins by stimulating other mechanisms, which increase the secretion of mucosal membranes. This is one of the balancing effects of herbs.

Herbs also increase the body's detoxification process, which in turn speeds healing and promotes healthy mucosal membranes.

Aspirin's disruptive mechanisms are illustrated in its effective depletion of a number of nutrients from the body. These include iron, potassium, folic acid, and vitamin C. According to Kauffman (2000), death rates among populations of aspirin users are significantly higher than non-aspirin populations.

In contrast, the botanical versions supply many of these nutrients. Botanicals not only relieve pain and boost the immune system. They also supply nutrients to balance the system.

In other words, white willow bark and meadowsweet—by nature's design—contain a biomolecular version of salicin, moderated by a variety of constituents to balance its effects. Subsequently, whole-plant salicin botanicals do not have a history of the negative side effects. Their molecular arrangements are synergistically oriented with a balance of constituents, which resonate with and stimulate our body's immune system while slowing the conversion of prostaglandins and leucotrienes to gradually ease inflammation. Unlike aspirin, willow and meadowsweet actually *promote* a healthy stomach lining, rather than cause gastrointestinal problems. In fact, traditional herbalists often recommend meadowsweet specifically for acid reflux, gastritis and ulcers.

Botanical pain relievers have the ability to gradually modulate the eicanosoid response in order to ease inflammation and pain. They also stimulate the body's own healing mechanisms to help solve the root problem.

Herbal medicines also stimulate detoxification and strengthen the liver. Nearly every medicinal botanical contains constituents that provide antioxidant and blood-purifying effects. They will thus neutralize toxic free radicals and stimulate glutathione scavenging. They will stimulate the immune system to respond more efficiently. In addition, many botanicals stimulate more efficient filtration and excretion among the kidneys, colon, liver, sweat glands and lungs to speed the removal of waste products from the blood and tissues.

In contrast, pharmaceutical chemicals typically burden the liver and bloodstream with toxicity. This means, frankly, that herbs are simply not comparable to pharmaceutical drugs. They are entirely different creatures. It would be like comparing a rocking chair to a helicopter.

Just as botanicals affect the body vastly different from pharmaceuticals, traditional health practitioners look at pain much differently than do medical doctors. Traditional health practitioners such as herbalists, naturopaths and acupuncturists are not focused upon naming the illness (diagnosis). They are focused upon the root cause of the imbalances that exist within the body, and thus seek to help rebalance the body's metabolism so that it will heal itself.

We must remember that plants are living organisms themselves. Therefore, they also have immune systems. They thus produce a number of biochemicals that protect them from invading bacteria, fungi, sun damage and injury. These same biochemicals become available to humans when we consume their leaves, bark and roots.

Because plants are stationary, they must protect themselves with their various biochemicals. This means the biochemicals they produce interact with environmental threats in the same way those biochemicals will interact with environmental threats within the human body.

One might wonder why there is not more information being made available about the many positive effects of botanical foods and medicines. There is one large glaring reason for the lack of rigorous clinical studies for many botanical products: Botanical medicine is simply not profitable enough for the financial appetites of most large scientific institutions. Researchers have to be paid, and the pharmaceutical giants are very generous with their support for research, so long as that research illustrates the effectiveness of their drugs.

The other reason relates to the media. A survey of broadcast television and large websites—with their many ad placements—illustrates the financial power pharmaceutical giants now wield over our media. Should a network or media outlet attempt to broadcast objective information about botanical medicines, they will likely be reined in pretty quickly.

At least for now, natural botanical plants cannot be patented. (Genetically engineered plants can, however. So we need to keep an eye on this.) If we consider that hundreds of thousands of people die each year from medications, while very few if any die of herbal supplement use, the numbers do not imply any safety issue with botanicals. Yet every day research institutions are warning people about the dangers of using herbal medications. Ironically, much of these warnings are about problems caused by the *interactions* between herbs and pharmaceuticals.

Let's look at a few key examples of pain-relieving and inflammation-reducing herbs that actually promote mucosal membrane health. For the first few, we'll show some of their pain-relieving properties along with digestive comfort effects. We'll also list some of the active constituents within the herb to illustrate our point about herbs having many biochemicals that balance and buffer each other.

This presentation of the science and traditional use of medical herbs is not simply the personal opinion of the author. Rather, this discussion utilizes the medical science and research of numerous researchers, scientists and physicians trained in herbal medicines. Here traditional clinical uses of herbal medicine have been derived from a number of *Materia Medica* texts from various traditions, as well as from documented histories of using these herbs upon significant populations over centuries—some even over thousands of years. Unless otherwise noted in the text, this information utilizes the following reference materials (see reference section for complete citation):

Bensky *et al.* 1986; Bisset 1994; Blumenthal 1998; Blumenthal and Brinckmann 2000; Bruneton 1995; Chevallier 1996; Chopra *et al.* 1956; Christopher 1976; Clement *et al.* 2005; Duke 1989; Ellingwood 1983; Fecka 2009; Foster and Hobbs 2002; Frawley and Lad 1988; Gray-Davidson 2002; Griffith 2000; Gundermann and Müller 2007; Halpern and

Miller 2002; Hobbs 2003; 1997; Hoffmann 2002; Hope *et al.* 1993; Jensen 2001; Kokwaro 1976; Lad 1984; LaValle 2001; Lininger *et al.* 1999; Mabey 1988; Mehra 1969; Mindell and Hopkins 1998; Murray and Pizzorno 1998; Nadkarni and Nadkarni 1908/1975; Newall *et al.* 1996; Newmark and Schulick 1997; O'Connor and Bensky 1981; Potterton 1983; Schulick 1996; Schauenberg and Paris 1977; Schulz *et al.* 1998; Shi *et al.* 2008; Shishodia *et al.* 2008; Tierra 1992; Tierra 1990; Tiwari 1995; Tisserand 1979; Tonkal and Morsy 2008; Weiner 1969; Weiss 1988; Williard 1992; Williard and Jones 1990; White and Foster 2000; Wood 1997.

Willow Bark *Salix alba, Salix spp.*

Traditional Uses and Characteristics of Willow Bark

The willow tree can grow to 75 feet tall, but many species are smaller trees and even shrubs. It has rough bark with narrow, glandular, pointed leaves and small yellow flowers. It grows along streams and fields—and often in neighborhood yards. There are some 450 species of the genus *Salix,* and most contain similar constituents. Willow species grow practically all over the world.

Willow bark has been used traditionally for over five thousand years for pain, rheumatism and inflammation. Sumerian clay tablets some 4,000 years ago documented using willow leaves to treat fever and rheumatism. The 2500-3000 B.C. *Ebers-Edwin Smith Surgical Papyrus*—translated by James Breasted in the 1920s—documented the use of willow by the "Father of Medicine," Imhotep. He used willow for healing wounds and inflammation. The ancient Chinese also used willow to treat pain, wounds, goiter, hemorrhaging, and rheumatic fever. The ancient Greek physicians also used willow. Hippocrates, Celsius, Pliny the Elder, and Galen all recommended willow for pain and inflammation. Early western European physician and herbalist Dioscoridies also documented its use for pain and inflammation.

Herbalists Steven Foster and Christopher Hobbs (2002) documented that willow has "confirmed anti-inflammatory, pain-reducing, fever-lowering and antiseptic properties." The bark was often traditionally used, but famous herbalist Nicholas Culpeper suggested the sap from inside the bark—which also contains salicylic acid—can be used to "provoke the urine" or to "clear the face and skin from spots and discolourings." The leaves have also been defused (steeped into a tea) or even eaten raw to alleviate headaches, arthritis, colds, flu and urinary tract infections. American Indians also chewed the bark to lower fevers, relieve sore throats and toothaches; and even to reduce tonsil inflammation.

Willow contains several salicin glycoside compounds. The salicin molecule will split off in the body, providing a good portion of willow's inflammation and pain reduction effects. Natural salicin from willow is slower acting than aspirin, but it does not come with aspirin's adverse gastrointestinal effects because of its constituent complex of buffers and digestive aid components. The bark is especially high in certain tannins, which help reduce gastrointestinal discomfort.

Rafaele Piria, a university professor in Pisa and Turin, isolated salicin from willow bark in 1828. As we have discussed, this led to salicylic acid's isolation from meadowsweet and subsequent development of aspirin seventy years later.

Dr. Michael Tierra recommends willow bark for fever, headache, sciatic pain, arthritis, rheumatic conditions and neuralgic pain. Dr. Jethro Kloss advocated it for various types of fevers, chills, acute rheumatism, eczema, gangrene, nosebleeds, open wounds, and as a replacement to quinine. North American Indians also prepared poultices from willow for rashes, sores, itching, and cuts. Winter Griffith, M.D. notes that it may reduce symptoms of gout. Dr. Kloss and others describe it as tonic (immune system stimulant), antiperiodic (preventing relapses), astringent (contracts or constricts tissues and reduces bleeding), antiseptic, anodyne (soothing—relieves pain), diaphoretic (induces sweating), diuretic (increases urination), and antipyretic (reduces fever).

(Kammerer *et al.* 2005; Wood 1997; Weiss 1988, Williard 1992; Schauenberg and Paris 1977; Potterton 1983; Lininger *et al.* 1999; Ellingwood 1983; Mabey 1988; Foster and Hobbs 2002; Griffith 2000)

Some Research on Willow Bark

Probably the first clinical study on willow bark was performed by Reverend Edward Stone of Oxfordshire. In the 1760s, he gave 1 dram (1.8 gram) to 50 patients with rheumatic fever, and cured them all to one degree or another (Vane 2000).

While salicylic acid has been shown to inhibit both cyclooxygenase enzymes, other flavonoids in willow have also been shown to inhibit or moderate both cyclooxygenase enzymes COX-1 and COX-2 (Li *et al.* 2008). In one review of randomized human clinical studies on willow bark, three studies confirmed results with analgesic (pain-relieving) effects similar (and not inferior) to rofecoxib for backache; and one confirmed analgesic effects for osteoarthritis (Vlachojannis *et al.* 2009).

In another study of willow and its constituents (Khayyal *et al.* 2000) performed at the Cairo University, it was found that willow extract produces the same or greater ability to inhibit COX enzymes, reduce inflammatory cytokines, reduce leukocyte infiltration and suppress prostaglandins as aspirin and celecoxib. Willow extract also showed a greater ability to reduce malondialdehyde (a reactive species causing toxicity) levels, and significantly reduced oxidative free radical species compared to celecoxib. They found that several polyphenols in willow were responsible for this radical scavenging ability. This of course confirms the combined effects we've been discussing with respect to botanicals.

In a randomized, placebo-controlled double-blind clinical trial by researchers from the University of Sydney (Chrubasik *et al.* 2001), 228 outpatients with acute low-back pain took either willow bark extract or COX-2 inhibitor drug rofecoxib. After four weeks, 60% of the 114 patients that took a 240 mg extract from willow bark experienced more than a 30% improvement using the Total Pain Index, while 60% of the 114 patients that took rofecoxib (now withdrawn from the market) also responded "well." In other words, the two groups responded practically identically. The authors noted that the primary difference between the two treatments was the cost—the willow bark being cheaper.

In a study from Eberhard Karls University in Germany (Biegert *et al.* 2004), 127 outpatients with osteoarthritis and 26 patients with rheumatoid arthritis were tested in two trials of six weeks. Randomized patients took a placebo, an arthritis drug, or 240 mg of salicin extracted from willow daily. In the OA group, those taking the willow extract averaged a 17% reduction in pain compared with 10% reduction in the placebo group. Among the RA patients, the mean pain reduction was 15% compared to 4% among the placebo group. It should be noted that this was a single extract of willow, salicin—less efficacious than the more active willow constituent, salicylic acid. In addition, a whole-herb extract containing the various other efficacious constituents would likely have fared better.

This was illustrated by a clinical trial from Germany's University of Tübingen (Schmid *et al.* 2001). Ten healthy volunteers took a whole willow bark extract with the equivalent of 240 mg of salicin in two doses three hours apart. Over the next 24 hours, the blood of the volunteers was tested for salicylates in the bloodstream. Salicylic acid was 86% of the total salicylate content in the blood. Salicyuric acid was 10%. Gentisic acid was 4%. The amount of salicylic acid in the blood corresponded to 87 mg of synthetic acetylsalicylic acid. The researchers concluded that, "The formation of salicylic acid alone is therefore unlikely to explain analgesic or anti-rheumatic effects of willow bark."

Researchers from the University of Freiberg (Chrubasik *et al.* 2001), tested three groups of patients who used either 240 mg of willow extract supplemented with pain medication, 120 mg of willow bark supplemented with pain medication, or only pain medication. Only 18% of the 224 control patients who used only pain medication were pain-free after 18 months. On the other hand, 40% of the 115 patients who used the 240 mg of willow extract plus pain medication were pain-free, and 19% of the 112 patients who used the 120 mg of willow extract were pain-free after 18 months.

In another randomized, double-blind study at the University of Tübingen (Schmid *et al.* 2001), 78 patients took either 240 mg of willow bark extract or placebo for two weeks. After the two week period, the average pain score (WOMAC standardized index) of the willow bark group was reduced by 14%, while the placebo group was reduced by 2%. The authors concluded that the study confirmed willow's analgesic effects.

Willow bark does cause a mild reduction in platelet aggregation like aspirin does, but nowhere near the sometimes-dangerous levels that aspirin produces. This is because willow bark contains a variety of other constituents that moderate these effects. In a study at the Rambam Medical Center in Israel (Krivoy *et al.* 2001), 51 patients were studied for platelet aggregating reduction—comparing willow bark extract with aspirin and a placebo. The mean platelet-aggregating factor from arachidonic acid was 78% (high baseline) in the placebo group. The aspirin group's platelet-aggregating factor was 13% in comparison. The platelet-aggregating factor was 61% for the willow bark extract group. This illustrated some blood thinning ability, but nowhere near the extreme reduction (that can cause internal bleeding) of aspirin.

In another double-blind study from Israel's Rambam Medical Center (Crubasik *et al.* 2000) published in the *American Journal of Medicine*, 210 low-back pain patients were given willow bark in either 120 mg doses (67 patients) or 240 mg doses (65 patients), while 59 patients were given a placebo. After four weeks, 39% of the high dose (240 mg) willow treatment group was pain-free. Meanwhile, 21% of the 120 mg willow group was pain-free and 6% (four) of the placebo group was pain-free after the four weeks.

How does this compare with the pharmaceutical industry's COX-inhibitors for pain reduction? In another randomized, double-blinded low-back pain study by some of the same researchers (Chrubasik *et al.* 2002), 183 patients took either 240 mg willow bark extract or rofecoxib for four weeks. Both the willow extract group and the rofecoxib group had an identical 44% decrease in pain. This is a second clinical trial illustrating willow bark extract's nearly identical effect of COX-2 inhibitor rofecoxib.

As mentioned, botanical medicines have multiple *positive* side effects. Illustrating this was a study by researchers from the University Hospital in Zürich (Hostanska *et al.* 2007) that tested willow bark on the proliferation of colon cancer cells. It was found that the whole extract and many of willow's constituents inhibited the growth of cancerous cells.

Meadowsweet *Spiraea ulmaria, Filipendula ulmaria, Spiraea betulifolia, Filipendula glaberrima, Filipendula vulgaris*

Traditional Uses and Characteristics of Meadowsweet

Also sometimes called *Queen of the Meadow,* this perennial bush grows throughout Europe and North America in damp grasslands and by streams in the forests. It has small, sweet-smelling white flowers that bloom in the summer. Its flowers, leaves and root extracts have been used to reduce fevers, aches, pains and inflammation for thousands of years. The Egyptians, Greeks, Romans and Northern Europeans were known to have utilized meadowsweet extracts for the treatment of rheumatism, infection of the urinary tract and abdominal discomfort. North American Indians used meadowsweet for bleeding, kidney issues, abdominal pain, colds and menstrual pain. Traditional herbalist Dr. Nicholas Culpeper wrote that meadowsweet "helps in the speedy recovery from cholic disorders and removes the instability and constant change in the stomach." [Cholic refers to increased bile acids.]

According to herbalist Richard Mabey, the tannin and mucilage content in meadowsweet moderate the adverse gastrointestinal side effects of isolated salicylates. For this reason, it is often used for heartburn, hyperacidity, acid reflux, gastritis and ulcers. Meadowsweet has also been used to promote the excretion of uric acid. A purified version of salicin was isolated from meadowsweet in 1830 by Swiss Johann Pagenstecher. This led to the production of acetylsalicylic acid by the Bayer Company, now known by its common name of aspirin. The root of the word aspirin, "spirin" is derived from meadowsweet's genus name *Spiraea*.

The tannins within meadowsweet have been documented to have beneficial effects upon digestion as well. Thus, meadowsweet is often recommended for digestive disorders such as indigestion, diarrhea and colitis. Meadowsweet is also often recommended for the removal of excess uric acid because of its diuretic and detoxifying effects. It has thus been used for kidney stones. Herbalist David Hoffman documents its ability to reduce excess acidity in the stomach and ease nausea. Meadowsweet has been described as astringent, aromatic, antacidic, cholagogue (increasing bile flow), demulcent (soothing and providing mucilage), stomachic (tonic to digestive tract), and analgesic. The German Commission E monograph suggests the flower and herb for pain relief.
(Gundermann and Müller 2007; Wood 1997; Weiss 1988, Miceli *et al.* 2009; Williard 1992; Schauenberg and Paris 1977; Potterton 1983; Ellingwood 1983; Mabey 1988; Lininger *et al.* 1999; Foster and Hobbs 2002; Griffith 2000; Hoffman 1990)

Some Research on Meadowsweet

Meadowsweet flower extracts exhibited liver-protective effects against toxic hepatitis. Meadowsweet was found to stimulate a normalization of liver enzymes, liver antioxidant effects. It also proved to normalize lipid peroxidation (cholesterol production) within the liver (Shilova *et al.* 2008).

Meadowsweet inhibited MMP-1 fibroblast T-cells, which promotes elastin production (Lee *et al.* 2007).

Meadowsweet extract was observed as hematoprotective (protects against liver damage) and exhibited significant antioxidant activity, with high levels of safety (Shilova 2006; Ryzhikov and Ryzhikova 2006).

It was observed being cytotoxic to cancer cells in research sponsored by the Russian Academy of Sciences (Spiridonov *et al.* 2005).

Meadowsweet's phenolic extracts were found to have significant antioxidant and free radical scavenging potential (Sroka *et al.* 2005; Calliste *et al.* 2001).

Meadowsweet extract decreased inflammation, which included suppressing proinflammatory cytokines, decreasing IL-2 synthesis, and eliminating hypersensitivity *in vivo* (Churin *et al.* 2008).

Meadowsweet's antioxidant capacity was one of the highest levels in one test of 92 different phenolic plant extracts (Heinonen 1999).

Meadowsweet showed significant inhibition of several bacteria (Rauha *et al.* 2000). It was also shown to be antimicrobial by Radulović *et al.* (2007). This makes it applicable to septic arthritis.

Meadowsweet extract also exhibited the ability to reduce blood clotting. During *in vivo* and *in vitro* research (Liapina and Koval'chuk 1993), meadowsweet was determined to have anticoagulant (reducing clotting) and fibrinolytic (breaking down fibrin) properties, making it useful for reducing arthritic scar tissue.

Meadowsweet's anticoagulant and fibrinolytic properties were considered similar to heparin in another study (Kudriasho *et al.* 1990).

Contrasting with NSAIDs, meadowsweet was also found to be curative and preventative for acetylsalicylic acid-induced ulcers in rats (Barnaulov and Denisenko 1980).

Furthermore, meadowsweet has been found to inhibit the growth of *H. pylori*—the microorganism thought to cause or contribute to the majority of ulcer disorders (Cwikla *et al.* 2009).

As far as side effects go, in a clinical study of 48 human patients with cervical dysplasia (small tumors) treated with a meadowsweet ointment, 67% (32 cases) had a reduction in the tumors and 52% (25 cases) had complete regression of the tumor. Ten patients were completely cured within a year (Peresun'ko *et al.* 1993).

Ginger *Zingiber officinalis*

Ginger is one of the most versatile food-spice-herbs known to humanity. In Ayurveda—the oldest medical practice still in use—ginger is the most recommended botanical medicine. As such, ginger is referred to as *vishwabhesaj*—meaning "universal medicine"—by Ayurvedic physicians. As mentioned earlier, an accumulation of studies and chemical analyses in 2000 determined that ginger has at least 477 active constituents. As in all botanicals, each constituent will stimulate a slightly different mechanism—often moderating the mechanisms of other constituents. Many of ginger's active constituents have anti-inflammatory and/or pain-reducing effects. Research has illustrated that ginger inhibits COX and LOX enzymes in a balanced manner. This allows for a gradual reduction of inflammation and pain without the negative GI side effects that accompany NSAIDs. Ginger also stimulates circulation, inhibits various infections, and strengthens the liver.

Ginger has therefore been used as a treatment for rheumatoid arthritis, respiratory ailments, fevers, nausea, colds, flu, hepatitis, liver disease, headaches and many digestive ailments to name a few. Herbalists classify ginger as analgesic, tonic, expectorant, carminative, antiemetic, stimulant, anti-inflammatory, and antimicrobial.

(Frawley and Lad 1986; Hobbs 1988; Newmark and Schulick 2000; Lininger *et al.* 1999; Hoffman 1990).

A Sampling of the Thousands of Studies on Ginger

In a six-week randomized, double-blind and placebo-controlled study by researchers from the Miami Veterans Affairs Medical Center and the University of Miami (Altman and Marcussen 2001), 261 osteoarthritis patients were either given ginger extract or a placebo for six weeks. After the study, 63% of the ginger group experienced a reduction in knee pain. The patients were also examined for standing knee pain and pain after walking. In the ginger group, pain after walking improved 173% more than the control group. The ginger group had significantly more reduced pain in each parameter, including the Western Ontario and McMaster Universities Arthritis Composite Pain Index. It should be noted also that 59 patients of the ginger group and 21 patients of the control group experienced mild gastrointestinal upset.

As for this mild stomach upset (not ulcers or bleeding), the logical rationale for this is the use of the ginger extract rather than fresh ginger. Whole ginger is clinically proven to reduce nausea, stomachache, ulcers and many other gastrointestinal problems. With at least 477 constituents, whole ginger has the ability to provide these effects along with the inflammation-reduction effects. Through extraction, many constituents are often lost. Some are sensitive to heat and light. Others are sensitive to ethanol or methanol extraction methods. Therefore, during the pulverization, dehydration and refining process used to make ginger extract, there is a great likelihood that many constituents will not remain in the extract. This is the major reason ginger has been classified into our food category rather than our herbal medicine section.

In other words, it is suggested that ginger be consumed only in its raw form. Fresh ginger root can be purchased at practically any grocery or health food store. It then can be washed like any other fresh food, and then grated onto a salad or other dish. If it is put onto a cooked dish, it is recommended that it be put in after the cooking. Just grate onto the food before serving. Ginger root can also be bitten into and chewed raw, and it can also make a nice tea—not steeped too long of course. It would seem this inexpensive food-medicine would be a *must* addition to meals for any chronic arthritis sufferer.

A randomized, double-blind and placebo-controlled study by researchers from the Tel Aviv University and Medical Center (Wigler *et al.* 2003) gave 29 arthritis patients ginger extract or a placebo. After six months of treatment, the ginger group "showed a significant superiority over the placebo group."

Cayenne *Capiscium frutescens or Capiscium annum*

This red pepper contains the alkaloid capsacin—known to reduce the amount of substance P in nerves, thereby reducing pain transmission. Cayenne also has the distinction of stimulating the production of mucosal membranes among the digestive tract and airways.

Capiscium contains capsaicinoids; various carotenoids such as zeaxanthin, beta-cryptoxanthin, and beta-carotene; steroid glycosides, vitamins A & C and volatile oils; and at least twenty-three flavonoids including quercetin, luteolin and chysoeriol. These constituents work together to provide a number of joint benefits. Cayenne is known to increase circulation; increase detoxification; stimulate appetite; increase liver and heart function; stimulate the immune system and increase metabolic function. It is also a recognized antibacterial and antiviral agent. Some consider cayenne's antiseptic abilities at the level of an antibiotic. Its actions have been described as carminative, alterative, hemostatic, anthelmintic, stimulant, expectorant, antiseptic and diaphoric.

Cayenne is also useful as a topical cream. In a review by the Faculty of Medicine at the University of Ontario (Gagnier *et al.* 2007) of studies from 1966 to 2003, it was concluded that when applied as a topical treatment, cayenne consistently reduced low-back pain more than placebo. For this reason, capiscium is now an active ingredient in a number of over-the-counter topical creams for arthritis and other aches.

Turmeric *Curcuma longa*

Turmeric can also either be considered a medicinal herb or a food-spice. It is a root (or rhizome) and a relative of ginger in the *Zingiberaceae* family. Just as we might expect from a botanical, turmeric has a large number of active constituents. The most well known of these are the curcuminoids. These include curcumin (diferuloylmethane), demethoxycurcumin and bisdemethoxycurcumin. Others include volatile oils such as tumerone, atlantone, and zingiberone, polysaccharides, proteins, and a number of resins.

These work together to stimulate the immune system along with mucosal secretions. For these reasons, turmeric is known for its anti-inflammation effects.

As stated in a recent review from the Cytokine Research Laboratory at the University of Texas (Anand 2008), studies have linked turmeric with "suppression of inflammation; angiogenesis; tumor genesis; diabetes; diseases of the cardiovascular, pulmonary, and neurological systems, of skin, and of liver; loss of bone and muscle; depression; chronic fatigue; and neuropathic pain."

Indeed, turmeric has been used for centuries for arthritis, inflammation, gallbladder problems, diabetes, wound-healing, liver issues, hepatitis, menstrual pain, anemia, and gout. It is considered alterative, antibacterial, carminative and stimulant. It also is known for its wound-healing, blood-purifying and circulatory powers, and has the ability to, as Dr. Tierra puts it, "relieve pains in the limbs." The research has illustrated that curcumin has about 50% of the effectiveness of cortisone, without its damaging side effects.

(Jurenka 2009; Frawley and Lad 1986; Newmark and Shulick 2000; Tierra 1990; Hobbs 1998; LaValle 2001)

A Sampling of Turmeric Research

A number of studies have proved over the past decade that turmeric or its constituents halt or inhibit both COX enzymes and LOX enzymes (Aggarwal and Sung 2009; Thampithak *et al.* 2009; Sompamit *et al.* 2009).

In a randomized, double-blind clinical study from the Medical College at India's University of Poona (Kulkarni *et al.* 1991), 42 osteoarthritis patients were given either a placebo or a combination of boswellia and turmeric. During and after three months of treatment, the boswellia and turmeric group experienced a significant drop in pain severity and disability score compared to the placebo group.

In a blinded, randomized study done at the UK's University of Reading (Bundy 2004), 500 human volunteers with irritable bowel syndrome took either one or two tablets of a standardized turmeric extract for 8 weeks. After the 8-week period, the prevalence of IBS dropped by 53% for the one-tablet group and 60% for the two-tablet group. Pain severity scores also dropped significantly. Because both arthritis and IBS are considered autoimmune inflammatory diseases, the relevancy seems appropriate.

In another study on 45 patients with peptic ulcers (Prucksunand 2001), ulcers were completely resolved and absent in 76% of the group taking turmeric powder in capsules.

Other studies have also shown similar positive gastrointestinal effects of turmeric. We can conclude that not only is turmeric a known anti-inflammatory, but its *positive* gastrointestinal side effects greatly contrast the negative GI side effects of NSAIDs.

Turmeric can certainly be taken in a capsule as the above studies mention. However, because turmeric is readily available as a delicious spice, there is every reason to conclude that adding it (along with ginger) to our daily meal-plans is appropriate for arthritis sufferers. This said, some herbalists, such as James LaValle, R.Ph, N.M.D., suggest that for best results turmeric should also be taken as a supplement.

Bupleurum

Bupleurum (*Bupleurum chinense* or *Bupleurum falcatum*) has also been called Hare's Ear, Saiko and Thorowax. Bupleurum belongs in the Umbelliferae family, and thus is related to fennel, dill, cumin, coriander and others—and exerts similar medicinal effects.

The root is typically used, and its constituents include triterpenoid saponins called saikosides, flavonoids such as rutin, and sterols such as bupleurumol, furfurol and stigmasterol. The saikosides in Bupleurum have been known to boost liver function and reduce liver toxicity. In general, Bupleurum appears to also stimulate detoxification.

Bupleurum is used to stimulate the spleen, purify the blood and rejuvenate the liver—and has been used to treat hepatitis. Bupleurum was studied by researchers at the Beijing University of Traditional Chinese Medicine (Chen *et al.* 2005) on 58 patients with spleen deficiency. After one month of treatment, tests showed that levels of epinephrine and dopamine were decreased and beta-endorphin levels had increased substantially among the Bupleurum-treated group. They concluded that Bupleurum significantly *"regulates nervous and endocrine systems."*

Szechwan Pepper

This is the fruit from *Zanthoxylum simulans* which is also sometimes referred to as *Fructus Zanthoxyli Bungeani* or *Pericarpium zanthoxyli bungeani* in traditional Chinese medicine. More precisely, this herb is also referred to as Sichuan pepper. The tree is also called Prickly ash, and is grown around the world. The small peppers that come from the Prickly ash tree can be dried and ground or used fresh.

Chuan Jiao is also referred to as Fagara, Sansho, Nepal pepper or Szechwan pepper.

Because it is very spicy and hot, it is often used in Sichuan dishes—known for their spiciness. Chuan Jiao contains limonene, geraniol and cumic alcohol, among with a number of other medicinal constituents.

In traditional Chinese medicine, Chuan Jiao is known to remove abdominal pain, vomiting, nausea and parasites—especially roundworm. It is also used as a skin wash for eczema, and has a mild diuretic effect.

Dang Gui (Dong Quai)

This is *Angelica sinensis,* also referred to as *Corpus radix angelicae sinensis* in traditional Chinese medicine. The roots and rhizomes are used. In Western herbology, it is sometimes referred to simply as Angelica. It is also called Dong quai.

This herb contains coumarins and a number of volatile oils. Thus it is known to lower blood pressure, relax tense muscles and improve circulation, as it inhibits platelet aggregation. It is also known as a potent anti-inflammatory, and is known to rejuvenate the adrenal glands.

Dong quai is also considered antispasmodic, which means it reduces hypersensitivity. It stimulates tolerance. It is a very popular herb for balancing the female reproductive system and irregular menstruation. It is considered a tonic in general, and has been used in traditional medicine for colds, fevers, inflammation, arthritis, rheumatic issues and anemia.

Chinese Licorice and Licorice

Glycyrrhiza uralensis is also called Chinese Licorice. It is not the common Licorice (*Glycyrrhiza glabra*) known in Western and Ayurvedic herbalism. However, the two plants have nearly identical uses and constituents. So this discussion also serves *Glycyrrhiza glabra.*

Chinese licorice is known in Chinese medicine as giving moisture and balancing heat to the lungs. It has thus been extensively used to stop coughs and wheezing. It is also known to clear fevers. Taken either internally or topically, it is known to ease carbuncles and skin lesions. It is also soothing to the throat and eases muscle spasms. The root is thus described as antispasmodic.

Researchers from New York's Mount Sinai School of Medicine (Jayaprakasam *et al.* 2009) extensively investigated the anti-asthmatic properties of *Glycyrrhiza uralensis*. They found that *G. uralensis* had five major flavonoids: liquiritin, liquiritigenin, isoliquiritigenin, dihydroxyflavone, and isoononin. Liquiritigenin, isoliquiritigenin, and dihydroxyflavone were found to suppress airway inflammation via inhibiting eotaxin. Eotaxin stimulates the release of eosinophils to asthmatic airways during inflammation.

Licorice also contains glactomannan, triterpene saponins, glycerol, glycyrrhisoflavone, glycybenzofuran, cyclolicocoumarone, glycybenzofuran, cyclolicocoumarone, licocoumarone, glisoflavone, cycloglycyrrhisoflavone, licoflavone, apigenin, isokaempferide, glycycoumarin, isoglycycoumarin, glycyrrhizin and glycyrrhetinic acid (Li *et al.* 2010; Huang *et al.* 2010).

One of its main active constituents, isoliquiritigenin, has been shown to be a H2 histamine antagonist (Stahl 2008). Chinese Licorice has been shown to prevent the IgE binding that signals the release of histamine. This essentially disrupts the histamine inflammatory process while modulating immune system responses (Kim *et al.* 2006).

Another important constituent, glycyrrhizin, is a potent anti-inflammatory biochemical. It has also been shown to halt the breakdown of cortisol produced by the body. Let's consider this carefully. Like cortisone, cortisol inhibits the inflammatory process by interrupting interleukin cytokine transmission. If cortisol is prevented from breaking down, more remains available in the bloodstream to keep a lid on inflammation.

This combination of constituents gives Licorice aldosterone-like effects. This means that the root stimulates the production and maintenance of steroidal corticoids. Animal research has confirmed that Licorice is anti-allergic, and decreases anaphylactic response. It also balances electrolytes and inflammatory edema (Lee *et al.* 2010; Gao *et al.* 2009).

Cinnamon

This is *Cinnamomum cassia*, also referred to as *Ramulus cinnamomi cassiae* in traditional Chinese medicine. It is commonly called cinnamon—a delicious culinary spice present in most kitchens.

Cinnamon is used in just about every traditional medicine. The bark is often used, although the twigs are also utilized. Its constituents include limonene, camphor, cineole, cinnamic aldehyde, gums, mannitol, safrole, tannins and oils.

According to Western herbalism, Ayurvedic medicine and traditional Chinese medicine, it is useful for colds, sinusitis, bronchitis, dyspepsia, asthma, muscle tension, toothaches, the heart, the kidneys, and digestion. It is also thought to strengthen circulation in general. Its properties are described as expectorant, diuretic, stimulating, analgesic and alterative. In other words, it is an immune-system modulator. It is also thought to dilate the blood vessels and warm the body according to these traditional disciplines.

Astragalus

Astragalus (*Astragalus mongholicus* or *Astragalus membranaceus*) root is a well-known immune system adaptogen. In other words, it strengthens the immune system, allowing it to become more tolerant. Astragalus has also been proven to be calming, anti-inflammatory and anti-microbial.

In Chinese medicine, Astragalus is known to treat *qi* deficiency. Remember, *qi* (or *chi*) is the vigor of the body, expressed in circulation, heat, detoxification and immunity. Thus, Astragalus invigorates the body. Astragalus is often used to treat exhaustion, adrenal deficiency, spleen deficiency and circulation issues. Laboratory and *in vivo* research has shown it can reduce blood pressure and increase circulatory health.

Astragalus contains a number of constituents, such as astragalosides, isoastragalosides, astramembrannin, afrormosin, catycosin, daucosterol, formononetin, ononin, pinitol, sitosterol, and various flavonoids, including methoxyisoflavone. It also contains two polysaccharide glucans, heteroglycans, and calycosin.

Researchers from China's Sichuan University (Wang *et al.* 2010) gave *Astragalus membranaceus* to 15 asthma patients and 15 healthy volunteers. They found that Astragalus reduced IL-4 cytokines and modulated the Th1/Th2 ratio, reducing pro-inflammatory processes—evidenced by changes in genetic signalling.

Researchers from Shanghai's Huashan Hospital of Fudan University (Xie *et al.* 2006) found that Astragalus reduced the production of TNF-alpha and inhibited NF-kappa B activity. This illustrated its adaptogenic properties and ability to inhibit inflammation.

Astragalus root may not be a major airway modifying herb as some others are, but its use as an adaptogen can support the powerful effects of airway-oriented herbs.

For example, researchers from China's Huai Ning County Hospital (Wang *et al.* 1998) studied the effects of a combination of *Astragalus membranceus, Codonpsis pilosula* and *glycyrrhiza uralensis* on 28 asthmatic patients for six weeks. After the treatment period, their lung functions, measured by FVC, FEV1 and PEF, were significantly improved. They also found that the herbs significantly decreased airway responsiveness following the treatment period.

Gold Thread

This is from the species *Coptis chinnensis.* It is often referred to as *Rhizoma coptidis* in Chinese medicine. Its common names include Gold thread or Golden thread. In Ayurveda, other species of *Coptis* spp. are also considered Gold thread.

Materia Medica of traditional Chinese medicine have documented that Gold thread removes heat associated with histamine responses affecting the eyes, throat and skin. It has also proved helpful for digestion. Applied topically, it has been used to calm skin rash, and has been used to treat boils and abscesses.

In Ayurveda, Gold thread is considered a bitter and tonic herb that reduces fever (antipyretic). It is also reputed to belong in the same category as Goldenseal.

Reishi

This is none other than *Ganoderma lucidum,* also known as Reishi—a popular medicinal mushroom. Reishi has been shown in numerous studies to significantly stimulate the immune system and moderate inflammation.

Reishi contains many constituents, including steroids, triterpenes, lipids, alkaloids, glucosides, coumarin glycoside, choline, betaine, tetracosanoic acid, stearic acid, palmitic acid, nonadecanoic acid, behenic acid, tetracosane, hentriacontane, ergosterol, sitosterol, ganoderenic acids, ganolucidic acids, lucidenic acids, lucidone and many more.

Ling Zhi strengthens immunity and modulates the body's tolerance and responses to allergens. Reishi has been shown to increase production of IL-1, IL-2 and natural killer cell activity. A number of studies have shown that Reishi can significantly lower IgE levels specific to allergens, and reduce inflammatory histamine levels. It has also been shown to improve lung function and has been used traditionally for bronchitis and asthma.

Recently, researchers from Japan's University of Toyama (Andoh *et al.* 2010) found that Reishi also relieves skin itching and rash *in vivo*.

Panex Ginseng

Panex ginseng is a traditional remedy for allergies and hypersensitivity with thousands of years of use. Panax ginseng will come in white forms and red forms. The color depends upon the aging or drying technique used.

The Ginseng in the FAHF formula is termed *Radix* Ginseng or Ren shen but it is *Panex ginseng*. Depending upon how the Ginseng is cured, there are several types of Ren shen.

When Ginseng is cultivated and steamed, it is called 'red root' or Hong Shen. Ginseng root will turn red when it is oxidized or processed with steaming. Some feel that red root is better than white, but this really depends upon its intended use, the age of the root, and how it was processed. Soaking Ginseng in rock candy produces a white Ginseng that is called Bai shen. This soaking seems odd, but this has been known to increase some of its constituent levels such as superoxide and nitric oxide. When the root is simply dried, it is called 'dry root' or Sheng shaii shen. Korean Red Ginseng is soaked in a special herbal broth and then dried.

There are a number of species within the *Panax* genus, most of which also contain most of the same adaptogens, referred to as gensenosides. Most notable in the *Panex* genus is American Ginseng, *Panax quinquefolius*.

Ginseng contains camphor, mucilage, panaxosides, resins, saponins, gensenosides, arabinose and polysaccharides, among others.

Eleutherococcus senticosus, often called Siberian Ginseng, is actually not Ginseng. While it also contains adaptogens (eleutherosides), these are not the gensenoside adaptogens within Ginseng that have been observed for their ability to relieve hypersensitivity.

Researchers from Italy's Ambientale Medical Institute (Caruso *et al.* 2008) tested an herbal extract formula consisting of *Capparis spinosa, Olea europaea, Panax ginseng* and *Ribes nigrum* (Pantescal) on allergic patients. They found that allergic biomarkers, including basophil degranulation CD63 and sulphidoleukotriene (SLT) levels were significantly lower after 10 days. They theorized that these biomarkers explain the herbal formulation's *"protective effects."*

Researchers from Japan's Ehime University Graduate School of Medicine (Sumiyoshi *et al.* 2010) tested *Panax ginseng* on mice sensitized to hen's eggs. After the oral feedings, they found that the Ginseng significantly reduced allergen-specific IgG Th2 levels. It also increased IL-12 production, and increased the ratio of Th1 to Th2 among spleen cells. In addition, it enhanced intestinal CD8, IFN-gamma, and IgA-positive counts. The researchers concluded that, *"Red Ginseng roots may be a natural preventative of food allergies."*

Ginseng has been found to stimulate circulation and improve cognition. It is also known to reduce fatigue, and stress. Herbalists also use it to improve appetite, and as a mild stimulant and potent antioxidant.

Black Plum

Prunus mume (Seib et Zucc) is also referred to as *Fructus pruni mume* in Chinese medicine. It is also called *Omae* in Korea, *Ume* or *Umeboshi plum* in Japan, which translates, quite simply, to 'Dark plum' or 'Black plum.' It is also referred to as Mume. It is, quite simply, the fruit of a special variety of plums.

This plum is treasured for its immune-stimulating properties. The Chinese *Materia Medica* describes it as able to alleviate coughing and lung deficiencies. It has a strongly astringent property, and thus helps to cleanse the digestive tract and halt diarrhea. Research documented in the *Medica* has indicated that it stimulates bile production, is antimicrobial, and has been able to relieve fever, nausea, abdominal pain and vomiting.

Tylophora

Tylophora indica—also called *Tylophora asthmatica*—has been researched over the past four decades, yet surprisingly has received little attention from many herbalists and media texts.

Tylophora is a perennial shrub native to Southern and Eastern India. The plant has traditionally been used to treat asthma, rheumatism and dermatitis. It is known as being emetic, expectorant, bronchodilating and diaphoretic.

Tylophora contains several medicinal alkaloids, including tylophorine. These and other alkaloids have been described as phenanthroindalizidines.

A crossover study by Indian researchers (Shivpuri *et al.* 1969) gave 110 asthmatic patients either raw Tylophora (leaf) or a placebo (spinach). After one week, 62% of the Tylophora group had moderate to complete symptom relief, while the placebo group experienced 28% relief in comparison. The researchers then treated the placebo group with Tylophora and gave the group treated first with Tylophora the placebo. This time, 50% of the new Tylophora group experienced moderate to complete relief of asthma symptoms, while 11% of the new placebo group reported relief.

Three years later the same researchers (Shivpuri *et al.* 1972) followed up this study by testing 103 asthmatic patients with an alcoholic extract of Tylophora leaves. This time, 56% of the Tylophora group reported moderate to complete relief of asthma symptoms, compared to 32% in the placebo group.

A few years later, another Indian research team (Thiruvengadam *et al.* 1978) gave 350 milligrams of Tylophora leaf powder or a placebo plus anti-asthmatic medications each day to 30 asthmatic patients for two weeks. The Tylophora group had a significant improvement in lung function and significantly reduced shortness of breath. They concluded that, *"there was a sustained rise in maximum breathing capacity (MBC), vital capacity (VC), and peak expiratory flow rate (PEFR) with the leaf (plant extract) as compared with the placebo."*

In another study, researchers (Gore *et al.* 1980) gave 11 patients with asthma, along with 18 healthy volunteers, 3-6 leaves of Tylorphora per day. They found that the Tylophora significantly reduced sneezing and nasal obstruction. They also found Tylophora increased breathing capacity that lasted almost 10 days after the treatment.

In this last study, the researchers hypothesized that Tylophora stimulated the adrenal gland to release cortisol, with possibly a muscle-relaxant effect to go along with it.

This possibility of Tylophora stimulating the adrenal gland was confirmed in animal studies over a decade later (Udupa *et al.* 1991).

Boswellia (Frankincense)

The medicinal Boswellia species include *Boswellia serratta, Boswellia thurifera,* and *Boswellia spp.* (other species). Boswellia contains a variety of active constituents, including a number of boswellic acids, diterpenes, ocimene, caryophyllene, incensole acetate, limonene and lupeolic acids.

The genus of *Boswellia* includes a group of trees known for their fragrant sap resin that grow in Africa and Asia. Frankincense was extensively used in ancient Egypt, India, Arabia and Mesopotamia thousands of years ago, as an elixir that relaxed and healed the body's aches and pains. The gum from the resin was applied as an ointment for rheumatic ailments, urinary tract disorders, and on the chest for bronchitis and general breathing problems. It is classified in Ayurveda as bitter and pungent.

Over the centuries, boswellia has been used as an internal treatment for a wide variety of ailments, including bronchitis, asthma, arthritis, rheumatism, anemia, allergies and a variety of infections. Its properties are described as stimulant, diaphoretic, antirheumatic, tonic, analgesic, antiseptic, diuretic, demulcent, astringent, expectorant, and antispasmodic.

Researchers from Germany's Tübingen Institute of Pharmacology (Gupta *et al.* 1998) gave placebo or 300 milligrams of Boswellia gum resin three times a day for six weeks to 80 long-time asthma patients. After the treatment period, 70% of the Boswellia group had significant reductions or a disappearance in asthma symptoms and episodes— compared to 27% among the control group. Forced expiratory flows, volume capacity and peak flows were significantly increased among the Boswellia group. The Boswellia group also displayed a significant reduction in inflammatory eosinophils.

In two studies, boswellic acids extracted from Boswellia were found to have significant anti-inflammatory action. The trials revealed that Boswellia inhibited the inflammation-stimulating LOX enzyme (5-lipoxygenase) and thus significantly reduced the production of inflammatory leukotrienes (Singh *et al.* 2008; Ammon 2006).

Another study (Takada *et al.* 2006) showed that boswellic acids inhibited cytokines and suppressed cell invasion through NF-kappaB inhibition.

In *in vivo* studies by researchers from the University of Maryland's School of Medicine (Fan *et al.* 2005), Boswellia extract exhibited significant anti-inflammatory effects. The report also concluded that, *"these effects may be mediated via the suppression of pro-inflammatory cytokines."*

In an *in vitro* study also from the University of Maryland's School of Medicine (Chevrier *et al.* 2005), boswellia extract proved to modulate the balance between Th1 and Th2 cytokines. This illustrated Boswellia's ability to strengthen the immune system and increase tolerance.

A similar-acting Ayurvedic herb is Guggul. Guggul is another gum derived from the resin of a tree—*Commiphora mukul.*

Coleus

Coleus forskohlii has been used in Ayurveda for acute bronchial conditions for thousands of years. Over the past few decades, several studies have shown that it can directly reduce conditions related to the mucosal membranes, including asthma and COPD. The central mechanism appears to be that Coleus stimulates cyclic AMP production. Deficiencies in cAMP have been observed amongst many asthmatics.

The central constituent in Coleus is forskolin. This isolated extract has been more specifically studied with clinical success for subduing asthmatic symptoms. In a study from

Manzanillo's Hospital del Instituto Mexicano del Seguro Social (González-Sánchez *et al.* 2006), 40 patients with mild asthma were given either 10 milligrams per day of forskolin capsules or two inhalations of sodium cromoglycate every eight hours for things times a day.

For the six month period, only 40% of the forskolin-treated patients had asthma attacks, versus 85% of the sodium cromoglycate-treated patients. Forced expiratory volumes (FEV1) were similar between the two groups after the treatment period. The researchers concluded: *"We conclude that forskolin is more effective than sodium cromoglycate in preventing asthma attacks in patients with mild persistent or moderate persistent asthma."*

For this reason, forskolin inhalers are often prescribed and utilized by physicians for asthmatics, and prominently so in Europe.

Marica (Black Pepper)

While *Piper nigrum* is considered Ayurvedic, it is probably one of the most common spices used in Western foods. In fact, the world probably owes its use of Black pepper in foods to Ayurveda.

Black pepper is used in a variety of Ayurvedic formulations because of its anti-inflammatory action. Ayurvedic doctors describe Black pepper as a stimulant, expectorant, carminative (expulsing gas), anti-inflammatory and analgesic. It has been used traditionally for rheumatism, bronchitis, coughs, asthma, sinusitis, gastritis and other histamine-related conditions. It is also thought to stimulate a healthy mucosal membrane among the stomach and intestines.

Black pepper used as a spice to increase taste is certainly not unhealthy, but it takes a significantly greater and consistent dose to produce its anti-inflammatory effects.

A traditional Ayurvedic prescription for gastroesophageal reflux or GERD, for example, is to take Black pepper in a warm glass of water on an empty stomach first thing in the morning over a period of time. This dose of Black pepper, according to Ayurveda, stimulates mucosal secretion, and purifies the mucosal membranes of the stomach and intestines.

Researchers from South Korea's Wonkwang University (Bae *et al.* 2010) found that the *Piper nigrum* extract piperine significantly inhibited inflammatory responses, including leukocytes and TNF-alpha.

Long Pepper

The related Ayurvedic herb, *Piper longum,* has similar properties and constituents as Black pepper. It is used to inhibit the inflammation and histamine activity that results in lung and sinus congestion. Like Black pepper, Long pepper is also known to strengthen digestion by stimulating the secretion of the mucosal membranes within the stomach and intestines. It is also said to stimulate enzyme activity and bile production. One study by researchers from India's Markandeshwar University (Kumar *et al.* 2009) found that the oil of Long pepper fruit significantly reduced inflammation.

Triphala

Triphala means *"three fruits."* Triphala is a combination of three botanicals: *Terminalia chebula, Terminalia bellirica* and *Emblica officinalis*. They are also termed Haritaki, Bihitaki and Amalaki, respectively. This combination has been utilized for thousands of years to rejuvenate the intestines, regulate digestion and create efficiency within the digestive tract.

The 'three fruits' also are said to produce a balance among the three doshas of *vata, pitta* and *kapha*. Each herb, in fact, relates to a particular *dosha:* Haritaki relates to *vata*, Amalaki relates to *pitta* and Bibhitaki relates to *kapha*. The three taken together comprise the most-prescribed herbal formulation given by Ayurvedic doctors for digestive issues.

This use has been justified by preliminary research. For example, in a study by pharmacology researchers from India's Gujarat University (Nariya *et al.* 2003), triphala was found to significantly reverse intestinal damage and intestinal permeability *in vivo*.

The traditional texts and the clinical use of triphala today in Ayurveda have confirmed these types of intestinal effects in humans.

We might want to elaborate a little further on Haritaki in particular. *Terminalia chebula* has been used by Ayurvedic practitioners specifically for conditions related to asthma, coughs, hoarseness, abdominal issues, skin eruptions, itchiness, and inflammation. It is also called He-Zi in traditional Chinese medicine.

Research has found that Haritaki contains a large number of polyphenols, including ellagic acids, which have significant antioxidant and anti-inflammatory properties (Pfundstein *et al.* 2010).

Bishop's Weed (Khella)

Trachyspermum ammiis is also called Khella or Khellin among Middle-Eastern herbalists. It is also referred to as Ajwain weed or *Ammi visnaga* among Ayurvedic practitioners and traditional herbalists. Some also refer to it as *Carum copticum,* Spanish toothpick, Toothpick weed, *Daucus visnaga* and Honeyplant. The plant is related to celery and parsley, and blooms with clusters of fragile white flowers. From the flower heads come a fruit and seeds known for their medicinal properties.

Bishop's weed has a long tradition of use in Ayurvedic medicine and Egyptian medicine, especially for asthma, coughs, bronchitis and hypersensitivity. Its use was mentioned in the *Ebers Papyrus*, written more than 3,000 years ago.

Often the fruit and seeds are crushed to produce a brown oil, which is called omam. The oil can also be infused into creams and tinctures. Omam water is also produced from Bishop's weed. To make omam water, the seeds are simply soaked in water.

Bishop's weed has been shown to inhibit histamine release. It also opens the bronchi and is considered spasmolytic (stops spasms), anti-cholinergic (blocks acetylcholine), and vagolytic (inhibits vagus nerve responses).

Khella's most important constituents include thymol, isothymol, pinene, cymene, cromoglycate, terpinene and limonene. The fruits contain coumarins and furocoumarins. Khellin and visnagin are considered the more active compounds in Bishop's weed.

Bishop's weed is also antimicrobial. Its antispasmodic traits may be due to its ability to dilate the bronchial passages and blood vessels without stimulation. These actions make it useful for allergies and inflammation response.

Khella's traditional uses thus include coughing, asthma, bronchitis, heart pain and muscle spasms. It has also been used for wound healing, headaches and urinary conditions. While side effects are few, Bishop's weed has been said to increase the skin's sensitivity to the sun.

There is little research on Bishop's weed proving its usefulness. However, sodium cromoglycate—one of its more active anti-asthmatic constituents—has been extensively studied and proven effective for both allergies and asthma.

Disodium cromoglycate was developed by Dr. Roger Altounyan, an asthma sufferer, based on Khella's sodium cromoglycate. Dr. Altounyan first isolated sodium cromoglycate from Khella, in other words. Today, disodium cromoglycate is often used in many cases as a drug for asthma and allergy patients as an alternative to steroids. Disodium cromoglycate has undergone extensive clinical drug studies, and is considered one of the more effective anti-asthmatic medications—one of the most prescribed drugs for asthma behind prednisone and prednisolone. Disodium cromoglycate stabilizes mast cells and smooth muscle fibers. This is effected through modulation of calcium and other ions involved in cell membrane permeability. This effect also alters the degranulation process, thus inhibiting histamine [and leukotrienes] (González Alvarez and Arruzazabala 1981).

As discussed previously, Khella has a number of other constituents besides sodium cromoglycate. Sodium cromoglycate is isolated from the constituent called khellin, which also contains benzopyran and dimethylmethylfuro. These and other constituents provide spasmolytic (halts spasms) properties that relax the smooth muscles around the airways.

Khella is a member of the carrot family. (Umbelliferae). It also looks very similar to carrot. Some have called it wild carrots. This is notable because carrots and similar tubers such as turnips and Gingers all support lung health, as we'll discuss further.

Bittersweet

Solanum dulcamara, a creeping shrub that grows along streams and bogs, has been used extensively in traditional Western herbal medicine for all varieties of allergic skin issues and inflammatory conditions. It has been used for rheumatism and circulatory problems. The alkaloid solamine and the glucoside dulcamarin have been recognized as its active constituents, but as we'll discuss, solasodine appears to be intricately involved in stimulating corticoid production (See Plant Corticoid section for discussion of the research.)

Perhaps it is for this reason that many traditional herbalists have recommended bittersweet in cases of allergic skin conditions and mucous membrane issues. We should note that another constituent, solanine, can be poisonous in significant amounts. Therefore, as in all herbal products, consultation with a health professional is suggested before use.

Coltsfoot

The leaves and flowers of *Tussilago farfara* combines soothing mucilage will expectorant action. It's constituents include saponins, tannin, alkaloid (senkirkine), zinc, potassium, calcium and of course the mucilage.

Traditional herbalists made syrups from coltsfoot, and also recommended it as a smoking herb. The fresh leaves have also been used as poultices for skin ulcers or sores, because of its soothing actions. Herbalists suggest moderate consumption of this herb.

Coriander/Cilantro/Parsley

Coriandrum sativum has documented throughout traditional medicines as an anti-allergy and antioxidant herb. The seeds are called Coriander, and the leaves are called Cilantro. Cilantro has been popularly used throughout Central America, Italy, and also Asia—where it is sometimes called Chinese parsley. Cilantro is the backbone ingredient—together with tomatoes and garlic—of salsa. It is related to Italian parsley, with many of the same constituents. Coriander is taken as fresh or juiced fresh, and it has been used by Ayurvedic practitioners primarily for allergic skin rashes and hay fever.

Fresh Italian parsley can readily be found in supermarkets and farmers' markets. While often used as a garnish (for looks and/or to clean the breath), a therapeutic quantity of parsley is about a *bunch*. A bunch of parsley is about two ounces or about ten stalks together with their branches and leaves. A *bunch* can be added to a salad or put into a soup. Parsley can be delicious with tomatoes, vinegar and olive oil. And of course, it can also freshen the breath.

Cumin Seed

Cuminum cyminum has a long history of use among European and Asian herbalists. It is described as antispasmodic and carminative, so it tends to soothe inflammatory responses. Like Fennel, Cumin has been used traditionally to ease abdominal cramping and gas.

Cumin seed contains mucilage, gums and resins. Traditional herbalists consider these constituents primarily responsible for Cumin's ability to help strengthen the mucosal membranes. This makes Cumin part of a strategy to rebuild the mucosal membranes of the airways.

Elecampane

The roots and branches of *Inula helenium* have been used for bronchial issues such as asthma, bronchitis and whooping cough for many centuries. It is often the go-to herb to control coughing. It is thus considered antitussive and carminative.

Elecampane contains several sesquiterpene lactones, including alantolactone. However, its soothing effects are likely produced by its relatively high mucilage content—which makes it useful for rebuilding mucous membranes. It also contains 44% inulin, so it is a good prebiotic.

The roots or branches are typically used by traditional healers. Herbalists typically recommend Elecampane use on a moderate basis, as larger doses can be irritating to the digestive system.

Evening Primrose

Another herb known by traditional herbalists to be beneficial for allergic skin responses is Evening primrose, or *Oenothera spp.* The seeds are rich in gamma-linolenic acid (GLA)—a fatty acid known to slow inflammatory responses of prostaglandins, especially those relating to skin hypersensitivity. The oil from Evening primrose can be applied directly onto the skin and/or taken internally. Evening primrose oil has thus been used successfully in cases of allergic eczema, for example.

Fennel

Foeniculum vulgare contains anetholes, caffeoyl quinic acids, carotenoids, vitamin C, iron, B vitamins, and rutins. Ayurvedic and traditional herbalists from many cultures have used Fennel to relieve digestive discomfort, gas, abdominal cramping, bloating and irritable bowels; and to treat asthmatic hypersensitivities. Fennel stimulates bile production. Bile digests fats and other nutrients, increasing their bioavailability.

One of Fennel's constituents, called anethole, is known to suppress pro-inflammatory tumor necrosis factor alpha (TNF-a). This inhibition slows excessive immune response. The combination of anethole and antioxidant nutrients such as rutin and carotenoids in Fennel also strengthen immune response while increasing tolerance.

Fennel is not appropriate for pregnant moms, because it has been known to promote uterine contractions. As with any herbal supplement, Fennel should be used under the supervision of a health professional. Those with birch allergies should also be aware that they may also be sensitive to Fennel. (The same goes for Cumin, Caraway, Carrot seed and a few others).

Grindelia

Grindelia camporum is a traditional western herb used specifically for asthmatic hypersensitivity, as well as bronchitis, skin irritations and other mucosal-related conditions. Its constituents include resins, saponins such as grindelin, volatile oils, alkaloids, selenium and tannins. The leaves and stems of the plant are used.

Grindelia has been described as antispasmodic, which means that it reduces or eliminates spasms. Grindelia more specifically has been documented to relax the smooth muscles around the airways and the airways in general. It is also reputed to help remove mucous from the bronchi, lower blood pressure, and slightly reduce the heart rate.

Grindelia has also been used to reduce hay fever hypersensitivity, and has become popular for reducing the skin's hypersensitivity to poison oak and hives from insect bites.

Herbalists recommend that Grindelia can be taken daily, but in small doses, because it can be toxic in large doses.

Job's Tears

Coix lachryma-jobi (L. var. ma-yuen Stapf) is an ancient grass/grain known to grow primarily in Asia. Native to the tropical regions of Southern Asia, it has been increasingly cultivated as an ornamental grass around the world.

Researchers from National Taiwan University (Chen *et al.* 2010) tested the anti-allergic activity of Job's tears in the laboratory. They found that an extract of Job's tears suppressed mast cell degranulation and inhibited histamine release. It also suppressed the release of inflammatory mediators IL-4, IL-6 and TNF-A—known to stimulate leukotrienes. The researchers concluded that Job's tears inhibited the body's physiological allergic response.

Ivy

Hedera helix L., also known as English Ivy or Common Ivy, grows throughout Europe, North America and Western Asia. It is known to climb walls and sides of buildings, and is the basis for the term "ivy league schools," as the aged buildings of some of these universities are covered with Ivy.

Ivy is also known for its expectorant properties. It has this been used to stimulate tearing and loosen phlegm and mucous of the bronchial passages.

Ivy has been the subject of a respectable amount of research for asthma. Pediatric researchers from Germany's Johann Wolfgang Goethe University (Hofmann *et al.* 2003) reviewed five randomized and controlled studies on Ivy, and selected three for analysis. They found that in all three studies, drops of Ivy extract significantly reduced airway resistance and improved respiratory function in children with chronic bronchial asthma.

They concluded that: *"extracts from dried ivy leaves are effective in the treatment of chronic airway obstruction in children suffering from bronchial asthma."*

Mallow

Malva silvestris grows throughout Europe and has had an extensive and popular reputation among Western and Middle Eastern traditional medicines as a demulcent herb: It soothes irritated tissues. Mallow contains polysaccharides, asparagine and mucilage—which stimulates a balance among the body's mucosal membranes. The leaves are typically used.

The mucilage is primarily composed by polysaccharides. These include beta-D-galactosyl, beta-D-glucose, and beta-D-galactoses.

Mallow has been used for sore throats, heartburn, dry sinuses, and irritable bowels.

This herb has also been used in decoctions by European herbalists for allergic skin responses and eczema. For this reason, Swiss doctors during the World Wars would apply mallow compresses onto skin rashes with good success.

Mallow's leaves, flowers and roots are all used. It is an emollient and demulcent, rendering the ability to soften and coat, while stimulating healthy mucous among the airways.

Mallow has been documented among traditional medicines to successfully treat GERD, sinusitis and asthma.

Marsh Mallow

Althaea officinalis, has similar properties and constituents as the *Malva verticillata* L (Mallow). It belongs in the same family, Malvaceaea, and has similar constituents.

Marsh mallow has also enjoyed an extensive and popular reputation among traditional medicines around the world. This is because it contains mucilage, which supports and stimulates a healthy mucosal membrane.

For this reason, Marsh mallow is considered a demulcent: it's leaves soothe irritated sore throats, heartburn, dry sinuses, and irritable bowels.

The leaves, flowers and roots are all used in healing. Marsh mallow is known to be emollient, which gives it properties that soften and coat practically any membrane within the body, including the sinuses, throat, stomach, intestines, urinary tract and of course, the airways.

The root of the Marsh mallow will contain up to 35% mucilage. It also contains a variety of long-chain polysaccharides. Extracts use cold water, so they dissolve the mucilage without the starches. For this reason, tea infusions for drinking and gargling using Marsh mallow often use cold water overnight, although it can also be steeped for 15-20 minutes using hot water.

Mullein

The leaves, flowers and herbs of *Verbascum theapsiforme* and *V. philomoides olanum* have been part of the traditional herbalist repertory for thousands of years. It is classified as a demulcent and expectorant, because it is known to soothe irritated airways and help clear thickened mucous.

Mullein's soothing and demulcent properties are due primarily to its mucilage content, which can be as high as 3%. Other constituents include saponins, which are believed to produce the expectorant properties of this herb.

Mullein has thus been used for centuries for hypersensitivity among the mucosal membranes, including coughing and bronchialspasm, skin irritations and ear infections. In all these cases, its effects have been considered soothing to epithelial cells.

Pine Bark Extract

Traditional herbalists have used pine bark extracts for respiratory conditions and other mucosal-related conditions for centuries. The process of extraction is complex, however. Pine bark contains numerous constituents that yield health benefits, but also contains a high-density tannin complex requiring careful purification.

Today's standard for pine bark extracts is an extract of French Maritime Pine (*Pinus pinaster*) called Pycnogenol®. This extract is produced using a process patented by the Swiss company Horphag Research, Ltd. The process renders a number of bioavailable procyanidolic oligomers (PCOs), including catechin and taxifolin, as well as several phenolic acids.

Pycnogenol® has undergone extensive clinical study and laboratory research. Today, Pycnogenol® has been the subject of nearly 100 human clinical studies, testing over 7,000 patients with a variety of conditions. This extract's unique layered proanthocyanidin content has been shown, among other things, to significantly reduce systemic inflammation.

For example, in a German study (Belcaro *et al.* 2008), Pycnogenol® lowered C-reactive protein levels—known to increase during systemic inflammation and allergies—after 156 patients were given 100 milligrams of Pycnogenol® or placebo for three months. The average CRP decrease went from 3.9 to 1.1 following the treatment period. This is a 354% reduction in this important systemic inflammation marker after only three months of use.

Pycnogenol® has also been shown to directly improve asthma symptoms and increase lung function. Researchers from Loma Linda University's School of Medicine (Lau *et al.* 2004) gave 60 asthmatic children from 6 to 18 years old Pycnogenol® or placebo for three months. The Pycnogenol® group experienced a significant reduction of asthma symptoms, and an increase in pulmonary function. Pycnogenol® also allowed the patients to reduce or discontinue the use of inhalers significantly more than the placebo group.

Researchers from the University of Arizona's School of Medicine (Hosseini *et al.* 2001) gave up to 200 milligrams of Pycnogenol® or a placebo to 26 asthma patients for four weeks. Then the researchers crossed over the two groups, and the placebo group took the Pycnogenol® and vice versa, for another four weeks. In both four-week periods, the Pycnogenol® treated groups showed significantly lower levels of leukotrienes as compared with the placebo groups. Forced expiratory volumes (FEV1) also were significantly improved for the Pycnogenol® groups over the placebo groups. The research also resulted in no adverse side effects.

In a study of allergic rhinitis to birch pollen, 39 allergic patients were given Pycnogenol® several weeks before the start of the 2009 birch allergy season. The treatment reduced allergic eye symptoms by 35% and sinus symptoms by 20%, compared to the placebo group. Better results were found among those who took Pycnogenol® seven to eight weeks before the birch pollen season began (Wilson *et al.* 2010).

In a study from the National Research Institute for Food and Nutrition in Rome, Italy (Canali *et al.* 2009), 150 milligrams of Pycnogenol® were given to six healthy adults for five days. After the five days, blood tests showed that Pycnogenol® interrupted the genetic expression of 5-lipoxygenase (5-LOX) and cyclooxygenase-2 (COX-2). It also inhibited phospholipase A2 (PLA2) activity. The Pycnogenol® supplementation program also reduced leukotriene production and altered prostaglandin levels. As discussed earlier, COX-2 and 5-LOX production is tied to inflammation processes, while leukotriene synthesis is tied specifically with asthmatic hypersensitivity.

Pycnogenol® also reduces histamine, another critical systemic inflammatory mediator as we've discussed. Researchers from Ireland's Trinity College (Sharma *et al.* 2003) found that Pycnogenol® inhibited the release of histamine from mast cells. The researchers commented that this effect appeared to be the result of the significant bioflavonoid content of Pycnogenol®.

Pycnogenol® has also been shown to reduce and inhibit NF-kB by an average of 15%. NF-kB is involved in the expression of asthmatic hyperreactive leukotrienes, as well as adhesion molecules. The matrix metalloproteinase 9 (MMP-9) enzymes known as conducive to asthmatic responses, is also reduced by Pycnogenol® (Grimm *et al.* 2006).

The bottom line is that Pycnogenol®, an extract bark of the French maritime pine tree, has been shown not only to reduce systemic inflammation in general through the radical scavenging abilities of procyanidolic oligomers. It has also been shown to directly affect asthmatic hypersensitivity and lung capacity by inhibiting inflammatory mediators that stimulate leukotrienes.

Red Algae

Red algae—from the *Rhodophyta* family—have been used for thousands of years to treat inflammation-oriented mucosal conditions, including bronchitis and allergic hypersensitivity.

Researchers from the National Taiwan Ocean University (Kazłowska *et al.* 2010) studied the ability of the red seaweed *Porphyra dentata*, to halt allergic responses. The researchers found that a *Porphyra dentata* phenolic extract suppressed nitric oxide production among macrophages using a NF-kappa-Beta gene transcription process. This modulated the hypersensitivity immune response on a systemic level. The phenolic compounds within the Red algae have been identified as catechol, rutin and hesperidin.

Skunk Cabbage

The root of *Symplocarpus foetidus* has also been used traditionally for asthma, as well as whooping cough and bronchitis. The herb has a funky odor, but it is considered a strong antispasmodic and expectorant. Antispasmodic means, again, that it relaxes the airways and the smooth muscles around the airways. Expectorant means that it helps clear mucous from the airways.

Skunk cabbage contains silica, iron, manganese, a resin, volatile oil and acrid principle—which causes its odor. It has sedative effects, and therefore is also used as a nervine, to calm nervousness.

Wild Pansy

This herb, botanical name *Viola tricolor,* has been used extensively in Western herbal medicine for skin and mucous membrane issues. Its wonderful colorful flowers are difficult to miss in grasslands across North America and Europe.

Wild pansy is known to be high in saponins, as many other anti-allergic herbs are. Saponins are the glycosides such as triterpenes—active compounds in many of the medicinal plants we've discussed in this chapter. Ginseng is a rich source of saponins, for example.

Wild pansy has a significant reputation in traditional herbal medicine of improving mucosal conditions like asthma, bronchitis and skin conditions. Today's its extracts are used in a number of popular herbal tonics, extracts, antitussives and dermatology medicines (Rimkiene *et al.* 2003).

Wild pansy's saponins are drawn out via simple tea infusion. This can be applied externally onto skin rashes, as well as taken internally.

Mucilage Seeds

A number of seeds are helpful for calming and settling the airways, including seeds such as Flax, Safflower, Rapeseed, Caraway, Anise, Fennel, Licorice seed, Black seed and others. Seeds contain basic compounds that offer mucilage, saponins and other polysaccharides that contribute to the health of the mucous membranes.

Not surprisingly, combinations or single versions of these seeds have been used in traditional medicine for centuries.

Pharmacology researchers from Cairo's Helwan University (Haggag *et al.* 2003) treated allergic asthmatic patients with an herbal blend containing Anise, Fennel, Caraway, Licorice, Black seed and Chamomile—all known for their mucosal-rebuilding effects. They found that the extract significantly decreased cough frequency and intensity. It also increased lung function, with higher FEV1/FVC percentages among the asthmatic patients, as compared to those who consumed a placebo tea.

Aloe

Aloe vera has been used traditionally for inflammation, constipation, wound healing, skin issues, ulcers and intestinal issues for at least five thousand years. Aloe's constituents include anthraquinones, barbaloins and mucopolysaccharides, which help replenish the mucosal membranes.

Ointments and Inhalants

It is no surprise that oils of these compounds tend to ease coughing and clear congestion when they are rubbed on the chest and neck. Herb-derived ointments that are applied to the skin of the neck and chest have been traditional treatments for asthmatics and chest congestion due to colds and bronchitis for thousands of years among traditional medicine cultures.

In the nineteenth and early twentieth centuries, these traditions were developed into commercial products, primarily as ointments containing menthol and camphor. They were eventually applied to vaporizers, chest rubs and in inhalants.

In a study from the hospital researchers from Toronto (Rynard *et al.* 1968), 65 patients with chronic respiratory conditions—20 of which had asthma—were treated with nightly vapor inhalations of a blend that included oils of Camphor, Garlic and Eucalyptus. Most patients experienced *"lasting improvement"* of symptoms after three to five months of treatment, while asthmatics *"felt relief from acute symptoms during the first three weeks,"* according to the researchers.

Of the 34 patients who completed the full treatment period of five months, 28 patients volunteered for follow-ups that extended for another 18 months after the treatment was completed. Of these, 19 patients remained healthy with no symptoms or respiratory episodes during the 18 months. Another three were *"much improved"* and two experienced a bout of pneumonia during the follow-up period but completely recovered. One had an upper respiratory infection but also recovered. In other words, only three previously chronic respiratory patients suffered further respiratory symptoms.

Researchers from New York's Albert Einstein College of Medicine (Reznik *et al.* 2004) studied the use of these commercial camphor-menthol rubbing ointments with 127 adolescent asthmatics. Those asthmatics who used the rubbing ointments had significantly fewer emergency hospitalizations and anaphylactic crises than those using medications alone.

Camphor

Camphor oil is derived from the camphor tree, which is native to Asia and Japan. The tree will grow from 50 to 100 feet tall, and will live for many decades. The oil has been used for thousands of years throughout Asia and the Middle East for anointing, healing and embalming.

Camphor oil is steam-extracted from the tree's wood and roots. Its central constituents include camphene, eugenol, cineole, pinene, phellandrene, limonene, terpinene, cymene, terpinolene, sabinene, furfural, safrole, linalool, terpinen, caryophyllene, borneol, piperitone, geraniol and cinnamaldehyde, among others.

This extensive list of components illustrates the complexity of camphor. It thus has many properties. It is considered anti-inflammatory, antiseptic, analgesic, carminative, diuretic, rubefacient and stimulating.

Camphor has been used traditionally for coughs, bronchial infections, colds, muscle pain and arthritis. It is either rubbed onto the skin, put into a compress or vaporized with steam. It is not consumed internally. Some consumed herbal formulations have utilized camphor oil, but these have only very tiny portions of camphor. Care must be taken by breastfeeding mothers applying camphor on the chest not to allow the baby to consume any.

Camphor research has typically concentrated on ointments formulated with camphor and menthol.

Eucalyptus

Eucalyptus is a large fragrant genus of trees that have primarily come from Australia, although they have been migrating to different regions over the past few hundred years. Today, California and many Pacific Rim countries are now home to eucalyptus species, as is the Mediterranean, Africa and many parts of Asia. The tree's bark and leaves are a source of a medicinal sap known for its decongestant and anti-inflammatory properties.

Eucalyptus oil is derived from this sap, and it is the 1.8-cineol called eucalyptol—a monoterpene—that is the key constituent of eucalyptus oil. Eucalyptol has been shown to suppress arachidonic acid metabolism as well as inhibit cytokine release from monocytes.

Researchers from Germany's Bonn University Hospital (Juergens *et al.* 2003) tested eucalyptus extract (eucalyptol) on 32 asthmatics dependent upon steroid medications.

The patients were given 200 mg 1.8-cineol (eucalyptol) orally three times daily in capsules or a placebo for twelve weeks. At the same time, the patients' oral steroid medications (prednisolone) were reduced by 2.5 mg increments every 3 weeks as appropriate with symptoms. The eucalyptus extract group was able to maintain a 36% controlled reduction in oral steroids after twelve weeks, compared to just 7% among the placebo group. The researchers concluded that the eucalyptus extract has *"significant steroid-saving effect in steroid-depending asthma."*

Mints and Menthol

The plants of the mint family include Peppermint (*Mentha piperita*), Watermint (*Mentha aquatica*), Spearmint (*Mentha spicata*), Pennyroyal (*Mentha pulegium*) and several others. They have a variety of common constituents, of which menthol is the most applicable to respiratory issues. Other active constituents of many mints will include menthylacetate, menthone, mentofuran, limonene, cineole, isomenthol, neomenthol, azulenes and rosmarinic acid.

Mint is well-known for its ability to settle digestion and ease flatulence. These effects are due to azulene's ability to relax the smooth muscles around the intestines. Azulene also relaxes the smooth muscles around the airways as well. Note that Chamomile also contains azulene.

Menthol is most known for its ability to clear congestion and expand the airways. It is the expectorant property of menthol that produces this effect. Menthol reduced coughing in a study from Britain's Leicester University Hospitals (Kenia *et al.* 2008) of 42 children.

Menthol also increases perceived nasal airflow. A study from researchers from the Tokyo Women's Medical College (Tamaoki *et al.* 1995) tested nebulized menthol on patients with mild asthma. The menthol group suffered less wheezing and used less bronchodilator medication.

A review of research from the UK's University of Wales (Eccles 1994) indicated that menthol's respiratory reflex effects may at least partially come from its ability to modulate calcium ion channels among the smooth muscles and their associated nerves.

Other Herbal Inhalants

These extracts also make for superb inhalant oils. Oils from camphor, menthol, and eucalyptus have been used alone in diffusers or in humidifiers for bronchial congestion of various types in traditional medicines. These also have been combined with other known bronchial inhalants in some traditional formulations, including:

- ➢ Benzoin tincture (resin of the bark of the Benzoin tree of the genus *Styrax*)
- ➢ Pine needle oil
- ➢ Canadian balsam extract from the Fir tree
- ➢ Mullein

Anti-inflammatory Herbal Spices

We've discussed how a few herbs can naturally reduce inflammation without disrupting our COX system and our mucosal membranes. A number of other herbs also contain anti-inflammatory properties. These work in different ways, and while they may or may not specifically modulate food sensitivities, they can help strengthen the immune system, and thus reduce the inflammatory process that provokes hypersensitivity. Thus, they can contribute to the modulation of the immune system, allowing us to begin tolerating foods that were not previously tolerated. Here is a quick overview of some of the most well-known (and most available) of these anti-inflammatory herbs:

Basil (*Osimum basilicum*) contains ursolic acid and oleanolic acid, both shown in laboratory studies to inhibit inflammatory COX-2 enzymes.

Garlic (*Allium sativum*) probably deserves a larger section, but that information could easily encompass a book in itself—as was well documented by Paul Bergner: *The Healing Power of Garlic* (1996). Garlic is an ancient medicinal plant with a wealth of characteristics and constituents that stimulate the immune system, protect the liver, purify the bloodstream, reduce oxidative species, reduce LDL lipid peroxidation, reduce inflammation, and stimulate detoxification systems throughout the body. This is supported by a substantial amount of rigorous scientific research.

Garlic is also one of the most powerful antimicrobial plants known. A fresh garlic bulb has at least five different constituents known to inhibit bacteria, fungi and viruses. Much of this antimicrobial capability, however, is destroyed by heat and oxygen. Therefore, eating freshly peeled bulbs are the most assured way to retain these antimicrobial potencies.

Cooked, aged or dehydrated garlic powder also has a variety of powerful antioxidants, but little of its raw antibiotic abilities. Garlic is also a tremendous sulfur donor as well. The combination of garlic's antibiotic, antioxidant, anti-inflammatory and immune-building characteristics make it a *must* spice-herb-food for any inflammatory condition.

Oregano (*Origanum vulgare*) contains at least thirty-one anti-inflammatory constituents, twenty-eight antioxidants, and four significant COX-2 inhibitors (apigenin, kaempherol, ursolic acid and oleanolic acid).

Rosemary (*Rosmarinus officinalis*) contains ursolic acid, oleanolic acid and apigenin—a few of the many constituents in this important botanical—shown to inhibit inflammatory enzymes in laboratory studies. Research has also shown that rosemary's volatile oils can halt airway constriction by inhibiting mast cell degranulation.

Other Mucosal Herbs

The list does not end here. Still other herbs have been used among traditional medicines throughout the world to reverse hypersensitivity among mucosal regions. Many of these also help purify the blood, strengthen the liver, strengthen the adrenals, strengthen the immune system and inhibit inflammation.

Comfrey, Aloe and Slippery elm, for example, aid the health of the mucosal membrane with their high mucilage and mucopolysaccharide content—while Cayenne, Nutmeg and Goldenseal stimulate the body's detoxification processes to clear catarrh.

Each has its special benefit, depending upon the specific mucosal region and weakness producing the symptoms; and each has shown clinical benefits among traditional medicines to improve the health of our mucosal membranes:

- Aloe (*Aloe vera*)
- Anise (*Pimpinella anisum*)
- Black sage (*Cordia curassavica*)
- Borage (*Borago officinalis*)
- Cayenne (*Capsicum* spp.)
- Chamomile (*Matricaria chamomilla*)
- Comfrey (*Symphytum officinale*)
- Duckweed (*Stellaria media*)
- Echinacea (*Echinacea purpurea*)
- Goldenseal (*Hydrastis canadensis*)
- Green Tea (*Camellia sinensis*)
- Guggul (*Commiphora mukul*)
- Lemongrass (*Cymbopogon citratus*)
- Nutmeg (*Myristica fragrans*)
- Shadon beni (*Eryngium foetidium*)
- Shandileer (*Leonotis nepetifolia*)
- Slippery elm (*Ulmus fulva*)
- Spurge (*Euphorbia hirta* L.)
- Stinging Nettle (*Urtica dioica*)
- Thyme (*Thymus serphyllum*)
- Tulsi (*Ocimum gratissimum*)
- Wild onion (*Hymenocallis tubiflora*)

Herbal Cough Syrups

As we've described earlier, coughing is a sign of irritation among our mucosal membranes. Either the membranes have been overloaded with a toxin or dead parts of microorganisms, or they have been thinned due to lack of health in general.

Herbal cough syrups have also been used with great success over the centuries to control coughing and open the airways. A wonderful cough syrup recipe adapted from the traditional healer Dr. Jethro Kloss is:

- Two teaspoons of dried Wild Cherry bark, two teaspoons of Mullein, one teaspoon of Ginger and one teaspoon of Coltsfoot are steeped in a quart of boiled water.
- After the herbs have been strained out, a cup of raw honey is added to the water. The mixture is boiled down to the consistency of syrup.
- A freshly-squeezed juice of one lemon is stirred in.
- The mix can be put into a small jar for immediate use (at room temperature). The rest can be stored in a mason jar in the refrigerator. However, cough syrups are always best warmed and served at room temperature.
- While Mullein and Wild cherry are key ingredients, the other two can be replaced by other mucous membrane herbs listed above, such as Slippery elm or Elecampane.

Herbal Techniques

We've discussed a long list of herbs that can help rebuild our mucosal membrane health. Choosing the right herb and/or formula for a particular case can thus be a little tricky. For this reason, a seasoned expert in herbal formulations can offer specific suggestions relating to ones constitution and precise level of sensitivities.

The choice of application will likely depend also upon the part of the body affected. While most of these medicinal herbs help stimulate mucosal membrane health in general, some benefit particular tissue systems better than others. Some, like mullein, will benefit the lungs, while ginger will benefit the digestive tract. Still, mullein will benefit the GI tract and ginger will benefit the lungs as well. So these kinds of crossovers occur, but at the same time, ginger is better for digestive issues than it is for lung issues.

Another example might be that Marsh mallow, Mallow and Mullein might be recommended in a case of GERD along with asthmatic symptoms, because GERD illustrates a weakness in the mucosal membranes.

Or perhaps, for issues where sinusitis presents along with asthmatic hyperreactivity, the herbalist may recommend the use of ventilation or ointment of camphor, menthol and eucalyptus along with anti-asthma herbs to clear the sinus passageways, speed the removal of mucous from the nasal region, and exert some antimicrobial effects that these bring.

Dosages and Methods

We have not detailed precise dosages in this section because there are many considerations when determining dosages. These include age, physical health, constitution, unique weaknesses, diet, lifestyle and other factors. Herbs should also be carefully matched, and some herbs and formulations have been known to interact with certain medications.

Therefore, it is suggested that herbs are chosen, formulated and dosed by an experienced herbalist. If there are any medications being used, the prescribing physician should be consulted.

This said, most of the herbs mentioned above, with the exception of essential oils, are safest when used as *infusions*. An infusion is simply the steeping of the fresh or dried root, bark, leaf, seed, stem or fruit in water. In the case of most herb leaves and stems, the water is brought to a boil, and the herb can be steeped for 5-10 minutes using a strainer or tea-ball. In the case of most roots, seeds and barks, the root can be steeped a little longer, for 10-20 minutes, depending on the herb. In some cases a seed, root or bark is better when it is soaked overnight in room temperature water.

Another strategy is to simply ingest a capsule or pressed tablet of a powdered version of the herb or herbal formulation. Liquid extracts are also available from many reputable herbal suppliers. In these cases, the literature accompanying these products should be closely examined for dosages and possible interactions.

A number of the formulations (or their derivatives) mentioned in this section are available as encapsulated, pressed tablets or liquid extracts, together with dosage suggestions. Before using this strategy, care should be taken to assure that the herbal formulation has been ultimately designed by a reputable herbalist. Most of the popular commercial brands of herbal formulations employ professional herbalists to design their formulations. Many will also name the herbalist on the marketing material or label of the product. These should be considered more trustworthy formulations.

Essential oils of herbs can also be rubbed into the skin of the chest region. We discussed this earlier in the case of camphor, menthol and eucalyptus rubs. Care should be taken not to ingest these; or rub these into the eyes, ears, nostrils or onto the breasts before or during breastfeeding. There are several reputable formulations of mentholated rubs with camphor on the market today.

By far the best approach is to have an herbalist formulate and recommend herbs specific to ones constitution, symptom severity, medication and lifestyle. In the alternative, a commercial formula (such as ones discussed in this chapter) blended or overseen by a reputable herbalist, together with instructions on the packaging, can be used. Remember, again, if taking medications, the prescribing physician should be consulted to avoid possible interactions. Also, very small doses, gradually building up to the suggested dose, are usually recommended in the beginning to test tolerances.

Food Choices

Our diets directly affect the strength of our mucosal membranes. Let's look at the research showing how our diets can affect our mucosal membranes, particularly of those of our airways:

In a study of 460 children and their mothers on Menorca—a Mediterranean island—medical researchers from Greece's Department of Social Medicine and the University of Crete (Chatzi *et al.* 2008) found that children of mothers eating primarily a Mediterranean diet (a predominantly plant-based diet) produced significantly lower rates of asthma among the children.

They found that mothers with a high Mediterranean Diet Score during pregnancy reduced the incidence of persistent wheeze among their children by 78%. Their children also had 70% lower incidence of allergic wheezing; and a 45% reduction in allergies among their children at age six (after removing other possible variables).

Another extensive predictive study was the International Study of Asthma and Allergies in Childhood (ISAAC). The study was conducted among eight Pacific countries, which included Samoa, Fiji, Tokelau, French Polynesia and New Caledonia. The research found that the major predicating factors in current asthma wheeze were regular margarine consumption, electric cooking, and maternal smoking. Factors that decreased asthma incidence included having two or more older siblings and being born within the country currently residing in.

Furthermore, they found that the risk factors for increased rhinoconjunctivitis included the regular consumption of meat products, butter, margarine and nuts; along with regular television viewing, acetaminophen use and second-hand smoke. Allergic eczema was also associated with regular meat consumption, pasta consumption and butter consumption; along with regular television viewing, acetaminophen use and second hand smoke. The researchers concluded that: *"Regular meat and margarine consumption, paracetamol [acetaminophen] use, electric cooking and passive smoking are risk factors for symptoms of asthma, rhinoconjunctivitis and eczema in the Pacific."*

The research from Sweden's Uppsala University discussed earlier (Uddenfeldt *et al.* 2010) studied the lifestyle and diets in 12,560 adolescents, adults and elderly adults with a follow-up period of 13 years, between 1990 and 2003. The researchers found that those eating a diet heavy with fruit and fish significantly reduced rates of asthma. In elderly persons, the rates were reduced by nearly 50%.

Medical researchers from Britain's University of Nottingham (McKeever *et al.* 2010) researched the relationship between diet and respiratory symptoms, including forced expiratory volumes. Their data was derived from 12,648 adults from the Monitoring Project on Risk Factors and Chronic Diseases in The Netherlands. They also included dietary patterns and lung function decline over a five-year basis.

They found that diets with higher intakes of meat and potatoes, and lower levels of soy and cereals, was linked to reduced lung function and lower expiratory levels (FEV1) levels. They also found that the heavy meat-and-potatoes diet produced higher levels of chronic obstructive pulmonary disease. They also found that a "cosmopolitan diet" with heavier intakes of fish and chicken (both of which are commonly fried) produced higher levels of wheeze and asthma.

Remember the research from the University of Athens (Bacopoulou *et al.* 2009). Here 2,133 children at ages seven and eighteen were studied. The daily consumption of fruit and vegetables significantly reduced the risk of asthma symptoms through age 18.

Researchers from the Johns Hopkins School of Medicine (Matsui and Matsui 2009) studied 8,083 people over two years old using data from the National Health and Nutrition Examination Survey (2005-2006). They found that among patients diagnosed by a doctor as having asthma and/or wheeze in the last year, higher blood levels of folate was linked to lower total IgE levels—a sign of reduced allergy and hypersensitivity (atopy). They also found a dose-dependent relationship between higher folate levels and doctor-diagnosed wheeze and/or asthma.

Good sources of folate include lettuce, spinach, lentils, beans, asparagus and other plant-based foods.

Researchers from Mexico's Institute of National Public Health (Romieu *et al.* 2009) followed 158 asthmatic children and 50 healthy children from Mexico City for 22 weeks. Diet, lung function testing and sinus mucous analysis was done every two weeks. Diets with greater amounts of fruits and vegetables resulted in lower levels of pro-inflammatory IL-8 cytokines. A diet that most closely trended towards the Mediterranean diet (index) resulted in better lung function tests. Children with the higher Mediterranean diet index scores also scored the highest in forced expiratory volume (FEV1) testing. The researchers concluded: *"Our results suggest that fruit and vegetable intake and close adherence to the Mediterranean diet have a beneficial effect on inflammatory response and lung function in asthmatic children living in Mexico City."*

Another study by researchers from the University of Crete's Faculty of Medicine (Chatzi *et al.* 2007) surveyed the parents of 690 children ages seven through 18 years old in the rural areas of Crete. The children were also tested with skin prick tests for 10 common allergens. This research found that consuming a Mediterranean diet reduced the risk of allergic rhinitis by over 65%. The risk of skin allergies and respiratory conditions (such as wheezing) was also reduced, but by smaller amounts. They also found that greater consumption of nuts among the children cut wheezing rates in half, while consuming margarine more than doubled the incidence of both wheezing and allergic rhinitis.

Nutrition researchers from Italy's D'Annunzio University (Riccioni *et al.* 2007) also studied the relationships between nutrition and bronchial asthma. They found significant evidence that inflammatory activity associated with the asthmatic hyperresponse relates directly to the production of reactive oxygen species. Furthermore, they determined that the damage done by these free radicals produces *"specific inflammatory abnormalities"* within the airways of asthmatics.

A related study by these researchers (Riccioni *et al.* 2007) tested 96 people—which included 40 asthmatics and 56 healthy control subjects—for blood levels of vitamin A and lycopene. They found that lycopene and vitamin A levels were significantly lower among the asthmatic patients versus the healthy controls. They concluded that: *"Dietary supplementation or adequate intake of lycopene and vitamin A rich foods may be beneficial in asthmatic subjects."*

As part of the International Study on Allergies and Asthma in Childhood (ISAAC), a contingent of researchers from around the world (Nagel *et al.* 2010) convened to analyze studies on asthma and diet conducted between 1995 and 2005 among 29 research facilities in 20 different countries. In all, the dietary habits of 50,004 children ages eight through twelve years old were analyzed.

This study revealed that those with diets containing large fruit portions had significantly lower rates of asthma. This link occurred among both affluent and non-affluent countries. Fish consumption in affluent countries (where vegetable intake is less) and green vegetable consumption among non-affluent countries were also associated with reduced asthma. In general, the consumption of fruit, vegetables and fish was linked with less lifetime asthma incidence among the entire population. Frequent consumption of beef burgers, on the other hand, was linked with greater incidence of lifetime asthma.

Researchers from Spain's University of Murcia (Garcia-Marcos *et al.* 2007) examined the effects of diet on asthma in 106 six and seven year-old children. Utilizing a Mediterranean diet score along with a survey of symptoms, they found that eating a predominantly Mediterranean diet decreased severe asthma symptoms among the girls. Diets high in cereal grains produced 46% lower incidence of severe asthma. Frequent fruit eating decreased rhinoconjunctivitis incidence by 24%. In contrast, diets higher in fast foods produced 64% greater incidence of severe asthma.

Meanwhile, research from the National Center for Chronic Disease and Prevention (Cory *et al.* 2010) indicated that only 11-30% of adult Americans eat the recommended amounts of fruits and vegetables—some of the lowest levels in the world.

Nutrition scientists from Korea's Kyung Hee University (Oh *et al.* 2010) studied the relationship between allergies, asthma and antioxidants. They found by testing 180 allergic and 242 non-allergic Korean children that higher serum levels of beta-carotene, dietary vitamin E, iron and folic acid were associated with lower incidence of atopic reactions among the children. These antioxidant nutrients are derived primarily from plant-based foods.

Many other studies have shown these associations between diet and asthma. Researchers from the Allergy and Respiratory Research Group Centre for Population Health Sciences at the University of Edinburgh's Medical School (Nurmatov *et al.* 2010) analyzed 62 international asthma studies for control protocols and study design. They found that 17 of 22 well-designed studies that compared dietary fruit and vegetable intake with asthma showed that higher fruit and vegetables in the diet lowered asthma incidence.

Their analyses found that asthmatic children had significantly lower levels of vitamin A; and that greater levels of vitamin D, vitamin E and zinc was *"protective for the development of wheezing outcomes."*

The researchers concluded that adequate intake of antioxidant vitamins including vitamins A, C, and E were critical to reducing free radicals and inflammatory abnormalities. They also determined that antioxidants are able to reduce damage from incoming bacteria, viruses, toxins and xenobiotics (pollutants to the body). The researchers referenced a number of other studies that successfully associated oxidative stress with bronchial inflammation and subsequent asthma development.

Researchers from Italy's University G. D'Annunzio Chieti (Riccioni and D'Orazio 2005) discovered in their research that persistent asthma is linked to an increase in reactive oxygen species. Their research also found that antioxidant nutrients such as selenium, zinc and other antioxidant vitamins have the potential to help reduce asthma symptoms and severity.

Consuming a predominantly plant-based diet (such as the Mediterranean diet), has clear results: It is linked with reduced allergy and asthma incidence and a reduction of conditions connected with mucosal membrane hyperactivity.

Dietary Strategies

Noting this research, we can see that a diet with plenty of plant-based foods, whether it be the Mediterranean diet, a vegetarian diet, vegan diet or a raw food diet, will help promote mucosal membrane health.

However, another element is required. This is the need for foods that add to our probiotics and nourish those probiotics that line our mucosal membranes.

Our definition of 'living' refers to:
- ✓ Foods that are cultured or fermented with probiotic microorganisms, whether yeasts or probiotic bacteria.
- ✓ Foods that are mixed with cultured or fermented foods.
- ✓ Grains or beans that have been sprouted.
- ✓ Plant-based foods that have been harvested whole and prepared as whole foods, with minimal cooking and processing.
- ✓ Supplements that contain probiotics and/or plant-based whole foods that have been minimally cooked or processed.

What are the mechanisms involved in this dietary approach?
A diet high in living foods will:

- increase antioxidant levels
- increase detoxification
- lower the burden on the body's immune system
- provide a host of bioavailable nutrients
- provide fiber, reducing LDL lipid peroxidation
- increase liver activity and strengthen the liver
- alkalize and help purify the blood
- provide the body with trace and macro minerals
- lower inflammation
- increase our body's resident probiotics

Probiotic Foods

As we've discussed at length, probiotics are key to mucosal membrane health. Probiotics also help us digest food and they secrete beneficial nutritional products. Unbelievably, probiotics are a good source of a number of essential nutrients. They can manufacture biotin, thiamin (B1), riboflavin (B2), niacin (B3), pantothenic acid (B5), pyridoxine (B6), cobalamine (B12), folic acid, vitamin A and vitamin K. Their lactic acid secretions also increase the assimilation of minerals that require acid for absorption, such as copper, iron, magnesium, chromium, selenium and manganese among many others.

Probiotics are also critical to nutrient absorption. They break away amino acids from complex proteins, and mid-chain fatty acids from complex fats. They help break down bile acids. They help convert polyphenols from plant materials into assimilable biomolecules. They also aid in soluble fiber fermentation, yielding digestible fatty acids and sugars. Among many other nutritive tasks, they also help increase the bioavailability of calcium.

Nutrients and Probiotics

Biotin	Produced by probiotics
Thiamin (B1)	Produced by probiotics
Riboflavin (B2)	Produced by probiotics
Niacin (B3)	Produced by probiotics
Pantothenic Acid (B5)	Produced by probiotics
Pyridoxine (B6)	Produced by probiotics
Cobalamine (B12)	Produced by probiotics
Folic Acid (B9)	Produced by probiotics
Vitamin A	Produced by probiotics
Vitamin K	Produced by probiotics
Copper	Probiotics increase bioavailability
Calcium	Probiotics increase bioavailability
Magnesium	Probiotics increase bioavailability

Iron	Probiotics increase bioavailability
Manganese	Probiotics increase bioavailability
Selenium	Probiotics increase bioavailability
Chromium	Probiotics increase bioavailability
Potassium	Probiotics increase bioavailability
Zinc	Probiotics increase bioavailability
Proteins	Probiotics break down for digestibility
Fats	Probiotics break down for digestibility
Carbohydrates	Probiotics break down and process
Sugars	Probiotics break down and process
Milk	Probiotics increase digestibility
Phytonutrients	Probiotics increase digestibility
Cholesterol	Probiotics bind to + reduce blood levels

Many of the nutrients found in vitamin supplements and supplemented foods are in fact produced by probiotics. Most commercial forms of vitamin B12, for example, are derived from the probiotics *Propionibacterium shermanii*, *Pseudomonas denitrificans* or *Streptomyces griseus*.

We should note here that not all probiotics produce the same nutrients. Some, in fact, will consume some nutrients that others manufacture. For example, *Lactobacillus bulgaricus* will produce folic acid in yogurt, and *Lactobacillus acidolphilus* will consume folic acid. At the end of the day, a mixture of probiotics will still have a net increase in nutrients, however. For this reason, most cultured dairy products have significantly higher nutrient contents than the milk or cream they were made with.

Probiotics also assist in peristalsis—the rhythmic motion of the digestive tract—by helping move intestinal contents through the system. They also produce antifungal substances such as acidophillin, bifidin and hydrogen peroxide, which counteract the growth of not-so-friendly yeasts. Probiotic hydrogen peroxide secretions are also oxygenating, providing free radical scavenging. In addition, they can manufacture some essential fatty acids, and are the source of 5-10% of all short-chained fatty acids essential for healthy immune system function.

An example of the extent of probiotics' ability to produce antimicrobials is the antibiotic streptomycin. This antibiotic, produced by the probiotic bacteria, *Streptomyces griseus* was discovered in 1943 by Selman Waksman.

Probiotics directly and indirectly break down toxins utilizing biochemical secretions and colonizing activities. Nutrients produced by probiotics have been found to have anti-tumor and anticancer effects within the body. Some probiotics can prevent assimilation of toxins like mercury and other heavy metals. Others will directly bind these toxins or will facilitate their binding to other molecules in order to remove them.

Probiotic nutrients are instrumental in slowing cellular degeneration and the diseases associated with it. Through their nutritive mechanisms, probiotics help normalize serum levels of cholesterol and triglycerides. Some probiotics even help break down and rebuild hormones.

Probiotic nutrients can also increase the productivity of the spleen and thymus—the key organs of the immune system.

Probiotics are necessary components to healthy digestion. Their populations dwell along and within the intestinal mucosal lining, providing a protective barrier to assist in the process of filtering and digesting toxins and other matter prior to these toxins encountering the intestinal wall cells. This mechanism helps maintain the brush barrier cells and keep the mucosal lining of our intestines from damage caused by foreign molecules coming from our foods and their metabolites. Damage to the brush cells of the intestinal lining is the prime cause for a number of irritable bowel disorders.

Illustrating probiotic production of one critical nutrient, Italian researchers (Strozzi and Mogna 2008) gave 23 healthy volunteers *Bifidobacterium adolescentis* DSM 18350, *B. adolescentis* DSM 18352, or *Bifidobacterium pseudocatenulatum* DSM 18353. Stool samples taken before and 48 hours after administration showed a significant increase of bioavailable folic acid from each of the probiotic strains.

Probiotics will also compete with pathogenic organisms for nutrients. Assuming good numbers, this strategy can check pathobiotic growth substantially. Nutrients produced by probiotics will also help stimulate the immune cell production, and normalize their activity during inflammatory circumstances.

Let's review some of the most available probiotic foods. These are fermented or cultured foods that are teeming with probiotic bacteria and yeasts. These include yogurt and kefir, but also raw cheeses, traditional cottage cheese, traditional sour cream, traditional buttermilk, traditional sauerkraut, lassi, amasake (Japanese sweet rice drink), traditional miso, traditional tempeh, traditional tamari, traditional soy sauce and traditional kombucha tea and others.

Other foods utilize probiotics in their preparation. Traditional sourdough bread and bauerbrot are good examples. Most bread, in fact, uses some sort of (often probiotic) yeast fermentation process to prepare the flour for baking. In these, however, the probiotics are likely all killed during baking.

Some of the foods mentioned here are preceded by the word "traditional" because sadly, many of today's versions are pasteurized or otherwise acidified enough to kill any viable probiotic colonies. Both cottage cheese and butter were originally probiotic foods, for example, when we used to eat dairy products from our local dairies or own farms. Today, these two foods are produced commercially without probiotics. Ironically, even many commercial yogurts are unbelievably pasteurized prior to shipping—killing off most if not all of their viable colonies.

Another example is tamari and soy sauce. Today, most commercial versions are brewed with solvents. Probiotics are no longer part of these processes, as were the traditional versions.

Here are a few probiotic foods (among many others) to consider adding to our diets:

Traditional Yogurt

Because yogurt is usually produced using *L. bulgaricus, S. thermophilus* and sometimes *L. acidophilus,* it is certainly a good source of probiotics. However, we should clarify again that pasteurization kills many probiotics. This means that commercial yogurts that pasteurize the yogurt after it has been cultured will have killed most or all of those colonies used to convert the milk to yogurt. Some producers pasteurize the milk first and then make the yogurt.

The best yogurt is made using raw milk. It is quite simple to make yogurt: After heating a pot of milk to 180 degrees F (82 C) momentarily, we can add a half-cup of starter (active yogurt from a previous batch or an active commercial yogurt) into the milk after it cools to about 105 degrees F (40 C). After stirring thoroughly, we can put the container in a warm, clean, dry place, with a clean towel or loose seal over the container. The mixture will sour and gel in about six to ten hours depending upon temperature. Then we can jar and refrigerate.

The ideal blend of probiotic species for a yogurt starter—one that was developed over the centuries by the Bulgarians—is a ratio of seven parts *S. thermophilus* to one part *L. bulgaricus.* This ratio produces the ideal sourness that is tasty yet tart. It also prevents the *L. bulgaricus* from outgrowing and overwhelming the *S. thermophilus.*

This later point is one of the reasons why yogurt starters that include *L. acidophilus* often fail to supply any *L. acidophilus* in the end product. *L. bulgaricus* is a hardy organism that will easily overtake *L. acidophilus* in a culture. The use of *L. acidophilus* in yogurt is not only wasteful, but possibly can result in an overly acidic flavor, as *L. bulgaricus* colonies swell with the lactic acid produced initially by *L. acidophilus.* In addition, it appears that *L. bulgaricus* produce small amounts of hydrogen peroxide—which knocks out the *L. acidophilus* colonies.

The moral of this also is not to expect much in the way of *L. acidophilus* in a commercial yogurt that blends *L. acidophilus* with *L. bulgaricus.*

Yogurt and other fermented dairy foods have little or no lactose. This is because the probiotics convert the lactose to lactic acid. The lactic acid is healthy for the intestinal tract, because it renders a medium that helps promote our own probiotic colonies. Lactic acid also offers a pleasing tart flavor to yogurt and other fermented dairy.

Traditional Kefir

Kefir is a traditional drink originally developed in the Caucasus region of what is now considered southern Russia, Georgia, Armenia and Azerbaijan. Here Moslem tribe leaders vigorously protected their kefir recipe, as it was considered an esteemed and regal food with healing properties. The secret recipe was eventually ransomed by a young beautiful female Russian emissary who was kidnapped by a local prince. She wrestled a few kefir grains from the secrecy of the prince's family as a settlement for her abduction. She brought kefir into the Moscow market shortly thereafter and it spread as a highly prized healing food all over Russia and Europe. Kefir also became a focus of Soviet research, discovering some of the surprising benefits of probiotics we have outlined in this book.

Kefir uses fermented milk mixed with kefir grains that resemble little chunks of cauliflower. One tablespoon of kefir grains can be mixed with whole milk and sealed in a jar at room temperature. The milk is fermented overnight in a warm location with the starter grains. Depending upon the temperature, milk and kefir grains, it will take 1-3 days to completely ferment. The jar should be opened and swirled one to two times a day. The grains are screened or filtered out and utilized for the next batch. Cow's milk is most used, but sheep's milk, goat's milk or deer milk can also be used.

Buttermilk

Buttermilk is a soured beverage that was originally curdled from cream. Traditional buttermilk utilized the acids that probiotic bacteria produce for curdling. Today, forced curdling is done using commercially available acidic products. Cream of tartar, lemon juice or vinegar is added to heated and stirred whole milk at a rate of one tablespoon per cup of milk, until the curdling starts. After standing for 15 minutes and stirring another 15, it is refrigerated. See the butter section for the traditional method.

Traditional Butter

Today commercial butter contains no probiotics. Traditionally, butter was made with the cow's natural probiotics. The raw milk sits for a half-day or day depending upon temperature, until the cream rises to the top. The cream is taken from the milk to be churned and aged; letting the probiotics convert lactose to lactic acid. This creates a mix of buttermilk and butter. The buttermilk is strained off, leaving the butter. The butter can be further dried of moisture and mixed with salt for taste. Again, the probiotics from the raw milk will have matured the butter and buttermilk naturally.

Traditional Cottage Cheese

Commercial cottage cheese is now made without probiotics. It was a probiotic process before dairy processors began to pasteurize the product and force the curdling with lactic acids. Again, probiotics also produce the lactic acids that were used to curdle the product in traditional cottage cheese making. Skim milk with cream and buttermilk is probably the easiest way to make cottage cheese at home today, using the curds off the cream separation. The probiotics arising from the buttermilk help curdle the thickened milk and cream before separating the curds. Salt is one of the secrets to making a tasty cottage cheese.

Traditional Kimchi

Kimchi is a fermented cabbage with a wonderful history from Korea. Kimchi was considered a ceremonial food served to emperors and ambassadors. It also was highly regarded as a healing and tonic food. There are a variety of different recipes of kimchi, depending upon the region and occasion.

Kimchi can be made by slicing and mixing cabbage with warm water, salt, ginger, garlic, red pepper, green onions, oil and a crushed apple. It is then put into a sealed jar(s) at room temperature for 24 hours, before putting into the refrigerator to continue the fermenting process (*Lactobacillus kimchii* is a typical colonizer). After several weeks of continued fermentation in the fridge, it is ready for eating.

Traditional Miso

Miso is an ancient food from Japan. A well-made miso will contain over 160 strains of aerobic probiotic bacteria. This is because the ingredients are perfect prebiotics for these probiotics.

Miso is produced by fermenting beans and grains. Soybeans are often used, but other types of beans are also used. Equal parts soaked and cooked soybeans and rice are mixed. A fungi spore (koji, or *Aspergillus oryzae*) and salt is added to the rice prior to mixing. The mixture is put into a covered container in a dark, dry, room-temperature location and stirred occasionally. It can take up to a year of aging like this for the fermentation to result in a tasty miso.

When other beans other than soy are used, they will produce different varieties of miso. Shiromiso is white miso, kuromiso is black miso, and akamiso is red miso. They are each made with different beans. There are also various other miso recipies, many of which are highly guarded by their makers.

Traditional Shoyu

Shoyu is a traditional form of soy sauce made by blending a mixture of cooked soybeans and wheat, again with koji, or *Aspergillus oryzae*. The combination is fermented for an extended time. The aging process for shoyu is dependent upon the storage temperature and cooking methods used, and is also guarded.

Traditional Tempeh

Tempeh is an aged and fermented soybean food. It is extremely healthy and contains a combination of probiotics and naturally metabolized soy. Tempeh is made by first soaking dehulled soybeans for 10-12 hours. The beans are then cooked for 20 minutes and strained. The dry, cooked beans are then mixed with a tempeh starter containing *Rhyzopus oryzae, Rhizopus oligosporus* or both. The mixture is shaped and flattened (about a half-inch high) and put into a warm (room temperature) incubation container for a day or two. The cake will be full with white mycelium (fungal roots) when it is ready. It can then be eaten raw, baked, or toasted.

Other beans other than soy are also sometimes used to make tempeh. The trick is in getting good starter colonies.

Traditional Kombucha Tea

Kombucha tea is an ancient beverage from the orient. Its use dates back many centuries; and was used by China and Taiwanese emperors. Its use was later popularized in Russia, and then in Eastern Europe, where its reputation grew. A quality kombucha tea will contain a number of probiotics, including *Acetobacter xylinum, Acetobacter xylinoides, Glucobacter bluconicum, Acetobacter aceti, Saccharomycodes Ludwigii, Schizosaccharomyces pombe,* and *Picha fermentans*—and other yeasts in the *Schizosaromyces* genus. The fermenting of these organisms renders a beverage that is full of nutrients and enzymes as well as healthy biotics. Kombucha has enjoyed a reputation of being detoxifying and revitalizing. Many alternative health experts have described it as a tonic.

Kombucha is made by blending a black or green tea with sugar, kombucha starter culture, and sometimes a bit of vinegar to create a slightly acidic environment. It is critical that a healthy starter be used. The mixture is then fermented in a warm, dry environment. It requires oxygen, yet will suffer from any toxins or bacteria from the air. Following a couple of weeks of fermentation, the product should be refrigerated to slow down growth and acidity.

Care should be taken to make sure the yeasts have adequately fermented the ethanols. Otherwise, the kombucha can be as high as 3-5% alcohol, and not healthy. Also be leery of a funky "mother." A kombucha mother might have been passed around for many years amongst those who have brewed their kombucha in their basements or other locales where molds and pathogenic bacteria could have joined and thus contaminated the mother.

Traditional Lassi

Lassi is a traditional and popular beverage from India—once enjoyed by kings and governors in ancient India. It is quite simple to make, as it is made with yogurt, fruit and spices. Quite simply, it is a blend of diluted yogurt with fruit pulp—often mango is used in the traditional lassi. A little salt, turmeric and sweetener give it a sweet-n-salty taste. Other spices are also sometimes used. Sugar is often added in today's versions, but honey and/or fruit are preferable.

Traditional Sauerkraut

Sauerkraut is a traditional German fermented food. It is made quite simply, by blending shredded cabbage and pickling salt (12:1, or 3 tablespoons of salt per five pounds of cabbage). The mixture is covered with water and put into a covered bowl or container. It is then stored in the dark in this semi-airtight cover for a month to two months at room temperature. Then it should be stored in the refrigerator in an enclosed container for a month or two to complete the fermentation of the cabbage. Probiotic bacteria such as *Lactobacillus plantarum* and *L. brevis* will typically overtake the early-growth bacteria during fermentation. This is a testament to the power of probiotics.

There are a number of other wonderful fermented foods that can be included into a probiotic-rich diet. This sampling illustrates the general techniques of fermentation. As we can see here, bacteria and fungi in our foods are not necessarily bad. To the contrary, if cultured correctly, they can be healthy for us, and may even help prevent infection from their more lethal cousins.

Most of these foods are traditional and even ancient foods that have been passed down through generations over thousands of years. This does not mean that we cannot be creative, however.

For example, there is a lot that can be done with yogurt. We've all heard of frozen yogurt, and certainly that is one. But yogurt in some cultures, such as among Indians, is eaten with every meal. It is eaten with and in salads, and rice dishes. Yogurt is creamy and delicious, and can make for an excellent salad dressing with a little oil and vinegar and dill. It can also be added to nearly every sauce to make the sauce creamy and delicious.

Kefir and lassi cultures can be added to nearly every combination of beverage, including smoothies and shakes.

Just about every vegetable can be pickled. Pickles using brine with probiotics are delicious and healthy. We can pickle peppers, olives and so many other foods.

Fermented beverages are now the rage among healthy foods. There are now many fermented beverages, including kombucha and others.

Raw vs. Pasteurized Milk

This naturally brings us to the topic of milk, since there are many reports that indicate that dairy may not be so healthy—and not conducive to detoxification processes.

To the contrary, numerous experiments have shown that raw milk, and dairy containing probiotics such as yogurt is not only healthy, but stimulates the immune system and fights off disease.

First let's consider a study by researchers at Switzerland's University of Basel (Waser *et al.* 2007). The researchers studied 14,893 children between the ages of five and 13 from five different European countries, including 2,823 children from farms, and 4,606 children attending a Steiner School (known for its farm-based living and instruction). The researchers found that drinking farm milk was associated with decreased incidence of allergies and asthma. Why?

Raw milk from the cow can contain a host of bacteria, including *Lactobacillus acidophilus, L. casei, L. bulgaricus* and many other healthy probiotics. Cows feed from primarily grasses will have increased levels of these healthy probiotics. This is because a grass diet provides prebiotics that promote the cow's own probiotic colonies. Should the cow be fed primarily dried grass and dried grains, probiotic counts will be reduced, replaced by more pathogenic bacteria. As a result, most non-grass fed herds must be given lots of antibiotics to help keep their bacteria counts low. Probiotics, on the other hand, naturally keep bacteria counts down.

As a result, the non-grass fed cow's milk will have higher pathogenic bacteria counts than grass-fed cows. This means that the milk itself will also have high counts. When the non-grass-fed cow's milk is pasteurized, the heat kills most of these bacteria. The result is a milk containing dead pathogenic bacteria parts. These are primarily proteins and peptides, which get mixed with the milk and are eventually consumed with the milk.

In other words, pasteurization may kill the living pathogenic bacteria, but it does not get rid of the bacteria proteins. This might be compared to cooking an insect: If an insect landed in our soup, we could surely cook it until it died. But the soup would still contain the insect parts—and proteins.

Now the immune system of most people, and especially infants with their hypersensitive immune system, is trained to attack and discard pathogenic bacteria. And how does the body identify pathogenic bacteria? From their proteins.

In the case of pasteurized commercial milk, our immune systems will readily identify heat-killed microorganism cell parts and proteins and launch an immune response against these proteins as if it were being attacked by the microorganisms directly. This was shown in research from the University of Minnesota two decades ago (Takahashi *et al.* 1992).

It is thus not surprising that weak immune systems readily reject pasteurized cow's milk. In comparison, healthy cow raw milk has fewer pathogenic microorganisms and more probiotic organisms. This has been confirmed by tests done by a California organic milk farm, which compared test results of their raw organic milk against standardized state test results from conventional milk farms.

In addition, pasteurization breaks apart or denatures many of the proteins and sugar molecules. This was illustrated by researchers from Japan's Nagasaki International University (Nodake *et al.* 2010), who found that when beta-lactoglobulin is naturally conjugated with dextran-glycylglycine, its allergenicity is decreased. A dextran is a very long chain of glucose molecules—a polysaccharide. The dextran polysaccharide is naturally joined with the amino acid glycine in raw state. When pasteurized, beta-lactoglobulin is separated.

This is not surprising. Natural whole cow's milk also contains special polysaccharides called oligosaccharides. They are largely indigestible polysaccharides that feed our intestinal bacteria. Because of this trait, these indigestible sugars are called prebiotics.

Whole milk contains a number of these oligosaccharides, including oligogalactose, oligolactose, galactooligosaccharides (GOS) and transgalactooligosaccharides (TOS). Galactooligosaccharides are produced by conversion from enzymes in healthy cows and healthy mothers.

These polysaccharides provide a number of benefits. Not only are they some of the more preferred foods for probiotics: Research has also shown that they reduce the ability of pathogenic bacteria like *E. coli* to adhere to our intestinal cells.

These oligosaccharides also provide environments that reduce the availability of separated beta-lactoglobulin. This is accomplished through a combination of probiotic colonization and the availability of the long-chain polysaccharides that keep these complexes stabilized.

This reduced availability of beta-lactoglobulin has been directly observed in humans and animals following consistent supplementation with probiotics (Taylor *et al.* 2006; Adel-Patient *et al.* 2005; Prioult *et al.* 2003).

It is not surprising, given this information, that people with many conditions have benefited from withdrawing from pasteurized milk and cheese. Raw milk, yogurt, kefir, goat's milk and cheese, along with soy and almond milk, are great alternatives.

What About Casein and Beta-lactoglobulin?

In a number of studies, the milk protein casein has been shown to be implicated in a number of conditions, including cancer (Campbell and Campbell 2006).

In addition, beta-lactoglobulin has been implicated in allergies.

For example, Japanese researchers (Nakano *et al.* 2010) found that casein and beta-lactoglobulin were the main allergens in cow's milk—as confirmed by other research. They also found that 97% of 115 milk allergy children had casein-specific IgE antibodies, while 47% had IgE antibodies against beta-lactoglobulin (beta-LG).

However, fermented dairy and probiotic-rich raw dairy presents an altogether different casein and beta-lactoglobulin molecular structure than does pasteurized milk.

When milk is heated to extremely high degrees, the surfaces of casein micelles—minute fat globules about 100 nanometers in diameter—become harder, and more stable. They move within the fluid but remain in a highly rigid state. Other molecules within the milk do not affect these casein micelles. Thus, the consumption of these rigid casein micelles results in a macromolecule—large protein the body does not easily break down.

However, when dairy is fermented, these casein molecules become destabilized by the probiotics. Once a particular acidity is reached in the milk culture, the casein molecules will become sticky, and they will become congealed—observed as "curdling."

As this curdling takes place—driven by the conversion of lactose to lactic acid by probiotic bacteria—an interesting combination occurs. The destabilized casein micelles react with the beta-lactoglobulin whey protein, which produces a *beta-lactoglobulin-kappa-casein complex.* This neutralizes both the effects of separated beta-lactoglobulin molecules and the casein micelles within the body. In other words, both of these proteins—which spawn radicals in the body—become neutralized through the enzymatic processes driven by probiotic bacteria.

As this occurs, another whey protein, called lactoferrin, also undergoes degradation. This process liberates an immune-stimulating derivative called lactoferricin. This lactoferricin released during the degradation of lactoferrins is also produced by probiotic bacteria, most notably *Streptococcus thermophilus* and *Lactobacillus delbrueckii* ssp. *bulgaricus* (Paul and Somkuti 2010).

Thus we find that these whey-casein components and their derivatives create an altogether different combination of elements than pasteurized milk. They also maintain known antimicrobial components such as lactoferricin and other bacteriocins.

Supplementing with Probiotics

The main consideration in probiotic supplementation is consuming *live* organisms. These are typically described as "CFU" which stands for *colony forming units.* In other words, live probiotics will produce new colonies once inside the intestines. Heat-killed ones are not as beneficial, although they can also stimulate the immune system. So the key is keeping the probiotics alive while in the capsule and supplement bottle, until we are ready to consume them. Here are a few considerations about probiotic supplements:

Capsules: Vegetable capsules contain less moisture than gelatin or enteric-coated capsules. Even a little moisture in the capsule can increase the possibility of waking up the probiotics while in the bottle. Once woken up, they can starve and die. Enteric coating can minimally protect the probiotics within the stomach, assuming they have survived in the bottle. Some manufactures use oils to help protect the probiotics in the stomach. In all cases, encapsulated freeze-dried probiotics should be refrigerated (no matter what the label says) at all times during shipping, at the store, and at home. Dark containers also better protect the probiotics from light exposure, which can kill them.

Powders of freeze-dried probiotics are subject to deterioration due to increased exposure to oxygen and light. Powders should be refrigerated in dark containers and sealed tightly to be kept viable. They should also be consumed with liquids or food, preferably dairy or fermented dairy. Powders can also be used as starters for homemade yogurt and kefir.

Caplets/Tablets: Some tablet/caplets have special coatings that provide viability through to the intestines without refrigeration. If not, those tablets would likely be in the same category as encapsulated products, requiring refrigeration.

Shells or Beads: These can provide longer shelf viability without refrigeration and better survive the stomach. However, because of the size of the shell, these typically come with less CFU quantity, increasing the cost per therapeutic dose. Another drawback may be that the intestines must dissolve this thick shell. An easy test is to examine the stool to be sure that the beads or shells aren't coming out the other end whole.

Lozenges: These are one of the best ways to get probiotics directly into the mucosal membranes of our mouth, sinuses, throat and airways. A correctly formulated chewable or lozenge can inoculate the mouth, nose and throat with beneficial bacteria to compete with and fight off pathogenic bacteria as they enter or reside in our mouth, nose, throat and airways of the lungs.

Probiotic supplements that survive well among the mucous membranes of the airways, sinuses and oral cavity include *L. reuteri, L. rhamnosus, L. plantarum, L. paracasei, and Streptococcus salivarius.* As we discussed in the research, several of these, notably *L. reuteri,* have been shown to increase airway health and decrease lung infections.

However, most of the probiotics in a lozenge will not likely survive the stomach acids and penetrate the intestines. (Therefore, intestinal probiotics in one of the forms above are recommended in addition to probiotic lozenges.)

As the research showed in the last chapter (see topic on oral probiotics), lozenges are an excellent way to help prevent new infections and sore throats during increased exposures. The bacteria in a good lozenge or chewable will allow the probiotics to colonize around our gums and throat, fending off microorganisms that threaten their welfare.

This type of supplement should still be kept sealed, airtight and cool. Refer to the author's book *Oral Probiotics* for detailed information regarding species, strategies and additional research on these probiotics.

Liquid Supplements: There are several probiotic supplements in small liquid form. One brand has a long tradition and a hardy, well-researched strain. A liquid probiotic should be in a light-sealed, refrigerated container. It should also contain some dairy or other probiotic-friendly substrate, giving the probiotics some food while awaiting delivery to the intestines.

Probiotic Hydrotherapy: This method of supplementation is a great way to implant live colonies of probiotics into the lower colon. Colon hydrotherapy (or colonic) is one of the healthiest things we can do for preventative and therapeutic health in general. Colon hydrotherapy is performed by a certified colon hydrotherapist who uses specialized (and sanitary) equipment to flush out the colon with water. This colon flushing usually takes about 30 minutes. Once the process is complete, the hydrotherapist can "insert" a blend of probiotics into the tube and "pump" the probiotics directly into our colon. Colon hydrotherapy is a wonderful treatment recommended for most anyone, especially those with disorders related to systemic inflammation.

Colonic treatments are relatively inexpensive, compared with their benefit. Two to three colonics a year are often recommended for ultimate colon health. Those with sensitive or irritable bowels should consult with their health professional before submitting to a colonic, however.

Probiotic Dosage: A good dosage for intestinal probiotics for prevention and maintenance can be ten to fifteen billion CFU (*colony forming units*) per day. Total intake during an illness or therapeutic period, however, will often double or triple that dosage. Much of the research shown in this text utilized 20 billion to 40 billion CFU per day, about a third of that dose for children and a quarter of that dose for infants. (*B. infantis* is often the supplement of choice for babies.)

Supplemental oral probiotic dosages can be far less (100 million to two billion), especially when the formula contains the hardy *L. reuteri*.

People who must take antibiotics for life-threatening reasons can alternate doses of probiotics between their antibiotic dosing. The probiotic dose can be at least two hours before or after the antibiotic dose. (Always consult with the prescribing doctor.)

Remember that these dosages depend upon delivery to the intestines. Therefore, a product that passes into the stomach with little protection would likely not deliver many colonies to the intestines. Such a supplement would likely require higher dosage to achieve the desired effects.

Prebiotic Foods

One of the most important factors in establishing a healthy environment for our probiotic colonies is making sure they have the right mix of nutrients available. The nutrients our probiotic families favor are called prebiotics. In other words, some foods are particularly beneficial for *bifidobacteria, lactobacilli* and other probiotic populations. These are the oligosaccharides, fructooligosaccharides, galactooligosaccharides, and transgalactooligosaccharides—also referred to as inulin, FOS, GOS and TOS. Even two or three grams of one of these prebiotics will dramatically increase probiotic populations assuming healthy colonies. Inulin, FOS, GOS and TOS are also antagonistic to toxic microorganism genera such as *Salmonella, Listeria, Campylobacter, Shigella* and *Vibrio*. These and other pathogenic bacteria tend to thrive from refined sugars as opposed to the complex saccharides of inulin, FOS, GOS and TOS.

Oligosaccharides are short stacks of simple yet mostly indigestible sugars (from the Greek *oligos*, meaning "few"). If the sugar molecule is fructose, the stacked molecule is called a fructooligosaccharide. If the sugar molecule is galactose, the stacked molecule is called a galactooligosaccharide. These molecules are very useful for human cells and probiotics because they can be processed directly for energy as well as be combined with fatty acids to create cell wall structures and cellular communication molecules. These nutrients also provide energy and nourishment to our probiotic colonies.

The oligosaccharides inulin and oligofructose are probably the most recognized prebiotics. Inulin is a naturally occurring carbohydrate used by plants for storage. It has been estimated that more than 36,000 plant species contain inulin in varying degrees (Carpita *et al.* 1989). The roots often contain the greatest amounts of inulin.

Commercial sources of inulin include Jerusalem artichoke, agave cactus and chicory. Chicory, the root of the Belgian endive, is known to contain some of the highest levels of both inulin at 15-20%, and oligofructose at 5-10%. Inulin from agave has been described as highly branched. This gives it a higher solubility and digestibility than inulin derived from Jerusalem artichoke or chicory.

Notable prebiotic FOS-containing foods include beets, leeks, bananas, tree fruits, soybeans, burdock root, asparagus, maple sugar, whole rye and whole wheat among many others. Bananas contain one of the highest levels of FOS. Bananas are thus a favorite food for both humans and probiotics.

GOS and TOS are natural byproducts of milk. They are produced as lactose is enzymatically converted or hydrolyzed within the digestive tract. This process can also be done commercially. Before much of the recent research on prebiotics was performed, nutritionists simply thought of GOS and TOS as indigestible byproducts of milk.

Another element in plant foods providing prebiotic nutrition for probiotics is the polyphenol group. Polyphenols are groups of biochemicals produced in plants such as lignans, tannins, reservatrol, and flavonoids. There is some uncertainty as to which of these are most helpful to probiotic populations.

Some prebiotics have interesting side effects. For example, there seems to be a relationship between oligofructose inulin and calcium absorption. Inulin has been shown to improve calcium absorption by 20%, and yogurt supplemented with TOS has increased calcium absorption by 16% (van den Heuvel *et al.* 2000)

Galactooligosaccharides have another side effect that is important to note. Dr. Kari Shoaf and fellow researchers at the University of Nebraska (Shoaf *et al.* 2006) found in laboratory tests that galactooligosaccharides reduce the ability of *E. coli* to attach to human cells within tissue cultures. This effect was isolated from GOS' ability to nourish probiotics. This means that GOS provides more than nutrition to our probiotic colonies. This once considered useless indigestible nutrient also helps keep *E. coli* and other pathogenic bacteria from attaching to our cells. A nice package deal indeed.

FOS and GOS have been known to cause digestive disturbance in rare cases. Such a digestive disturbance is likely caused by dysbiosis, however.

Conclusively, a preponderance of scientific literature indicates that probiotics thrive from a diet of plant-based natural foods with plenty of phytonutrients, while overly processed, sugary and meat diets tend to promote pathogenic bacteria and their disease-causing endotoxins.

Yeasts and Yeast Derivatives

Baking yeast and brewer's yeast are common yeasts that are primarily derived from an organism called *Saccharomyces cerevisiae*. In most applications, the yeast is not eaten alive, however. It is *heat-killed* prior to eating. This simply means that it is cooked to a temperature that kills off the viable organisms. This doesn't mean that living *S. cerevisiae* organisms are toxic or anything. In reasonable colony sizes, they are perfectly docile, and even healthy to our bodies because they produce nutrients that our bodies use.

For baking, brewing and supplementation, the heat-killed version of this organism can be very healthy, because when it is alive, it produces a variety of nutrients and immune factors that are left behind in whatever food it was used to ferment.

Just before these yeasts die during heating or baking, they will release intense immune factors in an attempt to protect themselves. These immune factors also help protect our bodies, by stimulating our body's detoxification processes and boosting our immune system. In addition, some of their nutrients, such as B-vitamins produced by yeasts, will donate methyl groups to our liver's glutathione radical-neutralizing processes.

Furthermore, because the biofactors that yeasts produce tend to be acidic, they will lend a tart flavor to the food. This of course lends the flavoring that we relish among our traditional probiotic foods such as cottage cheese, pickles, and so many other foods as we discussed above.

This is the case for sourdough bread, for example. Sourdough bread is not only delicious. It is healthy, even if it is made with white flour (for best results, try whole wheat sourdough bread). Fermented brews such as beer and wine Originally, all the fermented brews such as ginger ale and root beer, were all made using probiotic fermentation.

Yeast Supplements

Baking yeast and Brewer's yeast, Nutritional Yeast and EpiCor®, are all derived from an organism called *Saccharomyces cerevisiae*. This organism is used in brewing and baking. It is thus considered a healthy organism, and acts in a territorial manner to repel organisms and toxins that are seen as foreign to their territories.

For this reason, EpiCor®, Brewer's Yeast or Nutritional Yeast come in dehydrated forms. In other words, the yeast colonies are killed by heat. This heat-killing preserves their nutrients, yet prevents their overgrowth in the body. (However, a person who has mold allergies might still have a reaction to heat-killed yeast because those proteins are still present.)

So what is the difference between EpiCor®, Brewer's Yeast and Nutritional Yeast? The answer lies in their unique processes of fermentation.

Brewer's Yeast is a byproduct of the brewing industry, thus it typically does not have the higher levels of nutrients that the other two have. Brewer's yeast still has a variety of nutrients, including many trace elements (such as chromium and selenium), B vitamins (but typically not B12 as many assume), many antioxidants and proteins.

Nutritional Yeast will typically produce more of these same nutrients, because it has been prepared in such a way that both stresses the yeasts more, and preserves more of their nutrients. Nutritional yeast will contain chromium and selenium, as well as thiamin, riboflavin, niacin, vitamin B6, folate, vitamin B12, pantothenic acid, magnesium, zinc, and a number of amino acids. It is a great protein source, with 50% protein by weight.

EpiCor® is another yeast derivative that is produced using a proprietary method. EpiCor®, however, may have even more enhanced levels of certain nutrients, which include those mentioned above, along with nucleotides and possibly additional antioxidants and immune factors. The reason that EpiCor® may have additional immune factors is because during fermentation, the yeast is *stressed*. Like any organism, when it is stressed, it produces immune factors to protect itself.

After EpiCor® has been stressed, it is then heat-killed, dehydrated and powdered, rendering those immune factors and nutrients.

EpiCor® has been the subject of focused research, which has found that it significantly lowers systemic inflammation.

In one study (Robinson *et al.* 2009), 500 milligrams of EpiCor® or a placebo was given to 80 healthy volunteers with seasonal grass allergies during pollen season. After six and twelve weeks, the EpiCor® group experienced a significant reduction of allergy symptoms compared to the placebo group.

Other EpiCor® studies have shown that it increases salivary IgA (mucosal immunity), and reduces serum IgE (pro-allergy sensitivity).

Red Yeast Rice: The yeast *Monascus purpureus,* when fermented with rice, becomes what is known as red yeast rice. Red yeast rice has been shown in research to lower LDL cholesterol (Liu *et al.* 2006). The mechanism renders red yeast the ability to help prevent lipid peroxidation in the body. Red yeast rice has been used in China for over a thousand years. However, red yeast rice use as a supplement has been questioned by the FDA and pharmaceutical industry. This might have something to do with the fact that correctly fermented red yeast rice can be a significant source of the constituent monacolin K, the primary active ingredient of the statin drug lovastatin.

While there are others, these yeast products have been shown to maximize the body's antioxidant capacities, increase tolerance, and stimulate detoxification processes. They also have considerable research backing up these claims.

Vinegars

Vinegars are excellent living foods that stimulate the body's living purification systems. Vinegar made from apples, grapes or other fruits also contain a variety of antioxidants, as well as acetic acid, which helps stimulate a good environment for our body's own probiotics, and one that repels pathogenic microorganisms.

There are a variety of different types of vinegars, depending upon the raw material used. In all cases, the raw material of a healthy vinegar will be a plant source, fermented by a healthy yeast culture. The yeast culture will convert the sugars of the plant source (and added sugars if used) to alcohol. As the alcohol is fermented further, it is oxidized by the zymase enzymes in the yeast, which convert to alcohol to carboxylic acetic acids. These acetic acids are the main constituent of vinegar, and what gives vinegar its tartness.

To speed up the process, alcohols are often used commercially to make vinegars. These include cheaper or turned wines, distilled alcohol (from wood or grain) and other spirits. The conversion of alcohol to vinegar is much quicker because the first step (sugar to alcohol) has already been made.

Fresh vinegar is typically made by crushing whole apples, grapes, potatoes, barley or other fruits or grains - even pears, bananas and others - into a mash. Sugar can be added to speed up the process, typically at a ratio of one-to-four of mash.

Brewer's yeast (*Saccharomyces cerevisiae*) can then be added for fermentation. One-quarter of a yeast cake will typically inoculate a liter of the mash. Alternatively, a "mother" of fresh vinegar that has been retained from a previous vinegar can be used. Such a "mother" will likely contain more yeast species than just the *S. cerevisiae* yeast, and possibly even some probiotic bacteria. The amount needed depends upon the strength of the "mother," but one cup of the mother (from the top center of the previous batch) per liter should probably do it.

The mix is then put aside in a warm place, with the jar covered by a cloth to let in oxygen. The period of fermentation depends upon the sugar content and the temperature stored. The vinegar may be strained or unstrained. Unstrained retains more living yeasts.

Balsamic vinegars will ferment for years in oak barrels, for example. An apple vinegar might take 60 days to nine months. Care should be taken that the alcohol levels are reduced down to well below .5% (legal alcohol limit). Higher acetic acid levels will mean lower alcohol levels. Testing with a round piece of fine marble (5/6 of marble weight reduction equates to acetic acid levels). Look for 30-32 grams reduction per marble piece, after vinegar loses sour taste for a 5% acetic acid vinegar.

Vinegar can be used in salads, for pickling vegetables and other creative recipes. It can also simply be taken by the teaspoon. A traditional raw cider is the Bragg's brand of apple cider vinegars (no financial affiliation).

Alcohol Warning

A key point to remember regarding fermented beverages is that unless the alcohol level is fermented down to a level below .5%, it will be considered an alcoholic beverage. Alcohol is unhealthy for body. Alcohol is ethanol, which is highly toxic to the liver. Alcohol damages the liver. This means that the liver will produce less enzymes and filter the blood poorly. This leaves the body in a state of increased toxicity. Over time this can produce severe liver disease, which can result in death.

Often people consider that because wines and other spirits are made from natural ingredients, they must be healthy. For example, resveratrol from wine is touted as being healthy. Resveratrol, however, comes from the grapes themselves. While red wine certainly will also contain resveratrol, the alcohol content of the wine can do more damage than the resveratrol can help.

As for those reputed to have been drinking a glass or two of wine every day and remain seemingly healthy, yes, the liver can certainly manage a minimal amount of alcohol every day. This doesn't mean that the alcohol is healthy for the liver. There have been a few studies that have indicated the possibility that a drink or two of wine every day may increase longevity. This type of epidemiological research, however, is highly questionable, notably because those who have a glass or two of wine everyday may also well be doing something else—such as socializing while drinking or reducing stress levels—that might also account for their longevity. Other studies have shown that socializing and reducing stress levels also extend life.

The bottom line is that the research showing that the liver is damaged by alcohol consumption is irrefutable. For example, Canadian scientists (Rehm et al. 2010) reviewed seventeen studies that analyzed the relationship between alcohol and cirrhosis of the liver. They found that all of them linked alcohol consumption with liver disease and death from liver disease. They also found that the same amount of alcohol consumption produces a higher incidence of liver disease among women.

Alcohol also damages our probiotic colonies.

Antioxidants

When we harvest a fresh plant-based food and eat it with minimal storage, processing and cooking, we are deriving significant benefits from the living organism that produced the food. Because living organisms defend themselves against toxins throughout their lives, by eating fresh whole foods or whole foods minimally cooked, our bodies can utilize the same elements the plant utilized to protect itself against toxins.

This in turn stimulates our immune systems, and also provides direct free radical protection. This is because antioxidants are designed to neutralize toxins.

As we've discussed, a plethora of research has confirmed that damage from free radicals is implicated in many health conditions. Free radicals from toxins damage cells, cell membranes, organs, blood vessel walls and airways—producing systemic inflammation—as the immune system responds to an overload of tissue damage.

Free radicals are produced by synthetic chemicals, pathogens, trans fats, fried foods, red meats, radiation, pollution and various intruders that destabilize within the body. Free radicals are molecules or ions that require stabilization. They reach stabilization by 'stealing' atoms from the cells or tissues of our body. This in turn destabilizes those cells and tissues—producing damage.

Antioxidants serve to stabilize free radicals before our cells and tissues are robbed—by donating their own atoms. A diet with plenty of fruits and vegetables supplies numerous antioxidants. Although antioxidants cannot be considered treatments for any disease, many studies have proved that increased antioxidant intake supports immune function and detoxification. These effects allow the immune system to respond with greater tolerance.

Antioxidant constituents in plant-based foods are known to significantly repel free radicals, strengthen the immune system and help detoxify the system. These include *lecithin* and *octacosanol* from whole grains; *polyphenols* and *sterols* from vegetables; *lycopene* from tomatoes and watermelons; *quercetin* and *sulfur/allicin* from garlic, onions and peppers; *pectin* and *rutin* from apples and other fruits; *phytocyanidin flavonoids* such as *apigenin* and *luteolin* from various greenfoods; and *anthocyanins* from various fruits and oats.

Some sea-based botanicals like kelp also contain antioxidants as well. Consider a special polysaccharide compound from kelp called *fucoidan*. Fucoidan has been shown in animal studies to significantly reduce inflammation (Cardoso *et al.* 2009; Kuznetsova *et al.* 2004).

Procyanidins are found in apples, currants, cinnamon, bilberry and many other foods. The extract of *Vitis vinifera* seed (grapeseed) is one of the highest sources of bound antioxidant *proanthocyanidins* and *leucocyanidines* called *procyanidolic oligomers* or PCOs.

Pycnogenol® also contains significant levels of these PCOs. Blueberries, parsley, green tea, black currant, some legumes and onions also contain PCOs and similar proanthocyanidins.

Research has demonstrated that PCOs have protective and strengthening effects on tissues by increasing enzyme conjugation (Seo *et al.* 2001). PCOs have also been shown to increase vascular wall strength (Robert *et al.* 2000).

Oxygenated carotenoids such as *lutein* and *astaxanthin* also have been shown to exhibit strong antioxidant activity. Astaxanthin is derived from the microalga *Haematococcus pluvialis,* and lutein is available from a number of foods, including spirulina.

Most of these phytonutrients specifically modulate the immune system. For example, the flavonoids *kaempferol* and *flavone* have been shown to block mast cell proliferation by over 80% (Alexandrakis *et al.* 2003). Sources of kaempferol include Brussels sprouts, broccoli, grapefruit and apples.

Furthermore, *resveratrol* from grapes and berries modulate nuclear factor-kappaB and transcription/Janus kinase pathways—which strengthens immunity. Good sources of resveratrol include peanuts, red grapes, cranberries and cocoa (wine is not advisable for cleansing as we'll discuss later).

Nearly every plant-food has some measure of phytonutrients discussed above and more. These phytonutrients alkalize the blood and increase the detoxification capabilities of the liver. They help clear the blood of toxins.

Foods that are particularly detoxifying and immunity-building include fresh pineapples, beets, cucumbers, apricots, apples, almonds, zucchini, artichokes, avocados, bananas, beans, collard greens, berries, casaba, celery, coconuts, cranberries, watercress, dandelion greens, grapes, raw honey, corn, kale, citrus fruits, watermelon, lettuce, mangoes, mushrooms, oats, broccoli, okra, onions, papayas, parsley, peas, whole grains, radishes, raisins, spinach, tomatoes, walnuts, and many others.

These plant-based foods are also our primary source of soluble and insoluble fiber. Diets with significant fiber help clear the blood and tissues of toxins, and lipid peroxidation-friendly LDL cholesterol. Fiber is also critical to a healthy digestive tract and intestinal barrier. Fiber in the diet should range from about 35 to 45 grams per day according to the recommendations of many diet experts. Six to ten servings of raw fruits and vegetables per day should accomplish this—which is even part of the USDA's recommendations. This means raw, fibrous foods should be present at every meal.

Good fibrous plant sources also contain healthy *lignans* and *phytoestrogens* that help balance hormone levels, and help the body make its own natural corticoids. Foods that contain these include peas, garbanzo beans, soybeans, kidney beans and lentils.

Plant-based foods provide these immune-stimulating factors because these very same factors make up the plants' own immune systems. For example, the red, blue and green flavonoid pigments in plants and fruits help protect the plant from oxidative damage from radiation. The proanthocyanidins in grains like oats, for example, help protect the oat plant from crown rust caused by the *Puccinia coronata* fungus. So the same biochemicals that stimulate immunity in humans are part of plants' immune systems.

These same whole food phytonutrients also neutralize oxidative radicals in our bodies—the reason they are called antioxidants. How do we know this? Scientists can measure the ability of a particular food to neutralize free radicals with specific laboratory testing. One such test is called the *Oxygen Radical Absorbance Capacity Test* (ORAC). This technical laboratory study is performed by a number of scientific organizations that include the USDA, as well as specialized labs such as Brunswick Laboratories in Massachusetts.

Research from the USDA's Jean Mayer Human Nutrition Research Center on Aging at Tufts University has suggested that a diet high in ORAC value may protect blood vessels and tissues from free radical damage that can result in inflammation (Sofic *et al.* 2001; Cao *et al.* 1998). These tissues, of course, include the airways. Research has confirmed that consuming 3,000 to 5,000 ORAC units per day can have protective benefits.

ORAC Values (100 grams) of Selected (raw) Fruits (USDA, 2007-2008)

Cranberry	9,382	Pomegranate	2,860
Plum	7,581	Orange	1,819
Blueberry	6,552	Tangerine	1,620
Blackberry	5,347	Grape (red)	1,260
Raspberry	4,882	Mango	1,002
Apple (Granny)	3,898	Kiwi	882
Strawberry	3,577	Banana	879
Cherry (sweet)	3,365	Tomato (plum)	389
Gooseberry	3,277	Pineapple	385
Pear	2,941	Watermelon	142

There is tremendous attention these days on two unique fruits from the Amazon rain forest and China called *açaí* and *goji berry* (or wolfberry) respectively. A recent ORAC test documented by Schauss *et al.* (2006) gives açaí a score of 102,700 and tests documented by Dr. Paul Gross gives goji berries a total ORAC of 30,300. However, subsequent tests done by Brunswick Laboratories, Inc. gave these two berries 53,600 (açaí) and 22,000 (goji) total-ORAC values.

In addition, we must remember that these are the dried berries being tested in the latter case, and a concentrate of acai being tested in the former case. The numbers in the chart above are for fresh fruits. Dried fruits will naturally have higher ORAC values, because the water is evaporated—giving more density and more antioxidants per 100 grams.

For example, in the USDA database, dried apples have a 6,681 total-ORAC value, while fresh apples range from 2,210 to 3,898 in total-ORAC value. This equates to a two- to-three times increase from fresh to dried. In another example, fresh red grapes have a 1,260 total-ORAC value, while raisins have a 3,037 total-ORAC value. This comes close to an increase of three times the ORAC value following dehydration.

Part of the equation, naturally, is cost. Dried fruit and concentrates are often more expensive than fresh fruit. High-ORAC dried fruits or concentrates from açaí or gogi will also be substantially more expensive than most fruits grown domestically (especially for Americans and Europeans). Our conclusion is that local or in-country grown fresh fruits with high total-ORAC values produce the best value. Local fresh fruit offers great free radical scavenging ability, support for local farmers, and pollen proteins we are most likely more tolerant to.

By comparison, spinach—an incredibly wholesome vegetable with a tremendous amount of nutrition—has a fraction of the ORAC content of some of these fruits, at 1,515 total ORAC. Spinach, of course, contains many other nutrients, including proteins lacking in many high-ORAC fruits.

Dehydrated spices can have incredibly high ORAC values. For example, USDA's database lists ground Turmeric's total ORAC value at 159,277 and oregano's at 200,129. However, while we might only consume a few hundred milligrams of a spice per day, we can eat many grams—if not pounds—of sweet colorful fruit every day.

Quercetin Foods

A number of foods and herbs that reduce inflammation and toxicity contain quercetin. This is no coincidence. Multiple studies have shown that quercetin inhibits the release of inflammatory mediators histamine and leukotrienes. Foods rich in quercetin include onions, garlic, apples, capers, grapes, leafy greens, tomatoes and broccoli. In addition, many of the herbs listed earlier contain quercetin as an active constituent. Many of the herbs listed in the herbal section also contain quercetin. Onions, garlic and apples contain some of the highest levels.

Quercetin stimulates and balances the immune system. In an *in vivo* study, four weeks of quercetin reduced histamine levels and allergen-specific IgE levels. More importantly, quercetin inhibited anaphylaxis responses (Shishehbor *et al.* 2010).

Cairo researchers (Haggag *et al.* 2003) found that among mast cells exposed to allergens and chemicals in the laboratory, quercetin inhibited histamine release by 95% and 97%.

Over the past few years, an increasing amount of evidence is pointing to the conclusion that foods with quercetin slow inflammatory response and autoimmune derangement. Researchers from Italy's Catholic University (Crescente *et al.* 2009) found that quercetin inhibited arachidonic acid-induced platelet aggregation. Arachidonic acid-induced platelet aggregation is seen in allergic inflammatory mechanisms.

Researchers from the University of Crete (Alexandrakis *et al.* 2003) found that quercetin can inhibit mast cell proliferation by up to 80%. Onions have also been shown *in vivo* tests to reduce bronchoconstriction.

Organic foods contain higher levels of quercetin. A study from the University of California-Davis' Department of Food Science and Technology (Mitchell *et al.* 2007) tested flavonoid levels between organic and conventional tomatoes over a ten-year period. Their research concluded that quercetin levels were 79% higher for tomatoes grown organically under the same conditions as conventionally-grown tomatoes.

Root Foods

It is no coincidence that many antioxidants are roots, such as ginger, turmeric, onions, garlic, beets, carrots, turnips, parsnips and others. These root foods are known for their ability to alkalize the bloodstream and stimulate detoxification. They are also known to help rejuvenate the liver and adrenal glands.

Beets, for example, contain, among other nutrients, betaine, betalains, betacyanin and betanin. They also contain generous portions of folate, iron and fiber. One of the primary fibers in beets is pectin, which is also found in apples. Pectin has a unique soluble and insoluble fiber content that maximizes the attachment of radical-producing LDL cholesterol in the intestines. Pectin also attaches to many other toxins, drawing them out of the body as well.

Meanwhile, betaine is known as stimulating liver health. Betaine has been shown to reduce liver injury (Okada et al. 2011). Betaine is also considered healthy for the bile ducts, because it helps draw out toxins. Beets are delicious foods that can be grated into salads, juiced, steamed, baked and simply eaten raw. Red beets are typically considered the healthiest, but pink and white beets also contain betaine.

We should note that while beets contain significant amounts of betaine, other betaine-rich foods include broccoli, spinach and some whole grains.

Each of the root foods listed above contain unique constituents that support liver health, detoxification and consequently, mucosal health.

Greenfoods

A greenfood is a category of foods that are considered nutritionally superior than the typical fruits and vegetables. As a result, they are great strategies for increasing mucosal health. Greenfoods include the wheat grasses, sprouts, algae, and sea vegetables.

Greenfoods provide practically every nutrient imaginable, including enzymes, minerals, trace elements, essential and non-essential amino acids, vitamins, antioxidants and various phytonutrients. Many will provide over 1,000 nutrients.

A big benefit of greenfoods is their alkalinity. This gives them the ability to neutralize radicals and lipid peroxides, and help balance the pH of our various mucosal systems.

Much of this alkalinity comes from greenfoods' bioavailable mineral content. Many of these minerals are also colloidal. They tend to be hydrophobic, and maintain a positive electrical charge—rendering them alkaline.

Cereal Grasses

Wheat grass is the young grass of the wheat species, *Triticum aestivum*. In addition to a plethora of vitamins, minerals, amino acids, phytonutrients, metabolic enzymes—including superoxide dismutase and cytochrome oxidase—wheat grass maintains up to 70% chlorophyll.

Early research by Dr. Charles Schnabel, Dr. George Kohler and Dr. A.I. Virtanen in the 1925-1950 era found that cereal grasses like wheatgrass achieved their highest nutrient content at around 18 days—right before the first jointing.

Wheat grass can increase blood hemoglobin levels. Wheat grass tablets decreased blood transfusion needs by 25% among 20 children requiring frequent blood transfusions in a recent study.

Barley grass maintains similar properties. Research has found that barley grass is a potent free radical scavenger; significantly reduces total cholesterol and LDL-cholesterol; and inhibits LDL oxidation. Barley grass juice powder can have 14 vitamins, 18 amino acids, 15 enzymes, 10 antioxidants, 18 minerals and 75 trace elements.

Another cereal grass is Kamut grass. The khorasan wheat has higher protein levels than most wheat varieties, and contains higher zinc, selenium and magnesium content. Selenium is known for stimulating glutathione activity as we've discussed.

Sprouts

Sprouts and their powders are nutritional powerhouses. They have exponential nutritional value, well above the nutrient content of their seeds or the fully-grown plants. This was confirmed in the 1970s experiments by former Hippocrates Health Institute Director of Research, Viktoras Kulvinskas, M.S. Kulvinskas, who found that ascorbic acid levels in soybean sprouts increased from zero to 103 milligrams per 100 grams by day six—about the ascorbic acid content found in lime juice. These levels fall off significantly within days.

Each plant has a different nutrient peak. Ascorbic acid content in broad bean sprouts—used to cure scurvy during World War I—peaks in three days, after which the levels fall off.

Many believe that sprouts produce this greater antioxidant content to defend themselves against threats from the soil.

Great nutritional sprouts include wheat grass sprouts, barley, oats, beans, broccoli and cabbage. The latter two provide a class of nutrients called glucosinolates. These glucosinolates yield sulfur compounds and indole-3 carbinols. Both have shown to have significant anticarcinogenic and anti-inflammatory effects in the body.

Seed selection is critical. A good quality seed will germinate at least 50%. Heirloom seeds often germinate at much higher rates.

Sea Grasses

Kelps might be called seaweeds, but these phytonutrient powerhouses are anything but weeds. About 1,500 species of sea kelps flourish, many in the North Pacific and North Atlantic oceans.

Most kelps are stationary, and sustainably harvested in the wild. This means they must be allowed to regrow to guarantee future harvests. *Ascophyllum nodosum* kelp contains an impressive array of vitamins—more than many vegetables. They include over 60 essential minerals, amino acids and vitamins. They also contain growth promoters, according to kelp researchers.

Most kelps also contain fucoidan, a sulfated polysaccharide. Laboratory studies have indicated fucoidan has anti-tumor, anticoagulant and anti-angiogenic effects. It down-regulates Th2 (inhibiting allergic response), inhibits beta-amyloid formation (implicated in Alzheimer's), inhibits proteinuria in Heymann nephritis and decreases artery platelet deposits.

Other kelps include dulse, sargassi seaweed, *Undaria pinnatifida,* sea palm and others.

Spirulina

Spirulina use dates back to the Aztecs. A good source of carotenoids, vitamins (including vegan B12 according to independent laboratory tests) and minerals, spirulina contains all essential and most non-essential amino acids, with up to 65% protein by weight. It also contains antioxidant phytonutrients such as zeaxanthin, myxoxanthophyll and lutein. It also will contain antioxidant carotenoids, vitamins and minerals.

Spirulina also contains phycobiliprotein, a unique blue pigment anti-inflammatory and antioxidant. Research has showed that phycobiliproteins can protect the liver and kidney from toxins. They are also anti-viral, and stimulate the immune system.

In one study from the University of California-Davis, 12 weeks of 3000 milligrams of Hawaiian spirulina per day significantly increased hemoglobin concentration and mean corpuscular hemoglobin among 30 adults over the age of 50. IDO (indoleamine 2,3-dioxygenase) enzyme activity—a sign of increased immune function—was also higher among the subjects.

Chlorella

More than 800 published studies have verified the safety and efficacy of *Chlorella pyrenoidosa*. Chlorella's reputation of drawing out heavy metals and other toxins make it a favorite among health practitioners.

Chlorella maintains considerable vitamins minerals, and phytonutrients—including chlorella growth factor (CGF), known to stimulate cell growth. It is also a complete protein, with about 60% protein by weight and every essential and non-essential amino acid. Clinical studies have shown that chlorella stimulates T-cell and B-cell activity and contributes to the improvement of fibromyalgia, ulcerative colitis and hypertension. Another study showed that chlorella increases IgA levels and lowers dioxin levels in breast milk.

Chlorella's tough cell wall must be broken down mechanically to allow these nutrients' bioavailability. Our digestive enzymes cannot digest these outer cell walls. For this reason, quality chlorella growers will pulverize this tough outer cell wall.

Haematococcus and Astaxanthin

Another greenfood algae is *Haematococcus pluvialis,* known for its high astaxanthin content. Astaxanthin is a strong carotenoid similar to beta-carotene. For this reason, astaxanthin is one of the most powerful natural antioxidants known. It also has anti-inflammatory effects, and has been used for eye health, joint healthy, muscle soreness, cardiovascular health, and skin health. It can also protect against damage from UV radiation.

Blue-Green Algae from Klamath Lake

Aphanizomenon flos-aquae or AFA, grows on the pristine waters of Klamath Lake in Oregon. Commercial AFA harvesting began in the early 1980s. This rich volcanic Klamath Lake gives AFA a good source of protein and all the essential and non-essential amino acids. It also has many vitamins, minerals and phytonutrients. AFA contains about 60% protein by weight, and at least 58 minerals at ppm levels, along with significant chlorophyll content.

One of the more exciting phytonutrient compounds discovered in AFA is phenylethylamine (PEA). PEA has been called the 'love molecule,' as it serves to increase positive moods. PEA is also found in chocolate. AFA has significantly more PEA, however.

Aloe Vera

While aloe has long been known for its skin irritation and wound healing abilities, science on its internal use is still emerging.

Aloe is now used for gastrointestinal health, immune support and cardiovascular health, as well as the health of the skin and mucosal membranes.

Aloe may also help prevent kidney stones. A study published in the *Journal of the Thailand Medical Association* found that 200 grams of fresh aloe gel a day significantly decreased urinary oxalate excretion.

In addition, a study from London's Queen Mary School of Medicine on 44 active ulcerated colitis patients found that internal aloe use resulted in clinical improvement. And double-blind, randomized research using Aloecorp's Qmatrix processed aloe has shown that it reduces oxidative stress markers and stimulates the immune system.

Aloe can be taken as a juice or a gel.

Mucosal pH Balance

This discussion of nutrients should also include the reflective effects of a healthy diet: The proper acid-alkaline balance among the mucosal membranes, blood, urine and intercellular tissue regions. The reference to acidic or alkaline body fluids and tissues has been made by numerous natural health experts over the years. Is there any scientific validity to this?

Many nutritionists condemn an acidic metabolism and loosely call appropriate metabolism as a *state of alkalinity*. Strictly speaking, however, an alkaline environment is not healthy. The blood, interstitial fluids, lymph and urine should be *slightly acidic* to maintain the appropriate mineral ion balance. Let's dig into the science.

Acidity or alkalinity is measured using a logarithmic scale called pH. The term pH is derived from the French word *pouvoir hydrogene*, which means 'hydrogen power' or 'hydrogen potential.' pH is quantified by an inverse log base-10 scale. It measures the proton-donor level of a solution by comparing it to a theoretical quantity of hydrogen ions (H+) or H_3O+.

The scale is pH 1 to pH 14, which converts to a range of 10^{-1} (1) to 10^{-14} (.00000000000001) moles of hydrogen ions. This means that a pH of 14 maintains fewer hydrogen ions. It is thus *less acidic* and *more alkaline* (or basic).

The pH scale has been set up around the fact that water's pH is log-7 or simply pH 7—due to water's natural mineral content. Because pure water forms the basis for so many of life's activities, and because water neutralizes and dilutes so many reactions, water was established as the standard reference point or neutral point between what is considered an acid or a base solution. In other words, a substance having greater hydrogen ion potential (but lower pH) than water will be considered acidic, while a substance with less H+ potential (higher pH) than water is considered a base (alkaline).

Now the solution with a certain pH may not specifically maintain that many hydrogen ions. But it has the same *potential* as if it contained those hydrogen ions. That is why pH is hydrogen power or hydrogen potential.

In human blood, a pH level in the range of about 6.4 is considered healthy because this state is slightly more acidic than water, enabling the bodily fluids to maintain and transport minerals. It enables the *potential* for minerals to be carried by the blood, in other words. Minerals are critical to every cell, every organ, every tissue and every enzyme process occurring within the body. Better put, a 6.4 pH offers the appropriate *currency* of the body's fluids: This discourages acidosis and toxemia, maintaining a slight mineralized status.

The pH of our mucosal membranes should be lower, depending upon the epithelial region. In the stomach, it should range between 1 and 3 pH, while the saliva should range between 5.8 and 6.2. These lower levels are more acidic, which give our epithelial cells more protection against invaders.

Internal tissues need more alkalinity, and when the internal tissues and glands are more alkaline, they have more ionic potential to produce more acids. Acidosis is produced with greater levels of carbonic acids, lactic acids, and/or uric acids among the joints and tissues. These acids are readily oxidizing, which produces free radicals. However, an overly alkaline state can precipitate waste products from cells, which also floods the system with radicals. For this reason, *toxemia* results from either an overly acidic blood-tissue content or an overly alkaline blood-tissue content. In other words, pH *balance* is the key.

Ions from minerals like potassium, calcium, magnesium and others are usually positively oriented—with alkaline potential. But to be carried through a solution, the solution must have the pH potential to carry them.

Besides being critical to enzymatic reactions, these minerals bond with lipids and proteins to form the structures of our cells, organs and tissues—including our airways, nerves and mucosal membranes.

Natural health experts over the past century have observed among their patients and in clinical research that an overly acidic environment within the body is created by a diet abundant in refined sugars, processed foods, chemical toxins and amino acid-heavy animal foods. More recently, research has connected this acidic state to toxemia. The toxemia state is a state of free radical proliferation, which damages cells and tissues. It is also a state that produces systemic inflammation, because the immune system is over-worked as it tries to remove the cell and tissue damage.

As mentioned earlier, animals accumulate toxins within their fat tissues. They are bioaccumulators. Thus, animals exposed to the typical environmental toxins of smog and chemical pollutants in their waters and air—along with pesticides and herbicides from their foods—will accumulate those toxins within their fat cells and livers. And those who eat those animals will inherit (and further accumulate) these accumulated toxins. In addition, animals secrete significant waste matter as they are being slaughtered.

Plants are not bioaccumulators. While they can accumulate some pesticides and herbicide chemicals within their leaves and roots, they do not readily absorb or hold these for long periods within their cells. This is because many environmental toxins are, as mentioned, fat soluble. Because plants have little or no fat, they can more easily systemically rid their tissues of many of these toxins over time.

Further, as the research has shown, a diet heavy in complex proteins—which contain far more amino acids than our bodies require—increases the risk and severity of mucosal hypersensitivity. Amino acids are the building blocks of protein. A complex protein can have tens of thousands of amino acids. While proteins and aminos are healthy, a diet too rich in them will produce deposits in our joints and tissues, burdening our immune system.

As we discussed in the last chapter, research also reveals that diets rich in red meats discourage the colonization of our probiotics, and encourage the growth of pathogenic microorganisms that release endotoxins that clog our metabolism and overload our immune system. Diets rich in red meats also produce byproducts such as phytanic acid and beta-glucuronidase that can damage our intestinal cells and mucosal membranes within the intestines. Greater levels of cooked saturated fats also raise cholesterol levels, especially lipid peroxidation-prone low-density lipoproteins (LDL).

The complexities of digesting complex proteins produce increased levels of beta-glucuronidase, nitroreductase, azoreductase, steroid 7-alpha-dehydroxylase, ammonia, urease, cholylglycine hydrolase, phytanic acid and others. These toxic enzymes deter our probiotics and produce systemic inflammation. Not surprisingly, they've been linked to colon cancer.

By contrast, plant-based foods contain many antioxidants, anti-carcinogens and other nutrients that strengthen the immune system and balance the body's pH. Plant-based foods also discourage inflammatory responses. Plant-based foods feed our probiotics with complex polysaccharides called prebiotics. They are also a source of fiber (there is little fiber in red meat)—critical for intestinal health.

Nutrition researchers from Portugal's University of Porto (Barros *et al.* 2008) studied the diets and asthma severity among 174 asthmatic adults. They used symptoms, lung function and exhaled nitric oxide to gauge asthma severity and control among the patients. After eliminating factors related to medications, age, sex, education and other factors; they found that those whose asthma was controlled had a 23% higher aMED Score (a diet score denoting higher intake of fruits, vegetables, fiber and healthy oils) and drank less alcohol—compared to more severe asthmatics.

They also found that significant adherence to the Mediterranean diet reduced the risk of uncontrolled asthmatic episodes by 78%. They concluded: *"High adherence to traditional Mediterranean diet increased the likelihood of asthma to be under control in adults."*

The Mediterranean diet does not completely eliminate meat, but it is focused on more plant-based foods, healthier oils and less red meat. However we configure our diet, there are choices we can make at every meal. The research shows that the greater our diet trends toward the Mediterranean diet, the lower our toxic load will be and the stronger our immunity will be. This will allow us to better combat and eventually lower systemic inflammation.

This is also not a condemnation of dairy. Milk is a great food, assuming it contains what nature intended: probiotics. Real milk is inseparable from probiotics, and when probiotics are killed off by pasteurization, milk becomes a dubious food.

Mucosal Fats

The types of fats we eat directly nourish our mucosal membranes.

These come from low-processed plant-sources that maintain high levels of what the plant utilized for its own development and procreation (as most healthy plant fats come from the seeds of plants). A few of the healthy fats come from algae sources, as we'll discuss.

The fat balance of our diet is critical to our mucosal systems because these membranes are made of different lipids and lipid-derivatives like phospholipids and glycolipids. An imbalanced fat diet therefore can lead to weak cell membranes, which leads to cells that have restricted or inconsistent pores. The cell membrane pores allow nutrients in to the cells and waste out of the cells. Unhealthy fats also lead to weaker cell membranes that are more prone to damage by oxidative radicals—producing more cell damage and more toxicity in the body.

An example of this is the International Study of Asthma and Allergies in Childhood (ISAAC) conducted among eight Pacific countries, which included Samoa, Fiji, Tokelau, French Polynesia and New Caledonia. The research found that margarine consumption was one of the leading predicating factors in current asthma and wheezing among children.

Furthermore, they found that the risk factors for increased rhinoconjunctivitis included the regular consumption of meat products, butter and margarine among others. Allergic eczema was also associated with regular meat consumption and butter consumption among others.

Here is a quick review of the major fatty acids and the foods they come from:

Major Omega-3 Fatty Acids (EFAs)

Acronym	Fatty Acid Name	Major Dietary Sources
ALA	Alpha-linolenic acid	Walnuts, soybeans, flax, canola, pumpkin seeds, chia seeds
SDA	Stearidonic acid	hemp, spirulina, blackcurrant
DHA	Docosahexaenoic acid	Body converts from ALA; also obtained from certain algae, krill and fish oils
EPA	Eicosapentaenoic acid	Converts in the body from DHA

Major Omega-6/7 Fatty Acids (EFAs)

Acronym	Fatty Acid Name	Major Dietary Sources
LA	Linoleic acid	Many plants, safflower, sunflower, sesame, soy, almond especially
ARA	Arachidonic acid	Meats, salmon
PA	Palmitoleic acid (7)	Macadamia, palm kernel, coconut
GLA	Gamma-linolenic acid	Borage, primrose oil, spirulina

Major Omega-9 Fatty Acids

Acronym	Fatty Acid Name	Major Dietary Sources
EA	Eucic acid	Canola, mustard seed, wallflower
OA	Oleic acid	Sunflower, olive, safflower

Major Saturated Fatty Acids

Acronym	Fatty Acid Name	Major Dietary Sources
Lauric	Lauric acid	Coconut, dairy, nuts
Myristic	Myristic acid	Coconut, butter
Palmitic	Palmitic acid	Macadamia, palm kernel, coconut, butter, beef, eggs
Stearic	Stearic acid	Macadamia, palm kernel, coconut, eggs

Essential fatty acids (EFAs) are fats the body does not form. Eaten in the right proportion, they can also lower inflammation and speed healing. EFAs include the long-chain polyunsaturated fatty acids—and the shorter chain linolenic and linoleic polyunsaturates. EFAs include omega-3s and omega-6s. The omega-3s include alpha linolenic acid (ALA), docosahexaenoic acid (DHA) and eicosapentaenoic acid (EPA). EPA and DHA are found in algae, mackerel, salmon, herring, sardines, sablefish (black cod). The omega-6s include linoleic acid, (LA), gamma-linolenic acid (GLA) and arachidonic acid (ARA). The term *essential* was originally given with the assumption that these types of fats could not be assembled or produced by the body—they must be taken directly from our food supply.

This assumption, however, is not fully correct. While it is true that we need *some* of these from our diet, our bodies can readily convert LA to ARA, and ALA to DHA and EPA as needed. Therefore, these fats can be considered essential in the sense that they are not generated by the body, but we do not necessarily have to consume each one of them.

Monounsaturated fats are high in omega-9 fatty acids like oleic acid. A monounsaturated fatty acid has one double carbon-hydrogen bonding chain. Oils from seeds, nuts and other plant-based sources have the largest quantities of monounsaturates. Oils that have large proportions of monounsaturates such as olive oil are known to lower inflammation when replacing high saturated fat in diets. Monounsaturates also aid in skin cell health and reduce atopic skin responses.

Monounsaturated fatty acids like oleic acid have been shown in studies to lower heart attack risk, aid blood vessel health, and offer anti-carcinogenic potential. They are typical among Mediterranean diets, which have been shown to reduce heart disease risk and cancer risk—related to their lower levels of lipid peroxidative radicals. The best sources of omega-9s are olives, sesame seeds, avocados, almonds, peanuts, pecans, pistachio nuts, cashews, hazelnuts, macadamia nuts, several other nuts and their respective oils.

Polyunsaturated fats have at least two double carbon-hydrogen bonds. They come from a variety of plant and marine sources. Omega-3s ALA, DHA and EPA simply have longer chains with more double carbon-hydrogen bonds. ALA, DHA and EPA are known to lower inflammation and increase artery-wall health. These *long-chain* omega-3 polyunsaturates are also considered critical for intestinal health.

The omega-6 fatty acids are the most available form of fat in the plant kingdom. Linoleic acid is the primary omega-6 fatty acid and it is found in most grains and seeds.

Saturated fats have multiple fatty acids without double bonds (the hydrogens "saturate" the carbons). They are found among animal fats, and tropical oils such as coconut and palm. Milk products such as butter and whole milk contain saturated fats, along with a special type of healthy linoleic fatty acid called CLA or *conjugated linoleic acid.*

The saturated fats from coconuts and palm differ from animal saturates in that they have shorter chains. This actually gives them—unlike animal saturates—an antimicrobial quality.

Medium chain fatty acids like coconut and palm oils have been shown in human studies to lower lipoprotein-A concentrations in the blood while having fibrinolytic (plaque and clot reduction) effects (Muller et al. 2003).

Trans fats are oils that either have been overheated or have undergone hydrogenation. Hydrogenation is produced by heating while bubbling hydrogen ions through the oil. This adds hydrogen and repositions some of the bonds. The "trans" refers to the positioning of part of the molecule in reverse—as opposed to "cis" positioning. The cis positioning is the bonding orientation the body's cell membranes work best with. Trans fats have been known to be a cause for increased radical species in the system; damaging artery walls; contributing to inflammation, heart disease, high LDL levels, liver damage, diabetes, and other metabolic dysfunction (Mozaffarian *et al.* 2009). Trans fat overconsumption slows the conversion of LA to GLA.

Conjugated linoleic acid (CLA) is a healthy fat that comes from primarily from dairy products. CLA is also a trans fat, but this is a trans fat the body works well with—it is considered a healthy trans fat.

Researchers from St Paul's Hospital and the University of British Columbia (MacRedmond *et al.* 2010) gave 28 overweight adults 4.5 g/day of CLA or a placebo for 12 weeks in addition to their medications. After the twelve weeks, those in the CLA group experienced significantly better lung function compared to the placebo group. The CLA group also experienced a significant reduction of weight and BMI compared with the control group. The CLA group also had lower leptin/adiponectin ratios—associated with balanced metabolism.

Other research has also found that CLA can reduce lipid peroxidation and provide better balance among lipids (Noone et al. 2002).

Arachidonic acid (ARA): ARA is considered an essential fatty acid, and research has shown that it is vital for infants while they are building their intestinal barriers. However, ARA is pro-inflammatory and stimulates pro-inflammatory mediators like leukotrienes. Too much of it as we age thus burdens our immune systems, pushing our bodies towards systemic inflammation and slower detoxification.

Red meats provide the highest levels of arachidonic acid. Because arachidonic acid stimulates the production of pro-inflammatory prostaglandins and leukotrienes in an enzyme conversion process, too much ARA leads to a greater level of toxicity, producing more inflammation.

Interestingly, carnivorous animals cannot or do not readily convert linoleic acid (found in many common plants) to arachidonic acid, but herbivore animals do convert linoleic acid to arachidonic acid, as do humans. This conversion—on top of a red meat-heavy diet—produces high arachidonic acid levels. In contrast, a diet that is balanced between plant-based monounsaturates, polyunsaturates and some saturates (such as the Mediterranean diet) will balance arachidonic acids with the other fatty acids.

Gamma linoleic acid (GLA): A wealth of studies have confirmed that GLA reduces or inhibits the inflammatory response. Leukotrienes produced by arachidonic acid stimulate inflammation, while leukotrienes produced by GLA block the conversion of polyunsaturated fatty acids to arachidonic acid. This means that GLA lowers inflammation, and promotes a healthy immune system.

A healthy body will convert linoleic acid into GLA readily, utilizing the same delta-6 desaturase enzyme used for ALA to DHA conversion. From GLA, the body produces *dihomo-gamma linolenic acid,* which cycles through the body as an eicosinoid. This aids in skin health, healthy mucosal membranes, and down-regulates inflammatory hypersensitivity.

In addition to conversion from LA, GLA can also be obtained from the oils of borage seeds, evening primrose seed, hemp seed, and from spirulina. Excellent food sources of LA include chia seeds, seed, hempseed, grapeseed, pumpkin seeds, sunflower seeds, safflower seeds, soybeans, olives, pine nuts, pistachio nuts, peanuts, almonds, cashews, chestnuts, and their respective oils.

The conversion of LA to GLA (and ALA to DHA) is reduced by trans fat consumption, smoking, pollution, stress, infections, and various chemicals that affect the liver.

Docosahexaenoic acid (DHA) obtained from algae, fish and krill, has significant therapeutic and anti-inflammatory effects according to the research. DHA is also associated with stronger cell membranes, and lower levels of lipid peroxidation.

It appears that the anti-inflammatory effects of DHA in particular relate to a modulation of a gene factor called NF-kappaB. The NF-kappaB is involved in signaling among cytokine receptors. With more DHA consumption, the transcription of the NF-kappaB gene sequence is reduced. This appears to reduce inflammatory signaling (Singer *et al.* 2008).

DHA readily converts to EPA by the body. EPA degrades quickly if unused in the body. It is easily converted from DHA as needed. Our bodies store DHA and not EPA.

Because much of the early research on the link between fatty acids and inflammatory disease was performed using fish oil, it was assumed that both EPA and DHA fatty acids reduced inflammation. Recent research from the University of Texas' Department of Medicine/Division of Clinical Immunology and Rheumatology (Rahman *et al.* 2008) has clarified that DHA is primarily implicated in reducing inflammation. DHA was shown to inhibit RANKL-induced pro-inflammatory cytokines, and a number of inflammation steps, while EPA did not.

The process of converting ALA to DHA and other omega-3s requires an enzyme produced in the liver called delta-6 desaturase. Some people—especially those who have a poor diet, are immune-suppressed, or burdened with toxicity such as cigarette smoke—may not produce this enzyme very well. As a result, they may not convert as much ALA to DHA and EPA.

For those with low levels of DHA—or for those with problems converting ALA and DHA—low-environmental impact and low toxin content DHA from microalgae can be supplemented. Certain algae produce significant amounts of DHA. They are the foundation for the DHA molecule all the way up the food chain, including fish. This is how fish get their DHA, in other words. Three algae species—*Crypthecodinium cohnii, Nitzschia laevis* and *Schizochytrium spp.*—are in commercial production and available in oil and capsule form.

Microalgae-derived DHA is preferable to fish or fish oils because fish oils typically contain saturated fats and may also—depending upon their origin—contain toxins such as mercury and PCBs (though to their credit, many producers also carefully distill their fish oil). However, we should note that salmon contain a considerable amount of arachidonic acid as well (Chilton 2006).

Thus, the DHA derived from fish sources, because it requires increased levels of filtering and processing to remove PCBs and mercury, would not be considered a living source of DHA, as it is too far removed from the living source. Algae-derived DHA is a wholesome source, as it is derived directly from living algae. Algae-derived DHA also does not strain sensitive fishery populations.

Algal-DHA also decreases pro-inflammatory arachidonic acid levels. One study (Arterburn *et al.* 2007) measured pro-inflammatory arachidonic acid levels within the body before and after supplementation with algal DHA. It was found that arachidonic acid levels decreased by 20% following just one dose of 100 milligrams of algal DHA.

For those who consider fish the superior source of DHA: In a study by researchers from The Netherlands' Wageningen University Toxicology Research Center (van Beelen *et al.* 2007), all three species of commercially produced algal oil showed equivalency with fish oil in their inhibition of cancer cell growth. Another study (Lloyd-Still *et al.* 2007) of twenty cystic fibrosis patients concluded that 50 milligrams of algal DHA was readily absorbed, maintained DHA bioavailability immediately, and increased circulating DHA levels by four to five times.

In terms of DHA availability, algal-DHA is just as good as fish. In a randomized open-label study (Arterburn *et al.* 2008), researchers gave 32 healthy men and women either algal DHA oil or cooked salmon for two weeks. After the two weeks, plasma levels of circulating DHA were bioequivalent.

Alpha-linolenic acid (ALA) is the primary omega-3 fatty acid the body can most easily assimilate. Once assimilated, the healthy body will convert ALA to omega-3s, primarily DHA, at a range of about 7-40%, depending upon the health of the liver. One study of six women performed at England's University of Southampton (Burdge *et al.* 2002) showed a conversion rate of 36% from ALA to DHA and other omega-3s. A follow-up study of men showed ALA conversion to the omega-3s occurred at an average of 16%.

We should include that ALA, which comes from plants, has been shown to halt or slow inflammation processes, similar to DHA. In studies at Wake Forest University (Chilton *et al.* 2008), for example, flaxseed oil produced anti-inflammatory effects, along with borage oil and echium oil (the latter two also containing GLA).

Furthermore, flaxseed has been recommended specifically for toxicity and inflammation for centuries. This is not only because of its omega-3 levels: it is also because flaxseed contains mucilage, which helps strengthen our mucosal membranes.

The healthy fat balance: In a meta-study by researchers from the University of Crete's School of Medicine (Margioris 2009), numerous studies showed that long-chain polyunsaturated omega-3s tend to be anti-inflammatory while omega-6 oils tend to be pro-inflammatory.

This, however, simplifies the equation too much. Most of the research on fats has also shown that most omega-6s are healthy oils. Balance is the key.

Research has illustrated that reducing animal-derived saturated fats reduces inflammation, cardiovascular disease, high cholesterol and diabetes (Ros and Mataix 2008). All of these relate to toxicity, because as we've discussed, lipid peroxidation lies at the root of these conditions.

The relationships became clearer from a study performed at Sydney's Heart Research Institute (Nicholls *et al.* 2008). Here fourteen adults consumed meals either rich in saturated fats or omega-6 polyunsaturated fats. They were tested following each meal for various inflammation and cholesterol markers. The results showed that the high saturated fat meals increased inflammatory activities and decreased the liver's production of HDL cholesterol; whereas (good) HDL levels and the liver's anti-inflammatory capacity were increased after the omega-6 meals.

What this tells us is that the omega-3/omega-6 story is complicated by the saturated fat content of the diet and subsequent liver function. High saturated fat diets increase (bad) LDL (lipid peroxidation) content and reduce the anti-inflammatory and antioxidant capacities of the liver. Diets lower in saturated fat and higher in omega-6 and omega-3 fats encourage antioxidant and anti-inflammatory activity.

We also know that diets high in monounsaturated fats—such as the Mediterranean diet—are also associated with significant anti-inflammatory effects. Mediterranean diets contain higher levels of monounsaturated fats like oleic acids (omega-9) from foods like olives and avocados (and their oils); as well as higher proportions of fruits and vegetables, and lower proportions of saturated fats.

High saturated fat diets are also associated with increased obesity, and a number of studies have shown that obesity is directly related to inflammatory diseases—including allergies as we've discussed. High saturated fat diets and diets high in trans fatty acids have also been clearly shown to accompany higher levels of inflammation—illustrated by increases in inflammatory factors such as IL-6 and CRP (Basu *et al.* 2006).

To maximize anti-inflammatory factors, the ideal proportion of omega-6s to omega-3s is recommended at about two to one (2:1). The western diet has been estimated by researchers up to thirty to one (30:1) of omega-6s to omega-3s. This large imbalance (of too much omega-6s and too little omega-3s) has also been associated with inflammatory diseases, including asthma, arthritis, heart disease, ulcerative colitis, Crohn's disease, and others. When fat consumption is out of balance, the body's metabolism will trend towards inflammation. This is because in the absence of omega-3s and GLA, omega-6 oils convert more easily to arachidonic acid. And remember, ARA is pro-inflammatory (Simopoulos 1999).

Noting the research showing the relationships between the different fatty acids and inflammation, and the condition of the liver (which can be burdened by too much saturated fat), scientists have logically arrived at a model for dietary fat consumption for a person who is either dealing with or wants to prevent inflammation-oriented conditions and toxicity:

Omega-3	20%-25% of dietary fats
Omega-6+Omega-9	40%-50% of dietary fats
Saturated	5%-10% of dietary fats
GLA	10%-20% of dietary fats
Trans fats	0% of dietary fats

Nuts, seeds, grains, beans, olives and avocados can provide the bulk of these healthy fats in balanced combinations. Walnuts, pumpkin seeds, flax, chia, soy, canola and algal-DHA can fill in the omega 3s. Healthy saturated fats can be found in coconuts, palm and dairy products. These foods are typical of the Mediterranean diet.

Traditional Antioxidant Food Recipes

This brings us to some traditional food recipes that provide superior antioxidant power. The science on quercetin, enzymes and antioxidants now gives some of these cleansing remedies significant credibility:

> *Lemon and honey:* This remedy is often blended with an herbal tea such as peppermint or chamomile. The combination of lemon juice and honey provide an alkalizing and cleansing effect.
> *Super salsa:* This Mexican dish provides cilantro, garlic, cayenne peppers and tomatoes to stimulate blood purification and
> *Honion syrup:* Equal parts chopped onions and raw honey provides constituents to stimulate the immune system.
> *Horseradish syrup:* Equal parts grated horseradish and honey will clear the sinuses and open the airways, while providing an alkalizing effect.
> *Garlic syrup:* Garlic and raw honey combine two anti-microbials and immune-system boosters.
> *Super pickles:* Jerusalem Artichokes, celery and carrot, pickled in apple cider vinegar provide a great alkalizer and blood purifier.

- *Raw vegetable juices:* Juiced endive, celery and carrots. These feed us with immediate nutrients that stimulate our immune system and alkalize our blood.
- *Super soup:* Barley, celery, carrots, beets and ginger. These also provide significant blood alkalizing effects, liver cleansing and stimulate the immune system.
- *Super fruits:* Raw apricots, blueberries, blackberries, strawberries. These provide significant levels of antioxidants.
- *Miso soup:* Miso provides a fermented form of soybeans that stimulates immunity. This remedy has been a long-time favorite among Asian countries.
- *Turmeric curry dishes:* Ayurvedic cooking provides many traditional dishes steeped in spices that stimulate the immune system and provide antioxidants. Turmeric is a favorite that has shown to reduce cancer risk. This is only one type of spiced dish that Ayurvedic cooking provides. An Ayurvedic cookbook is suggested.

The Importance of Raw, Fresh Foods

Most nutrients are heat-sensitive. Vitamin C, fat-soluble vitamins A, E and B vitamins are reduced during pasteurization. Many fatty acids are transformed by high heat to unhealthy fats. Important plant nutrients, such as anthocyanins and polyphenols, are also reduced during pasteurization, along with various enzymes. Proteins are denatured or broken down when heated for long. While this can aid in amino acid absorption, it can also form unrecognized peptide combinations. In milk, for example, some of the nutritious whey protein, or lactalbumin, will denature into a number of peptide combinations that are not readily absorbed.

A 2008 study on strawberry puree from the University of Applied Sciences in Switzerland showed a 37% reduction in vitamin C and a significant loss in antioxidant potency after pasteurization. A 1998 study from Brazil's Universidade Estadual de Maringa determined that Barbados cherries lost about 14% of their vitamin C content after pasteurization. During heat treatment, vitamin C will also convert to dehydroascorbic acid together with a loss of bioflavonoids.

A 2008 study at Spain's Cardenal Herrera University determined that glutathione peroxidase—an important antioxidant contained in milk—was significantly reduced by pasteurization. In 2006, the University also released a study showing that lysine content was significantly decreased by milk pasteurization. A 2005 study at the Universidade Federal do Rio Grande determined that pasteurizing milk reduced vitamin A (retinol) content from an average of 55 micrograms to an average of 37 micrograms. A study at North Carolina State University in 2003 determined that HTST pasteurization significantly reduced conjugated linoleic acid (CLA) content—an important fatty acid in milk shown to reduce cancer and encourage good fat metabolism.

A 2006 study on bayberries at the Southern Yangtze University determined that plant antioxidants such as anthocyanins and polyphenolics were reduced from 12-32% following UHT pasteurization. Polyphenols, remember, are the primary nutrients in fruits and vegetables that render anti-carcinogenic and antioxidant effects.

One of the most important losses from pasteurization is its enzyme content. Diary and plant foods contain a variety of enzymes that aid in the assimilation or catalyzing of nutrients and antioxidants. These include xanthenes, lysozymes, lipases, oxidases, amylases, lactoferrins and many others contained in raw foods. The body uses food enzymes in various ways. Some enzymes, such as papain from papaya and bromelain from pineapples, dissolve artery plaque and reduce inflammation. While the body makes many of its own enzymes, it also absorbs many food enzymes or uses their components to make new ones.

Pasteurization also typically leaves the food or beverage with a residual caramelized flavor due to the conversion of the enzymes, flavonoids and sugars to other compounds. In milk, for example, there is a substantial conversion from lactose to lactulose (and caramelization) after UHT pasteurization. Lactulose can cause intestinal cramping, nausea and vomiting.

In the case of pasteurized juices, pasteurization can leave the beverage in a highly acidic state, which can irritate our mucous membranes and intestines.

As for irradiation, there is little research on the resulting nutrient content outside of a few microwave studies (which showed decreased nutrient content and the formation of undesirable metabolites). There is good reason to believe that irradiation may thus denature some nutrients.

Whole foods in nature's packages are significantly different from pasteurized processed foods. Fresh whole foods produced by plants contain various antioxidants and enzymes that reduce the ability of microorganisms to grow. The Creator also provided whole foods with peels and shells that protect nutrients and keep most microorganisms out. Microorganisms may invade the outer shell or peel somewhat, but the peel's pH, dryness and density—together with the pH of the inner fruit—provide extremely effective barriers to microorganisms and oxidation.

For this reason, most fruits and nuts can be easily stored for days and even weeks without having significant nutrient reduction. Once the peel or shell is removed, the inner fruit, juice or nut must be consumed to prevent oxidation and contamination—depending upon its pH and sugar content.

Whole natural foods also contain polysaccharides and oligosaccharides that combine nutrients and sugar within complex fibers. These combinations also help prevent oxidation and pathogenic bacteria colonization. With heat processing, however, the sugars are broken down into more simplified, refined form, which allows microbial growth and oxidation. Why? Because simple sugars provide convenient energy sources for aggressive bacteria and fungi colonies. By contrast, our probiotics are used to eating the complexed oligosaccharides in fibrous foods. In other words, heat-processing produces the perfect foods for pathogenic microorganism colonization.

As we discussed in the last chapter, pathogenic microorganisms provide the fuel for systemic inflammation. They can infect the body's (and airways') tissues directly, and/or their endotoxins—waste products—stream into our bloodstream to max out our immune system and detoxification processes. This causes systemic inflammation, and toxicity.

Healthy Cooking

While raw whole foods are often more wholesome to the body, some foods must be cooked to make them more digestible. These include most grains, beans, and some vegetables. Our section on Chinese medicine earlier illustrated that some herbs also require cooking to eliminate certain toxins.

The question is: how much cooking and processing do we need to do to our foods? How much cooking is necessary? Yes, cooking some foods often increases their digestibility. This is particularly important with grain-based foods and beans. Cooking these foods will help break down their fibers and complex carbohydrates into more digestible forms.

Also, many vegetables are more assimilable when they are cooked—or even better, steamed. Steaming vegetables in a pot with a covered lid will preserve most nutrients, while softening some of the fibers that hold the nutrients. Foods such as beets, asparagus, broccoli, rhubarb, squash and many others are delicious and nutritious after being steamed or lightly boiled in clean water.

Other plant foods are best eaten raw. These include lettuce, cucumbers, avocado, onions and many others. Because the nutrients in these foods are not so tightly bound within the cell walls of the plants, they can be destroyed by the heat and/or easily separated during cooking.

While the cell walls of plants do contain nutrients, they must be broken down during mastication and digestion. Some cell walls are tougher than others are, and require cooking or processing to break their cell walls. Chlorella—a blue-green algae—is a good example. Many nutrients in chlorella are bound within tightly-packed cell walls, so chlorella is more nutritious when the cell walls have been broken prior to ingestion.

A healthy diet strikes a balance between raw and cooked foods. A perfect way to accomplish this is a dinner that includes a salad topped with seeds, yogurt, olive oil and apple cider vinegar; and an entrée of cooked grains and/or beans with a nice sauce spiced with antioxidant herbs. Breakfast and lunch can include fresh fruit, nuts, raw cheese and fermented dairy; with lightly cooked grains such as oats and barley. Snacks can go raw with apples, nuts, raisins and seeds for sustained, slow-digesting energy and essential fats.

A plant-based food diet can be extremely creative and varied. It can also be extremely colorful and exotic. This is because there are so many different foods and spices to choose from. A flip through a Mediterranean diet cookbook will confirm this immediately.

A Few Mucosal-benefiting Nutrients

With that said, we should know that nearly every nutrient has a role in the body's immune system and mucosal integrity. Many of these specifically benefit the mucosal membranes, but many also support and balance other nutrients that provide mucosal benefits. Thus we can really list practically every nutrient here. Instead, we'll just list a few "heavy-hitters" that are known to significantly stimulate cleansing. Remember, however, that the body needs a balance of nutrients. Therefore, it is advisable to not focus on isolated nutrients, but rather on living nutrients combined (chelated) within natural supplement substrates.

Quercetin: We also discussed quercetin foods previously. Quercetin supplements may be appropriate if the diet is lacking in plant-based foods. As mentioned earlier, this flavonoid inhibits histamine and leukotrienes—inflammatory mediators—in the body.

Vitamin C is considered by researchers as one of the "first line of defense" antioxidants, because it is readily available to neutralize free radicals at mucosal membranes and tissue fluids. A number of studies have shown that vitamin C can reduce inflammation.

Vitamin C supplement doses aimed at reducing inflammation typically range from one to three grams per day. As mentioned, chelated versions and versions with bioflavonoids help the potency of vitamin C. Some health researchers have also noted that vitamin C and quercetin tend to work well together. This is why apples and onions are so healthy. While fruits and many vegetables offer readily-assimilable doses of vitamin C with bioflavonoids, vitamin C drink powders with chelated ascorbates also provide a good way to supplement extra vitamin C.

Lycopene: This phytonutrient, usually isolated from tomatoes, has been shown in some research to reduce inflammation. Best approach here is to consume tomatoes, which have been found to contain about 10,000 different nutrients.

Beta-carotene and other Carotenoids: These vitamin A precursors are essential antioxidants often lacking in many diets. Some research has shown that carotenoids can reduce radical damage to the eyes and other organs.

Vitamin E: Vitamin E supplementation has been shown to provide significant antioxidant benefits. As a result, studies have shown that vitamin E can help prevent cardiovascular disease, respiratory diseases and cognitive impairment.

A few recent studies on vitamin E have shown inconclusive findings, however. What is going on here?

Most people consider vitamin E a single nutrient. But there are actually at least eight forms of vitamin E. Four of them are tocopherols, which include alpha-tocopherol, beta-tocopherol, gamma-tocopherol, and delta-tocopherol. There are also four tocotrienol forms of vitamin E. This includes alpha-tocotrienol, beta-tocotrienol, gamma-tocotrienol, and delta-tocotrienol. The primary vitamin E form in most supplements is alpha-tocopherol.

Most of the research on vitamin E has utilized only alpha-tocopherols. Ongoing research has established that alpha-tocopherols do provide some benefits, but a mix of tocotrienols provide more benefit—especially with regard to cardiovascular health.

Diets can vary in terms of their vitamin E forms. Western diets are typically restricted to alpha-tocopherols and gamma-tocopherols. However, a mixed plant-based diet that includes coconut and palm foods, whole grain rice and other whole grains will render more of the tocotrienol forms.

The bottom line is that the E vitamins are essential antioxidants that help prevent lipid peroxidation—as discussed earlier.

Vitamin Bs: All the vitamin Bs are important to the body's mucosal systems. They are most known for donating methyl groups, used by the liver and glutathione to scavenge free radicals. We should also note that toxins and pharmaceuticals will reduce our stores of Bs. Also, many people lack the intrinsic factor that allows for B vitamin—especially B12—assimilation. For these people, many doctors have advised B12 shots.

Research has recently illustrated, however, that sublingual (under the tongue) B12 is absorbed just as readily into the blood as a B12 shot. There are several sublingual B vitamin supplements on the market today.

Magnesium, Sulfur, Zinc and Other Minerals

Minerals are critical to our detoxification and cleansing processes because they donate ions that neutralize radicals, and are part of key enzymes. Without enough of these important minerals, the body's metabolic systems slow down, due to the lack of enzymes.

Magnesium deficiency has been found to be at the root of a number of conditions, especially those related to anxiety, spasms and muscle cramping. Not surprisingly, inflammation can be significantly reduced with magnesium supplementation.

Magnesium, along with calcium, is critical for smooth muscle tone and nerve conduction. Magnesium is part of the calcium ion channel system. Magnesium regulates calcium infusion into the nerves, which helps keep them stabilized and balanced. This is why magnesium deficiencies within the calcium ion channel system causes overstrain among muscles. This translates to spasms, cramping and muscle fatigue.

If magnesium levels are low, the ion channels will be unstable, stimulating nerve hyperactivity. This nerve hyperactivity can cause changes in the flow of nutrients into cells and toxins out of cells. In other words, magnesium deficiency can result in toxemia.

Magnesium is also a critical element used by the immune system. A body deficient in magnesium will likely be immunosuppressed. Animal studies have illustrated that magnesium deficiency leads to increased IgE counts, and increased levels of inflammation-specific cytokines. Magnesium deficiency is also associated with increased degranulation among mast/basophil/neutrophil cells, which stimulates the allergic response.

Dr. Jabar from the State University of New York Hospital and Medical Center, notes the blood magnesium levels can help determine if magnesium supplements can help. Magnesium levels among red blood cells indicate whether magnesium will likely have any effects.

It is no surprise that magnesium has also been shown to benefit anxiety, as it helps balance nerve firing. Magnesium has also been shown to have anti-inflammatory effects when combined with dosing with larger (one gram or more) doses of vitamin C.

Foods high in magnesium include soybeans, kidney beans, lima beans, bananas, broccoli, Brussels sprouts, carrots, cauliflower, celery, cherries, corn, dates, bran, blackberries, green beans, pumpkin seeds, spinach, chard, tofu, sunflower seeds, sesame seeds, black beans and navy beans, mineral water and beets.

Calcium, is also critical for the functioning of nerves and muscles. Every cell utilizes calcium, evidenced by calcium ion channels present in every cell membrane. Therefore, calcium is necessary for healthy lungs and airways. Thus, calcium deficiency results in more than bone problems. Muscle cramping and airway constriction are also side effects of calcium deficiency. Low calcium levels also result in deranged nerve firing, which can produce anxiety and depression. Supplementing calcium should also be accompanied by magnesium supplementing. For example, a supplement with 1,000 mg of calcium can be balanced by 600 mg of magnesium along with trace minerals.

Good calcium foods include dairy, bok choy, collards, okra, soy, beans, broccoli, kale, mustard greens and others.

Zinc is another important mineral for toxemia. Researchers from Italy's INRAN National Research Institute on Food and Nutrition (Devirgiliis *et al.* 2007) have investigated the relationship between zinc and chronic diseases. Their research determined that an "imbalance in zinc homeostasis" can impair protein synthesis, cell membrane transport and gene expression. These factors, they explained, stimulate imbalances among hormones and tissue systems, producing inappropriate inflammation.

As zinc ions pass through the cell membrane, they assist the cell in the uptake of nutrients. Zinc transporters interact with genes to regulate the transmission of nutrients within the cell, and the pathways in and out of the cell. Zinc concentration within the cell is balanced by proteins called metallothioneins. These proteins require copper and selenium in addition to zinc. Metallothioneins are critical to the cell's ability to scavenge various radicals and heavy metals that can damage the cells. Deficiencies in metallothioneins have been seen among chronic inflammatory conditions, and even fatal diseases such as cancer.

Not surprisingly, research has also shown that zinc modulates T-cell activities (Hönscheid *et al.* 2009).

Good zinc foods include cowpeas, beans, lima beans, milk, brown rice, yogurt, oats, cottage cheese, bran, lentils, wheat and others.

Selenium: Research has shown that greater levels of lipid peroxidation (due to greater consumption of poor fats and fatty foods) decrease our body's levels of selenium. This is because selenium is a critical component of glutathione peroxidase—which reduces lipid peroxidation. Those with higher levels of lipid peroxidation tend to require more selenium because they exhaust this nutrient more readily, as we discussed earlier. While selenium supplements might offer generous amounts of selenium, one brazil nut will supply about 120 micrograms of selenium. This is 170% of the recommended daily value.

Sulfur: Research has also confirmed that dietary sulfur can significantly relieve inflammation and hypersensitivity. In a multi-center open label study by researchers from Washington state (Barrager *et al.* 2002), 55 patients with allergic rhinitis were given 2,600 mg of methylsulfonylmethane (MSM)—a significant source of sulfur derived from plants—for 30 days. Weekly reviews of the patients reported significant improvements in allergic respiratory symptoms, along with increased energy. Other research has suggested that sulfur blocks the binding of histamine among receptors.

Another study (Kim *et al.* 2006) of 50 patients with knee osteoarthritis given either 6 grams per day of MSM) or a placebo for 12 weeks found that after 12 weeks, the MSM group had significantly less pain and significantly more mobility than the placebo group.

Supplemental MSM is typically derived from plant sources. Good food sources of sulfur include avocado, asparagus, barley, beans, broccoli, cabbage, carob, carrots, Brussels sprouts, chives, coconuts, corn, garlic, leafy green vegetables, leeks, lentils, onions, parsley, peas, radishes, red peppers, soybeans, shallots, Swiss chard and watercress.

Potassium is lowered by many pharmaceutical medications, toxins and sweating. Low potassium levels will contribute to imbalances in blood pressure and the kidneys. These issues reduce our ability to cleanse toxins.

Good potassium foods include bananas, spinach, sunflower seeds, tomatoes, pomegranates, turnips, lima beans, navy beans, squash, broccoli and others.

Trace minerals: These should not be ignored in this discussion. Trace elements are important to nearly every enzymatic reaction in the body.

While minerals have been shown to provide therapeutic results, we must be careful about mineral supplements, especially those that provide single or a few minerals. Minerals co-exist in the body, and a dramatic increase in one can exhaust others as the body depletes the oversupply. Thus, an isolated macro-mineral supplement can easily produce a mineral imbalance in the body, which can produce a variety of hypersensitivity issues.

Better to utilize natural sources of minerals. These include, first and foremost, mineral-intensive vegetables. Nearly all vegetables contain generous mineral content in the combinations designed by nature. Best to eat a mixed combination of vegetables to achieve a healthy array of trace minerals.

Whole food mineral sources also contain many trace minerals in their more-digestible *chelated* forms. Chelation is when a mineral ion bonds with another nutrient, providing a ready ion as the body needs it.

Most organically-grown plant-based foods provide a rich supply of trace minerals, assuming we are eating enough of them. Other good sources of full spectrum trace minerals include natural mineral water, whole (unprocessed) rock salt, coral calcium, spirulina, AFA, kelp and chlorella. These sources will typically have from 60 to 80 trace elements, all of which are necessary for the body's various enzymatic functions. See the author's book, *Pure Water.*

We should also note that research by David Brownstein, M.D. (2006) has illustrated that whole unprocessed salt does not affect the body—high blood pressure, cardiovascular disease, diabetes and so on—as do refined salts (often called sodium).

These naturally-chelated mineral sources also prevent the side effects known for mineral supplements. For example, magnesium can easily produce diarrhea in the 2,000-5,000 milligram level. While this might be considered a minor side effect, diarrhea can also produce dehydration.

Numerous holistic doctors now prescribe full-spectrum mineral combinations for inflammatory conditions. Many have attested to their clinical successes in recommending minerals to balance the inflammatory response and stimulate healthy mucosal membranes. Full range supplements that have RDA levels of the macrominerals combined with trace levels of the other minerals can provide a good foundation. Eating more than 5-6 servings a day of fruits and vegetables can provide the rest.

Methylmethionine

Nature also provides nutrients from whole foods that can help rebuild our mucosal membranes. One of the more productive whole foods applicable to rebuilding our body's mucosal membranes is cabbage. Cabbage contains a unique constituent, s-methylmethionine, also referred to as vitamin U. Through a pathway utilizing one of the body's natural enzymes, called Bhmt2, s-methylmethionine is converted to methionine and then to glutathione in several steps.

In this form, glutathione has been shown to stimulate the repair of the mucosal membranes within the stomach, intestines and airways. Glutathione has also been shown to increase the health and productivity of the liver.

Raw cabbage or cabbage juice has been used as a healing agent for ulcers and intestinal issues for thousands of years among traditional medicines, including those of Egyptian, Ayurvedic and Greek systems. The Western world became aware of raw cabbage juice in the 1950s, when Garnett Cheney, M.D. conducted several studies showing that methylmethionine-rich cabbage juice concentrate was able to reduce the pain and bleeding associated with ulcers.

In one of Dr. Cheney's studies, 37 ulcer patients were treated with either cabbage juice concentrate or a placebo. Of the 26-patient cabbage juice group, 24 patients were considered "successes"—achieving an astounding 92% success rate.

Medical researchers from Iraq's University Department of Surgery (Salim 1993) conducted a double-blind study of 172 patients who suffered from gastric bleeding caused by nonsteroidal anti-inflammatory drugs (NSAIDs). They gave the patients either cysteine, methylmethionine sulfonium chloride (MMSC) or a placebo. Those receiving either the cysteine or the MMSC stopped bleeding. Their conditions became *"stable"* as compared with many in the control group, who continued to bleed.

Plants use s-methylmethionine to help heal cell membrane damage among their leaves and stems. This is reminiscent of antioxidants: Plants produce antioxidants to help to protect them from damage from the sun, insects and diseases. In other words, the very same biochemicals that protect plants also help heal our bodies.

Note that MMSC or cabbage juice does not inhibit the flow of gastric juices in the stomach to produce these effects as do acid blocking medications. Rather, they stimulate the body's natural production of mucous, which serves to protect the stomach's cells from the effects of acids.

Mucosal Hydration

As Dr. Jethro Kloss pointed out decades ago (1939), the average person loses about 550 cubic centimeters of water through the skin, 440 cc through the lungs, 1550 cc through the urine, and another 150 cc through the stool. This adds up to 2650 cc per day, equivalent to a little over 2-½ quarts (about 85 fluid ounces).

Meanwhile many have suggested drinking eight 8-oz glasses per day. This 64 ounces would result in a state of dehydration. In 2004, the National Academy of Sciences released a study indicating that women typically meet their hydration needs with approximately 91 ounces of water per day, while men meet their needs with about 125 ounces per day.

This study also indicated that approximately 80% of water intake comes from water/beverages and 20% comes from food. Therefore, we can assume a minimum of 73 ounces of fresh water for the average adult woman and 100 ounces of fresh water for the average adult man should cover our hydration needs. That is significantly more water than the standard eight glasses per day—especially for men.

The data suggests that 50-75% of Americans have chronic dehydration. Fereydoon Batmanghelidj, M.D., probably the world's foremost researcher on water, suggests a ½ ounce of water per pound of body weight. Drinking an additional 16-32 ounces for each 45 minutes to an hour of strenuous activity is also a good idea, with some before and some after exercising. More water should accompany temperature and elevation extremes, and extra sweating or fevers. Note also that alcohol is dehydrating.

A glass of room-temperature water first thing in the morning on an empty stomach can significantly help our mucosal membranes. Then we should be drinking water throughout the day. Our evening should accompany reduced water consumption, so our sleep is not disrupted by urination.

There are easy ways to tell whether we are dehydrated. A sensation of being thirsty indicates that we are already dehydrated. A person with mucosal hypersensitivity should thus be drinking enough water to not ever feel thirsty. Dark yellow urine also indicates dehydration. Our urine color should be either clear, or bright yellow if after taking multivitamins.

Drinking just any water is not advised. Municipal water and even bottled water can contain many contaminants that can burden the immune system, and damage our mucosal membranes. Care must be taken to drink water that has been filtered of most toxins yet is naturally mineralized. Research has confirmed that distilled water and soft water are not advisable. Natural mineral water is best. Please refer to the author's book, *Pure Water* for more information on water content, filters and water treatment options.

Water Therapy

The ancient physician Hippocrates was a proponent of hydrotherapy for respiratory and other mucosal-related conditions, and there have been many treatment successes among the many hydrotherapy treatment centers all over Europe, Asia and the U.S. over the centuries. Early nineteenth century physician Vincent Priessnitz from Austria popularized many types of modern water treatments, as did Father Sebastian Kneipp—a 19th century German monk. These included water compresses, cold-water therapy, contrast baths, hot baths, and warm baths.

Dr. Wilhelm Winternitz, an Austrian neurologist, observed one of Priessnitz's treatment centers and became one of the most celebrated proponents of water treatment in modern times. Dr. Winternitz designed a number of different water treatments and influenced American physicians such as Dr. John Harvey Kellogg, Dr. Jethro Kloss and Dr. Simon Baruch. Dr. Kellogg operated the famous Michigan Battle Creek Health Center for many years until it burnt down in 1902. The center utilized hydrotherapy as a key healing agent. Dr. Kloss ran his own clinic and also worked closely with the Battle Creek Center.

Despite its history of success, opposition to hydrotherapy came from pharmaceutical medicine circles in the decades that followed. Water cures became targeted by the new medical establishment, and many hydrotherapy treatment centers were shut down between 1920 and 1950. Hydrotherapy experienced a resurgence in the U.S. following World War II, when physical therapists found success in whirlpool treatment. Today hydrotherapy is widely used in various modalities, treatments, and physical therapy centers. Many hot springs and wellness spas are unmistakably similar to the hydrotherapy centers of years past. Today these centers draw millions of people seeking therapy and relaxation.

Research has also confirmed that living near or exercising in water significantly improves our mucosal health. For example, a number of studies have confirmed that swimming reduces asthma occurrence. In two studies investigating asthma incidence in children, it was determined that swimming significantly reduced asthma episodes and severity—at levels greater than those offered by other forms of exercise (Inbar *et al.* 1980).

Hot and Cold Water Techniques

Hot and warm water therapy increases circulation, relaxation and detoxification efforts. Let's review some of the techniques recommended:

Cold water showers or a quick cold water rinse off after a warm water shower is invigorating and stimulating to the immune system and nervous system. It also helps balance the body's thermoregulation systems, cool the body in hot weather, as well as heat the body (through muscle contraction) in cold weather.

These actions are produced by our blood vessels' response to cold water. Cold water constricts the blood vessels and leads to involuntary muscle contraction. This type of muscle contraction increases the body's immune function by pumping the lymphatic vessels. In other words, lymph flow is circulated by movement and muscle contraction.

The mechanism works like this: As cold water hits the skin, internal muscles autonomically contract. This effectively pumps or squeezes lymphatic vessels. When the lymph vessels are pumped, the lymphatic fluid speed is increased—much like our heart's pumping increases blood circulation.

Lymph circulation distributes macrophages, T-cells, B-cells and other immune factors throughout the body, enabling them to break down invading bacteria, viruses, and chemical toxins. This effectively speeds up our immune response. As our immune system is responding faster, our toxic load is decreased and our infective burden lightens.

Blood vessel constriction from cold water also stimulates the health of our blood vessels. This serves to increase blood vessel wall elasticity, especially when the cold shower follows a warm or hot shower.

German researchers (Goedsche *et al.* 2007) studied the treatments used of Dr. Kneipp on twenty patients with chronic obstructive pulmonary disease. Cold-water hydrotherapy was tested for immunostimulation, maximal expiratory flow, quality of life, and respiratory function. After ten weeks of three cold effusions and two cold washings on the upper body per day, IFN-gamma lymphocytes increased, quality of life increased, lung function improved and the frequency of respiratory infections decreased.

Many traditional healers have used cold water therapy with great success for asthmatic hypersensitivity. Additional cold water strategies include walking in a few inches to a few feet of cold water by a lake, river or ocean for at least a few minutes, building to up to 30 minutes a day.

Contrast baths reference a therapy of alternating hot water and cold water bathing. This therapy has been used with great success, and can be easily practiced at home by simply following a hot shower with a short cold one before toweling off.

Besides constricting blood vessels and stimulating lymph flow, a cold rinse at the end of a shower causes the skin pores to close. This leaves the body prepared to step out of the shower or bath. A cold rinse also reduces the potential of a basal cell chilling, which can stress the body. In other words, a cold rinse will better prepare the body for the temperature change.

Wet Sock hydrotherapy has been used for respiratory issues for centuries. The feet are soaked in hot water for 10-30 minutes while a pair of thin socks are soaked in cold, icy water. The feet are taken out of the hot water and the cold socks are wrung out and put on, with a pair of thick wool socks over top. This is followed by lying down or sitting with the feet up for an hour or two while relaxing.

Finnish sauna and plunge system: The Fins are famous for their wooden saunas, often built outside near a cold-water plunge. A vigorous sweat in the sauna immediately followed by the cold plunge stimulates the immune system dramatically. This ritual has also been a part of other cultures, including many North American Indian tribes, who used *sweat lodges* with great success. These cultures are known for their long lives and strengthened immunity. Infrared saunas are great modern devices for this purpose. Infrared saunas have the added benefit of quickly and safely dilating blood vessels.

Hot baths also have a great tradition of success among those with respiratory ailments. Hippocrates, known to western medicine as the father of medicine, stated that the hot bath *"…promotes expectoration, improves the respiration, and allays lassitude; for it soothes the joints and the outer skin, and is diuretic, removes heaviness of the heat and moistens the nose."*

Hot water calms the body and slows the heart rate, as the body's blood vessels relax and dilate in response to thermal radiation. A hot bath will open skin pores, allowing a detoxification and exfoliation of skin cells and their contents. For sore or damaged muscle tissues, the dilation of capillaries and micro-capillaries speeds up the process of cleansing the muscle cells of lactic and carbonic acids—the byproducts of inadequate respiration.

Recovery times from strenuous activity are typically reduced by the use of hot water therapy. Hot water is also *hydrostatic*—it gently massages the dermal layers. Hot water also slows internal organ activity, and relaxes the airway smooth muscles. This provides a soothing effect upon the innervations to these areas. The result is reduced stress and widened airways. This effect is increased when hot water is in motion—for example a hot tub.

Hot baths can also be medicated with a variety of mucosal herbs, as listed earlier. Simply make an infusion tea and pour it into the bath.

It should be noted that too much hot water for too long of a period can lead to cardiovascular stress. Hot water can also lead to heat exhaustion. For best results, hot water applications or saunas should be limited to about 10-15 minutes at the hotter levels.

Also, care should be taken to prevent chlorine and chlorine byproduct overload. The byproducts of chlorine breakdown are trihalomethanes (TTHM) and haloacetic acids (TAA5). Over-exposure to these can increase our toxin burden. Today there are healthier alternatives to chlorine, including bromine and salt water blends.

Hot Mineral Springs: From deep within the earth's surface come special waters of a thermal nature. Geothermal heat from volcanic magma creates a rich environment for charging aquifers with high temperatures and a variety of minerals. Many hot springs have a wholesome mixture of bicarbonates, iron, boron, silica, magnesium, copper, lithium, and many trace elements. Some contain exotic elements such as arsenic—believed to help heal skin issues and digestive issues. In other words, not all hot springs are alike.

Due to the earth's sulfur conveyor system, many of these hot spring waters are rich in sulfur in the form of hydrogen sulfide or sulfate. These can loosen phlegm and relax the airways.

Other mineral ions in hot springs have beneficial effects. Magnesium baths have been shown in studies to relax muscles and ease tension. Magnesium also strengthens arteries and relaxes the airway smooth muscles. Iron in hot springs has been associated with strengthening the immune system. Bicarbonates in hot springs—also called "soda springs"—have been associated with easing tension and aiding digestion.

Epsom Salt Bath: For those without a nearby hot springs, a simple bath can be easily turned into therapeutic waters. At home, we can duplicate a magnesium and sulfur mineral springs bath by adding natural mineral salts such as Epsom salts to our bath water. Epsom salts—originally named after the magnesium-rich waters of Epsom, England—are primarily magnesium sulfate, which will ionize in the water into magnesium ions and sulfur ions. As mentioned, ionic magnesium is beneficial to body tissues—relaxing the skin, reducing muscle tension, and lowering stress. Sulfur was also discussed above.

The Epsom salt bath can be supplemented with the addition of rock salt. Natural rock salt contains upwards of 80 minerals and trace elements, which can make the bath a nourishing soak for the entire body.

A drop or two of an essential oil such as lavender or rose oil into the bath will further support relaxation. Lavender oil in particular can significantly calm the nerves.

The skin is said to be the largest organ of the body and absorbs water quite readily. The skin is similar to a mucous membrane. Ancient seamen understood this fact well. When out to sea and dehydrated, seamen would soak their garments in seawater for survival.

For this same reason, our bath waters should not contain toxic chemical bubble baths, chemical-laden perfumed soaps, or heavily chlorinated water. The skin will readily absorb these toxins, putting an extra burden upon the liver and detoxification systems. Best to use clean water and only natural additives.

Steam baths are especially helpful for lung infections, sinus congestion, headaches and mucosal hypersensitivity. However, gradual immersion is suggested. The steam bath can be accomplished with a formal steam room, by the use of a humidifier, or simply with a hot bath in an enclosed room. A cool or coldwater rinse after is helpful for immune stimulation and temperature adjustment. Eucalyptus can be added to increase the expectoration effect. With this and all hot baths, water intake should be increased dramatically, depending upon duration.

Steams can also be done with a pan of boiled water steeped with anti-asthmatic herbs, or boiled potatoes. Just put a towel over the head and over the pan to breathe in the steam.

Humidified Air

As mentioned previously, the air is full of water in the form of vapor. When water is vaporized within our atmosphere, it is called humidity. Humidity levels are typically measured as *relative humidity*. This is the level of moisture the air can contain at a particular temperature. This means that 100% relative humidity indicates that this is the highest amount of moisture the air can contain at that temperature. Warmer temperatures can hold more vapor than colder temperatures, which is why hot humidity is especially uncomfortable.

Humidity levels can range from 100% percent at 100 degrees in the tropics to 25% at the same temperatures in the desert. At zero degrees F, however, 100% relative humidity is equivalent to only 4% humidity at room temperature. So cold temperatures are typically very dry, even at higher relative humidity levels.

As most of us have experienced, higher humidity during warm weather is uncomfortable. Too low of a humidity level will also be uncomfortable, as it will dry our skin and irritate our lungs. Our lungs are full of moisture, and a slightly humid environment is typically better for the lungs.

What this all means is that typical winters are too dry and summers are too humid in most places. This can be exacerbated indoors if we are not careful, creating an unhealthy indoor environment.

The trick is to create healthy indoor humidity levels. This does not mean reducing outdoor air levels, however. It is important that we have a constant flow of oxygen from nature into our indoor environment. Not only does this give us good oxygen content: It also reduces the amount of radon the house will contain. A closed up house attracts more radon than an open-air house because of the pressure gradient.

So how do we create a comfortable indoor humidity? Our bodies are most comfortable at 25% to 60% humidity at room temperature—with the upper range more conducive to better lung function. Indoor humidity can be affected by a house's building materials, ventilation systems, whatever air conditioning or heating units are in place, and human activity. Simply being in the house will increase its humidity. As we breathe, we send out about a cup of water into our environment every four hours—effectively raising the humidity level by 6-8%.

Most furnaces, fireplace fires and forced air heating units will dry the atmosphere. Most refrigerant air conditioners also dry the air as their evaporator coils draw water vapor. Swamp coolers or evaporative coolers increase the indoor humidity (and use less electricity). Also how we cook, take showers and use water in general will determine our indoor humidity levels. A shower will raise the humidity levels about as much as four hours of breathing.

To test our humidity level in the absence of a humidity gauge (advisable), we can watch the moisture levels on the surface of a glass of ice water. If little or no moisture forms immediately on the outside surface of the glass, our house is too dry. If we see moisture build up or mold on the ceilings, our house is likely too humid.

Changing our humidity is quite easy if it is too dry. A shower, humidifier or a room full of people will increase the humidity quite quickly. If the air is too moist, opening up all the windows (assuming it is dryer outside) is the simplest method. In a humid outside environment, we can reduce indoor plants, cook under an oven fan, and in general keep rotating the moist air out. Dehumidifiers are now available for extreme environments, but better to create our own dehumidifier by ventilating our home with fans and keeping windows open to move the moist air out.

Lung infections and most colds and flus respond well to moderately humid environments. Humid air will allow the lungs to detoxify more efficiently. For this reason, humidifiers and steam rooms can be extremely helpful for lung infections and bronchial congestion. Eucalyptus oil, peppermint oil and/or camphor can be put in the water or steam tray to increase lung clearance. Be aware, however, that too much humidity can also breed mold.

Sweating

Sweating is critical for the health of our skin's mucosal membranes because it helps clear and circulate our mucosal fluids. It also purges the body of toxins that often build up in other mucosal membrane regions.

The adult body has about 2.6 million sweat glands located throughout the body's skin cells. As exposure to chemicals has increased, our need for regular sweat is even greater. Our ancestors worked and sweated daily in order to survive. Today, many of us sit in our heat-controlled environments all day without ever breaking a sweat. This trend has suspiciously increased with the prevalence of asthma, allergies, and many other autoimmune diseases. University of Alberta researchers (2010) concluded in a study published in the *Archives of Environmental Contamination and Toxicology* that, *"induced sweating appears to be a potential method for elimination of many toxic elements from the human body."*

Typical methods of sweating include exercise, saunas and steam rooms. However, most people overlook the fact that outdoor work, walking or manual labor can produce a healthy sweat. Most people crank on the air conditioning at the slightest sign of heat. Sweating to cool off is a better strategy, as this will stimulate the turnover of toxins that burden our immune system.

Sweating outdoors in the summer heat also makes our body more heat tolerant, which allows us to live in warmer conditions in general. This means we can use the air conditioner less, which is better for our lungs and sinuses in the long run.

Exercise Strategies

For some of the same reasons, regular exercise will boost our immunity and increase our mucosal health. Exercise helps us circulate those mucosal membrane contents, by heavy breathing, sweating, and in general, body fluid turnover.

This is based on the fact that exercise increases circulation and detoxification, stimulates the immune system, pumps the lymphatic system and increases lung capacity. Exercise is one of the most assured ways to strengthen the immune system and thus increase tolerance. When we exercise, we contract muscles. Again, muscle contraction is what circulates (or pumps) lymph around the body through the lymph vessels. This is because the lymphatic system does not have a heart like the circulatory system has. The lymphatic system relies on muscle contraction for circulation—as we've discussed.

Lymph circulation is critical for mucosal health because immune cells circulating through the blood and lymph break down and carry out of the body those broken-down toxins and cell parts.

And of course, exercise also circulates oxygen and nutrients throughout the body. Exercise also stimulates the thymus gland, and speeds up healing of the intestinal cell walls. In all, exercise is one of the best and cheapest therapies available to boost immunity and tolerance.

All of these effects and more are produced by daily exercise and activity.

Choosing the Routine

Choosing the right type of exercise depends greatly upon the individual and situation. Good forms of exercise include swimming, walking, running, tennis, golf, baseball, basketball, softball, volleyball, surfing, racquetball and squash. While many say that running can induce more asthmatic episodes, this greatly depends on the person, their individual health, and weather conditions. In fact, many successful runners have been asthmatic at times. Same goes for swimmers and other sports. The bottom line is that these individuals were better for their exercise, not worse for it.

Many experts feel that sports involving water and warmer air are easier on the lungs, and sports like skiing or wintertime running can be more harsh on our airways.

Working out in a warmer, slightly humid environment is probably best. If that is not possible, then we can consider some accessories. If running or working out outside during the winter, we can wear a ski mask or scarf over the nose and mouth to reduce the cold air, for example. Breathing in through the nose will also help warm the air before it hits the lungs.

The morning also typically contains less air pollutants, so exercising during the morning may prove to cause less hypersensitivity.

Warming up before exercising is also important. A routine of stretching, jumping jacks, push-ups, knee bends and so on will increase circulation and prepare the body for rigorous exercise.

Days with longer exercise activity can alternate with shorter-burst activity. Shorter-burst activity increases lung function and increases tolerance. Longer, slower exercise produces more detoxification because there are fewer waste products being produced. For example, a person might alternate between walking, taking a hike in the woods, or slow swimming on one day, and play some basketball, soccer or do wind sprints the next. This can further be supplemented with abdominal and even weight (or isometric) training—both of which can increase breath control and respiratory health.

The bottom line is that it depends upon the individual. If a person enjoys a particular sport, they ought to pursue that sport. They will be better for it because they will more likely to continue that sport.

Manual Activity

Manual labor is shunned in modern western society, yet it is one of the best means to stay healthy. Manual labor works many muscle groups and stimulates detoxification. For most of us, there is always the choice of doing it ourselves or otherwise. A good example is weeding. While pulling weeds by hand or using the hoe to remove them requires virtually no expense or special skill, most westerners elect to spray the weeds with toxic chemicals. The election to spray not only eliminates the potential for exercise: It also exposes us to chemicals that add to our body's toxin load.

Active choices can also be as easy as taking the stairs instead of the elevator; walking to the next store rather than driving the car to the next parking lot; biking to work instead of driving; raking the leaves instead of using a leaf-blower—and so many other choices.

At the same time, the person with asthmatic hypersensitivity should not feel that we can just work out daily and not do anything else to improve our health. No. We still will need to eat the right foods, and partake in at least some of the other strategies we've outlined in this chapter and throughout this text. Using this information, we can increase our chances of achieving greater tolerance and increased immunity.

Breathing

Relearning to Breathe

Deep breathing is one of the best ways to increase both lung capacity and respiration efficiency. This is because it strengthens and enlarges the diaphragm, strengthens the supporting abdominal muscles, relaxes the smooth muscles of the airways, and helps reduce stress.

We will discuss a number of methods here, but we focus on two established techniques for healthy deep breathing:

Deep core breathing:
- ➢ Slowly push out the abdomen around the belly button. As the lungs fill, push out the upper abdomen. If lying down, a book may be placed on the abdomen to feel and see it rise.
- ➢ Continue pushing out until the lungs are full and the abdomen is fully pushed out.
- ➢ Top it off by expanding the rib cage to completely fill the lungs.
- ➢ Hold in position and relax for 3-7 seconds.

- Then push the air out by slowly contracting the upper abdominal muscles followed by contracting the lower abdomen as the lungs are completely emptied. This last step is called *flooring*.

Deep diaphragm breathing:
- Slowly push out at the top of the abdomen, enlarging the diaphragm to its capacity as the lungs fill.
- Follow by expanding the rib cage to fill out the lungs. Hold for 2-5 seconds.
- Then begin contracting the upper abdominal muscles to contract the diaphragm. This will begin pushing the air out.
- Slowly contract the diaphragm completely to force out as much air as possible.

Diaphragm breathing does not as completely fill or empty the lungs as deep core breathing does, but it is often more practical while sitting, walking or exercising. Core breathing can result in sleepiness, so it is best used at home in bed or on a comfortable sofa. Either method, if practiced daily for at least 15 minutes, can significantly increase our lung cavity capacity. We may begin to breathe deeper without trying. Placing a hand on the abdomen to feel its rise and fall can also help us center ourselves on our breathing.

In both methods, good breathing posture can be maintained. If sitting, the lower back can be arched slightly with the upper spine fairly straight and relaxed, and the back of the head in line with our lower spine. We can sit on the front of our 'sit bones' at the base of the pelvis, rather than the backside of our sit bones where the lower spine tends to curve outward. When we are sitting on the right part of our sit bones, our lower back will naturally arch.

If lying down on our back, a large pillow can be put under the knees, with the spine straight and a comfortable neck pillow that keeps the crown of the head aligned with the lower spine. Most *hatha-yoga* postures are also conducive to deep breathing exercises.

Keeping the Lungs Clear

Remember that the sinus cavity, pharynx, larynx, trachea and bronchi are all lined with epithelial cells covered with a thin fluid of mucous membrane and tiny hairs called cilia. Cilia trap foreign particles in the sticky, immune cell-rich mucous before they can enter the lungs. This should clear out most soot, debris, bacteria and viruses before they proceed further.

When toxic air (air pollution) or bacteria sneak past these defenses, the bronchial tree, alveoli and pleural cavity will swell with inflammation. The pleural cavity will also often leak fluids into the lung. These fluids, together with the swollen airways, effectively decrease lung capacity and air clearance.

For many, swollen and irritated air passages and pleura is constant, due to an overloading of air pollution, airborne chemicals, dust and microorganisms. Strategies to increase lung capacity and maintain healthy mucosal membranes are thus tantamount to reducing the impact of modern toxins.

Breathing Through the Nose

Scientists from University of North Carolina's Center for Environmental Medicine (Bennett *et al.* 2008) tested the effectiveness of breathing in through the nose among children and adults in both resting and exercising. They found that the noses of adults filter air better than the noses of children. They concluded: *"These results suggest that the lungs of children may be exposed to higher concentrations of inhaled, ambient particles than adults."*

It should be added that breathing in through the nose also does a number of other important things other than simply filtering air—which is certainly an important reason to do so. Following are some of the benefits for breathing through the nose, at least in the inward breath:

Breathing in through the nose warms the air before it hits our airways. The sinuses and turbinates are positioned to heat air through a channeling system that might be compared to a complex series of heating ducts. Instead of being in contact with air that is either significantly hotter or colder than our airways, we receive air that is close to our body temperature.

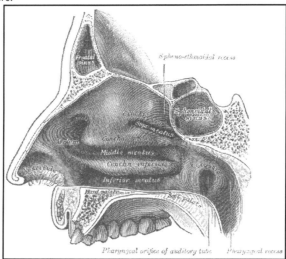

Breathing in through the nose also humidifies the air before it hits our airways. This is accomplished through the mucosal membranes of our turbinates, sinus cavity and pharynx. Direct air will typically be either too humid or too dry for our airways. Our turbinates and sinuses can intersperse just the right amount of water vapor into the air before it hits our airways.

Keeping the Sinuses Clear

This brings us to the logical conclusion that we need to keep the nasal passages clear. Obviously, keeping the sinuses and nasal passages clear is the key to breathing comfortably if we plan to breathe in through the nose. When the sinuses are clogged, our mucous membranes are not draining properly. Mucous needs to be swept out, and if the mucous is too thick or crustified with waste matter, it will narrow our available airways.

So how do we accomplish keeping the sinuses clear? Well, besides breathing in through the nose and general hygiene to help keep them clean—we might consider periodic nasal irrigation.

Nasal lavage is the first consideration. This can utilize a special Ayurvedic lavage device called the neti pot. Neti has been in practice for thousands of years. The pot is simply filled with warm weakly-salty water, and poured through each nostril. A small teapot can also be used.

The technique is to first mix about a quarter-teaspoon of non-iodized, refined salt to about a cup of lukewarm water. A pinch of baking soda may also be added, especially if the salt is iodized or otherwise burns in any way.

Lean forward, over the sink. With the chin level with the nose, turn the head sideways so the nose on a plane parallel with the ground as much as possible.

The water is lightly poured into one nostril, traveling around the septum and out the other nostril. There is no force or pressure involved. There is no snuffing in or pulling in. The solution is simply poured into one nostril, and out through the other. Just hold the head still while it pours out.

Nasal Irrigation: This can also be accomplished by gently pushing warm saline (water and salt) into each nostril using a soft squeeze bottle. Soft squeeze bottles designed for cleaning the nostrils are often available at most drug stores. After using the saline in the bottle, the bottle can be refilled. Care must be taken not to forcefully squirt the water through, which can get water into the upper sinuses.

Another technique is to sniff the water up the nose and back down through to the pharynx and throat, where it is spit out into the sink. This can provide a more complete cleansing of the pharynx and sinuses, but should not be overdone, and only if the sinuses are at least partially clear.

Nasal irrigation has been proven in research to aid in allergic conditions and sinusitis. For example, researchers from Taiwan's Chung Shan Medical University Hospital (Wang *et al.* 2009) gave nasal irrigation or not to 69 children with acute sinusitis. The saline irrigation group improved significantly better than the other group with regard to symptoms and quality of life.

Nasal irrigation was also effective in reducing sinus congestion, rhinorrhea, sneezing and nasal itching in a study by medical researchers from Italy's University of Milano (Garavello *et al.* 2010). In this study, 23 pregnant women with seasonal allergic rhinitis underwent either nasal irrigation or not for six weeks.

In another study, presented at the 50th Scientific Assembly of the American Academy of Family Physicians, Dr. Richard Ravizza and Dr. John Fornadley of Pennsylvania State University divided 294 students into three groups, one of which did nasal irrigation with salt water and the other two groups either took a placebo pill or did nothing. The nasal irrigation group experienced fewer colds during the treatment period compared to the other two groups.

To be fair, some have questioned whether daily regular nasal irrigation for long periods is necessarily good. In a study presented at a the American College of Allergy, Asthma and Immunology (Nsouli 2009), researchers tested 68 patients with a history of sinusitis, who had been using nasal irrigation daily. Of the total, 44 patients discontinued the irrigation while 24 continued the daily treatment. After a year, those who had discontinued the irrigation had 62% less sinusitis infections than the group who continued to use nasal irrigation daily. Dr. Tamal Nsouli commented that daily irrigation may deplete healthy mucous from the sinuses. As we've discussed, healthy mucous membranes also cover the sinuses, helping protect us from infection. Dr. Nsouli also commented that he is not opposed to irrigation for three or four times a week, but suggested avoiding daily irrigation for long periods.

We should note that the study details and protocol have yet to be published, and was only presented in abstract form at the conference. Diane Heatley, M.D., a Professor at the University of Wisconsin School of Medicine, questioned the report, stating, *"nasal irrigation has previously been proven safe and effective for treatment of sinus symptoms in both adults and children in a number of studies already published in peer-reviewed journals."*

An appropriate conclusion here is that regular nasal irrigation should still include some moderation. Using it during periods of congestion and sensitivity is certainly appropriate. Use after or during environmental conditions where there is an increased level of pollution and/or infectious agents is also appropriate. But we can remember that our mucous membranes also house important immune cells and probiotics, which help protect us. We don't want to flush those away needlessly.

Pollution Control

This naturally brings us to strategies to combat air pollution. We discussed the effects of air pollution in detail previously. There is certainly good reason to develop strategies to avoid air pollution. But how practical can these strategies be? Are we to wear a gas mask all day?

The best recommendation we find in some texts is simply to shut all the windows as much as possible. Is this really a solution? As we illustrated earlier, research has confirmed that indoor pollution is generally worse than outdoor pollution. What are we to do, then?

As we've discussed, ozone, particulate matter (soot) and carbon monoxide can damage mucosal membranes. Let's discuss a few strategies:

The Need for Fresh Air

First, we should clarify that there is little doubt that city living can damage our mucosal health. For example, a study done by the Arizona Health Care Cost Containment System (Smith *et al.* 2010) found that among 3,013 people, urban residents had a 55% greater likelihood of asthma than rural residents.

Living around or at least visiting a natural setting such as a forest or beach has many advantages. For example, researchers from Japan's Chiba University (Park *et al.* 2010) conducted 24 field experiments using 280 subjects among 24 forests throughout Japan. In each of the tests, six subjects walked through a forest, while another six walked through a city. The next day the six that walked the city would walk the forest and vice versa. The research concluded that forest environments reduce stress-related cortisol levels, lower heart rate, reduce blood pressure, lower anxiety and increase reaction time. The researchers concluded that: *"These results will contribute to the development of a research field dedicated to forest medicine, which may be used as a strategy for preventive medicine."*

Other studies have confirmed these results. One study found that people living in natural environments had lower levels of stress than those living in urban environments (Ulrich *et al.* 1991). Another, from Emory University, found that natural environments improve health conditions (Frumkin 2001).

Research has also found that even looking at natural environments, even in photos or through windows, enhances positive moods (Blood *et al.* 1999; Kaplan 2001).

All of these improvements, including lower stress levels, positive moods, lower blood pressure and reduced heart rate are all linked to mucosal health. Thus, we can conclude that living in a natural setting or spending some significant time in natural settings would be an important strategy to consider.

City Strategies

As much as we may want to, not everyone can pick up and move away from the city. In this case, focus can turn towards reducing immediate air pollutant exposure. We can make logical choices to reduce our exposure. This doesn't mean staying inside and closing all the windows either. It is important that we get enough sunshine and "fresh" air, and this requires us to go outside. We can simply use some common sense. For example, we can *avoid* the following:

- Running, walking or biking next to a freeway where soot and carbon monoxide levels are greatest.
- Hanging out downwind of a smoke-stack of an industrial plant known to throw toxins into the air.
- Sitting or standing downwind, or next to, an outdoor fire or gas stove for an extended period.
- Standing, sitting or walking next to someone spraying pesticides, herbicides or other chemicals.
- Frequenting tobacco-filled bars or other smoky places.
- Avoiding dusty areas such as construction sites, runways, racetracks, rodeos and other events that stir up lots of airborne particulates.

In addition, there are a number of proactive things we can do to reduce our airborne toxins. As discussed earlier, breathing in through the nose helps to filter out some particulates and other foreigners. This also warms the air. As we discussed, cold air can dry the mucous membranes, and thinned mucous membranes expose our airways to more airborne toxins.

If we live in an urban area with poor air quality we might consider exercising or getting outside during the morning, when the air quality is typically better. As temperatures rise, immediate ozone levels increase. We might also consider exercising near a lake, river, or ocean. Polluted air around water tends to disperse more quickly in the presence of wind, humidity, pressure gradients, and temperature differences around the water.

Out and out wearing of a face mask is typically not practical—although during an extreme situation, it is not a bad idea. More subtle strategies include wearing a scarf during winter months, and covering our mouth and nose with it when outside. In colder climates, a fleece ski mask could also help filter out some particulates.

These are but a few ways to prevent burdening our immune system with airborne toxins—but again, these cannot be our only strategy. We must also undertake reducing the *other, more controllable* immune system burdens to the greatest degree possible. This may also mean increasing the amount of antioxidants we consume in our diet. And let's not forget that the more antioxidants we eat, the better our ability to remove toxins will be. We can add to this the other strategies discussed—herbs, diet, detoxification and so on.

Home Pollution Strategies

Americans spend over 90% of their lives indoors, and indoor air pollution averages double to five times worse than outdoor pollution levels. In some cases, indoor pollution can be tens, even hundreds of times higher than outdoor pollutant levels.

The issue here is ventilation. While older homes might exchange all the air in the house every couple of hours—even up to twice an hour—modern energy-efficient homes exchange air well over five times slower. The average, in fact, is about .25 times per hour, meaning that it would take four hours to exchange all the air in the home. This problem has been termed the *tight building syndrome.*

Previously, we discussed *sick building syndrome.* Tight building syndrome can result in sick building syndrome, assuming that a tight building is not properly ventilated, or ventilated with a clean ventilation system. Or, quite simply, keeping windows open throughout the house. While this might be frowned upon by city dwellers, most indoor air is still quite worse than even big city air. Plus, as we'll explain further, circulating air removes particulates and other toxins as it moves.

For example, University of Glasgow researchers (Wright *et al.* 2009) found that ventilation increases lung function, but does little to reduce dust mite populations. They tested the homes of 120 asthmatic adults—who were allergic to *Dermatophagoides pteronyssinus* dust mites—using mechanical heat recovery ventilation systems (MHRV). This was in addition to conventional allergen avoidance measures in an attempt to reduce dust mite populations. After one year, the peak expiratory flow among the ventilator group was significantly better than the non-ventilator group. However, the ventilation systems *did not* reduce the mite levels within the houses.

So it is not the number of dust mites: It is the composition of the air itself, determined by circulation. A good ventilation system will circulate air while sending it through a filter. A good filter can remove endotoxins that mites produce, as well as the molds, bacteria, soot and other debris that commonly reside in our indoor air.

As we discussed in depth earlier, indoor air pollution is caused by fungi-laden basements, formaldehydes from furniture, asbestos and other building chemicals, household chemicals, volatile organic compounds, smoking, moldy ventilation systems, moldy dust-mite ridden carpets, and so on. Review the air pollutants sections of Chapter Three and Four for further details.

Air Filtration

These toxins can help overload our immune systems, especially if overloaded by other toxins and/or pathogens. In other words, it would be better to remove as many of these as possible before we breathed them in.

Air purifiers: These can significantly remove toxins from the air, as they draw air through a filter and then push the air out. Studies have shown that air purifiers can significantly increase the quality of life among asthmatics (Brodtkorb *et al.* 2010).

Electric ion generating machines generate negative ions. Ionizers have been reputed to remove dust and bacteria, yet this remains controversial. While dust and soot may be attracted to negative ions, they are likely to remain airborne, or possibly end up on floors or furniture to be picked up again.

The amount of ions generated by these machines may also be of concern. While outdoor air may range from 500 to 5,000 negative ions per cubic centimeter, and indoor air may only have a couple hundred per cubic centimeter, negative ion generators can easily pump out from ten thousand to ten million negative ions per cubic centimeter. At these higher levels—especially over a million—negative ions can become irritating to mucous membranes. They can irritate the throat, the eyes, and the lungs. Quite simply, our bodies were not designed for this level of negative ions.

Furthermore, a Cochrane review (Blackhall *et al.* 2003) of six good quality studies concluded that ionizers exerted no significant effects upon lung function, asthma symptoms or medication use among a total of 106 participants.

Ozone generators may be effective at removing bacteria, because bacteria require oxygen to live, and ozone depletes their oxygen levels. For this reason, a good ozone generator will often create a fresher smelling indoor environment. While ozone is not the same as smog, which has carbon or sulphur molecules connected to the molecules, ozone is an atmospheric response to smog, as ozone helps stabilize oxygen levels and clear out other molecules.

At the same time, higher ozone levels may also result in lung irritation and allergic response. As mentioned earlier, the FDA limits ozone generating machines in medical devices (used in hospitals and clinics) to emit no more than 50 parts per billion. The bottom line with both ionizers and ozone generators is that the atmosphere contains a fragile balance of components: It is not a random mixture. The level of ozone present in outdoor pollution reflects the atmosphere's cleansing process. In other words, the decision to use these machines should be made carefully, and the composition of fresh air is likely healthier than any machine-driven composition.

High-Efficiency Particular Arresting (HEPA) filters: It might be noted that neither the ozone nor ion generator systems have been shown to effectively remove dust, dander or allergens (unless the allergens are bacteria, which can be removed with ozone). A HEPA filter is a better strategy for removing dust, dander and other particulates. HEPA filters are designed to pick up over 99.9% of particulate sized .3 micron in size. Putting a HEPA filter on a simple air ducting system with a fan or heater will thus do wonders for removing dust, dander, and allergens.

Electrostatic air filters for forced air systems can be a good choice. These HEPA filters typically filter between ninety and a hundred percent of dander, mold, mites, dust, soot, and bacteria. Many of these filters come with the ability to clean and reuse, allowing us to clean them as often as needed—which should be at least monthly if use is constant.

Environmental filters are good alternatives, especially for cold urban environments. These draw in, filter and heat outdoor air. This maximizes circulation, ventilation and temperature control: The best of all worlds.

Pillowcase filters: This air filtration device is designed to filter the nighttime air through the pillowcase. One study (Stillerman *et al.* 2010) tested this with 35 adults who had allergic rhinoconjunctivitis and sensitivities to either dander or dust mites. The device was found to reduce 99.99% of allergen particulates greater than .3 microns within the patients' breathing zones. The patient group using the filtration device was found to have significantly fewer symptoms and better quality of life than the placebo group.

Natural Air Sanitation

We can also restrict the level of indoor pollutants by choosing to use household products with natural ingredients free as possible from chemical preservatives. This means using natural flooring and furniture, natural fragrance-free soaps and cosmetics, and cotton clothing. This also means buying fewer plastic household goods and more natural fiber goods. Should we change our purchasing behavior, we may also alter the behavior of those companies manufacturing these items.

When it comes to freshening up stale indoor air, pressurized aerosol air fresheners are not the way to go. They may contain various synthetic fragrances, benzyl ethanols, naphthalene, and formaldehydes among other undesirables. Various micro-particles are also created by these aerosols.

As mentioned in the trigger chapter, many aerosols and pump sprays also contain noxious propellants—many of which are also volatile organic compounds (VOCs). These include butane and propane. Despite their demand in the marketplace, aerosols are not required for survival: Humankind did just fine without them for thousands of years. An effective disbursing method is a simple spray bottle. An active ingredient—say lemon juice—can be diluted with water and lightly sprayed through a room to freshen it up nicely. There are, of course, many other uses for such a common spray bottle—effectively replacing propellant aerosols.

Beware of perfumes and colognes that may reside in the bathroom or on family members. And be careful of fashion magazines and men's magazines that insert fragrances into their pages and advertisements. These perfumes might smell nice, but they can also contain toxins that can burden the immune system in addition to harming our mucosal membranes.

Candles may smell nice, but they are often made with synthetic fragrances, hydrocarbon-based paraffin waxes, and lead or other heavy metal wicks. The combination often releases unhealthy black soot into our air. Beeswax candles with essential oils can provide good alternatives for the candle-loving household, combined, of course, with fresh air.

Healthy alternatives to toxic household cleaners include lemon, vinegar, borax and/or baking soda. Borax is a great scrubbing detergent for heavy household and yard cleaning jobs. Olive oil, lemon oil or beeswax make for good natural furniture polishes.

Cleaning surfaces with these will also significantly freshen indoor air as well. Rotting food and unclean surfaces create mildew and bacteria quite quickly. Fresh air is quite easy to achieve with clean surfaces. Dusting and wiping down flooring and walls with vinegar can be a good strategy. A small cup of vinegar or a box of baking soda placed in a corner can also absorb odors and airborne toxins. Non-septic friendly chlorine bleach or rubbing alcohol can be used sparingly to remove mold or other microorganisms.

As far as pesticides, there are also natural alternatives. These include clove oil, mints, orange oil, borax and others. Many pest control companies will now apply these alternatives upon request.

House Plants

A house full of indoor plants will do wonders for improving our indoor air quality. Placing between two and five plants in a hundred square foot room—depending upon the outside air—can significantly remove carbon and raise oxygen levels. Research from the *Mississippi Stennis Space Center* concluded that indoor plants absorbed and broke down formaldehydes, trichloroethylenes, benzenes and zylenes.

Better performing plants included the lady palm, the rubber plant, English ivy, and the areca palm plants. Toxin removal rates can range from 1,000 to 1,800 micrograms per hour. One study done in Norway (Fjeld *et al.* 1998) found 23% fewer complaints of fatigue and sinus congestion among workers working around plants.

Studies performed in Texas and at Washington State University found that cognition response and problem-solving were also significantly higher among people working around plants (Wolverton 1997).

It should be noted that potting soils of indoor plants can also harbor some molds, so care can be taken to dry out the soil between waterings, and keep some sunlight on the soil surface.

We can also create forests around our homes. This means planting and maintaining indigenous trees that provide oxygen, shade and soil health: Soils without good plant life and rooting systems become loose and dusty. Nearby outdoor plants can significantly decrease the carbon and toxins in our immediate circulating environment. This also means instead of tearing out trees and paving our courtyards, we can leave the trees or replant them. Living in a space surrounded by trees can also render more privacy, allowing us to keep our windows open more often.

Pros and Cons on Air Conditioning

Air conditioning offers benefits and downsides. On the benefit side, a good one can filter out pollens, soot, insect endotoxins and other potential toxins. This of course depends on the filter inside the air conditioner, and how often it is cleaned.

Filters not cleaned frequently can build up with fungi and bacteria that can significantly infect our airspace.

Most air conditioners reduce humidity as well. The problem with this massive reduction in humidity is that it can dry out the mucosal membranes in our airways. This, along with the cold air provided by many air conditioners, can stress our mucosal membranes.

Swamp coolers provide filtering and cooling, but add humidity. This can keep the airways more moist. However, swamp coolers can easily get infected with molds and bacteria: So they have to be cleaned periodically, perhaps every few weeks in the summer time, and definitely before using after the winter.

Practically every air conditioner creates condensation, which results in small droplets of water dripping around the unit or inside the unit. This can encourage fungi and bacteria growth around the walls and ventilation ducts of the system.

Air conditioning artificially cools down body temperature and airways. While this might be considered a good thing when it is hot outside, artificially cooling the body also stresses the body and the airways. The body must work harder to heat and humidify the air before it hits the lungs. This can stress the turbinates, the airway mucosal membranes, and the immune system.

Also note that car air conditioning systems typically intake air from around the car—full of traffic exhaust. The air can also contain exhaust from the car itself, or combustion byproducts from the engine. While screened through a filter, this air still contains toxins. We can periodically refresh the car's indoor air by stopping and rolling down the car windows.

Automobile air filters can also become filled with fungi and bacteria, so they can be periodically cleaned. Generally, people do not clean their car air filters. So it is safe to say that any older car has a significant build up of mold and other toxins within its air conditioner system and filters.

Noting these issues, it is probably more sustainable to simply minimize air conditioning and utilize fans when possible. Opening the car windows while driving also provides a fan of sorts. Fanned air on the skin helps cool the skin down without chilling the air. Remember that circulated air is typically cleaner than the same type of air when stagnant.

A fan strategy also allows our bodies to better acclimate to the outdoor temperatures. This is healthier for the body. Our bodies have cooling mechanisms that include sweating and relaxing. Both of these are healthy strategies. Sweating removes waste and toxins from the body, and relaxing takes pressure off the adrenal glands. We can conclude that sweating a little and relaxing a bit can also benefit our musocal membranes, especially among our skin and airways.

Natural Materials

Using nature's materials for floors, walls and furniture is also a good strategy. This means using stone, ceramic, wood, wool, cotton and so on. Practically every synthetic piece of furniture, wall covering or floor covering contains a host of chemicals, including formaldehyde, VOCs, insecticides, asbestos and fire retardants. While retarding fires is certainly commendable, these can also make us sick in the worst case, and add to our toxin load in the best case. Besides, stone can be a pretty good fire retardant.

Stone, ceramic tile or wooden floors can also be easily cleaned with vinegar and baking soda to safely eliminate dust and allergens. Wood can also be polished and cleaned with olive oil. Nowadays, most walls are sheet rock, which often contains chalks and asbestos that can slowly build up in the airways. Replacing them with wood siding is a possible strategy.

Outgassing

Outgassing (or offgassing) any new materials we buy is a good idea, regardless. To outgas a material, we can simply set it in the sun for a day before using it. This is a good idea for any new piece of furniture, wall covering, and anything else that may have been coated in VOCs or formaldehydes during manufacturing. Plastics may also be outgassed, but outgassing plastic in direct sunlight can also release additional monomer plasticizers.

Outgassing a new car might also be considered. That "new car smell" is more than just a nice smell. Leave the car in the sun for a few days or weeks with the windows open. For best results, always keep car windows cracked.

Ventilation

Air travels in currents. These currents are electromagnetic. Airflows will thus grab hold of air pollutants and channel them away. Air works much like water does, as it uses electrostatic forces to remove toxins. This means that our freshest air will be the air that flows through our environment. Stagnated air is polluted air. Moving air is typically cleaner and provides the best means to minimize toxicity. Circulating air also has the greatest tendency of maintaining normal atmospheric composition, humidity and pressure values.

Therefore, if possible, we might consider keeping our windows open at all times, even in the wintertime. When it is cold outside, we can crack the window barely—just enough to allow for some airflow. Fans can do the rest.

Work and School Pollution Strategies

Work and school environments are toxin traps. Why? Because they bring people and limited ventilation systems together under the same roof. They also host a number of toxins in building materials, carpets, desks, chairs, production materials, manufacturing exhaust, and whatever anyone brings in to work or school. This of course includes animal dander, dust mites, microorganisms and mold attached to people's clothing, hair and skin as they venture into the building.

This was illustrated in the New Zealand research discussed in Chapter Three, where cat allergens were found throughout schools, workplaces, theaters and airplanes.

While there is no way to eliminate these toxins, we can certainly take measures to lower our exposure, since as a whole, toxins from the workplace and school do contribute to our overall toxic load and burden upon our immune system. Furthermore, exposure to workplace toxicity in the form of manufacturing wastes, cleaners, gases and other chemical toxins can single-handedly make a person downright sick.

There are a number of policies and strategies among workplaces and schools that can reduce our exposures or toxic loads:

Hazardous Materials: Workplaces and schools typically utilize various chemicals and cleaning materials. Some workplaces use hazardous materials on a daily basis. These should be handled with care,to make sure that exposures are minimized.

According to United States Occupational Safety Code, *Manufacturer's Safety Data Sheets* (MSDS) are required for every chemical used by consumers, workers or cleaning professionals. These should be carefully read over to make sure that the material is being used in accordance with the MSDS. This means that enough ventilation is supplied. For most hazardous materials, this is the greatest risk: Hazardous materials are frequently used without the proper ventilation. These are toxins that can also cause illness and death, depending upon the chemical and exposure level.

HVAC: Our school and workplace should have a heating, ventilating and air conditioning system (also called HVAC) that is adequate for the population, space and environmental conditions. The more people, space and toxins present, the better the HVAC system needs to be. In the United States, these are typically determined by local, state or county building codes. When a building is designed, its HVAC must comply with the building code in place.

The standard codes are determined by The *American Society of Heating, Refrigerating and Air Conditions Engineers* (ASHRAE), who have developed the standards that most municipalities abide by. For example, the 1989 standards (6.2-1989) called for 15-20 cubic feet of fresh air to be brought in per minute (CFM) and per person occupying an indoor space. This means, for example, that an office with 10 people must have a system that pumps in 150-200 cubic feet of fresh air per minute.

This same calculation can be done for any school or other space.

In addition, building codes have changed over the years with respect to insulation. This means that if the building has been built in the past few decades, the building codes are tighter, and there will be likely less ventilation in general. This puts an extra strain on the HVAC system.

Windows are certainly a form of ventilation, but they should not be included in this calculation, because during cold or hot weather, the windows are often closed (though they should not be).

Any building needs to be checked with current code to make sure that the HVAC system matches the use and occupancy of the building. The building specifications designed by the architect before the building was built can easily be different from the building's current use. There may be many more workers or children in the building than originally specified for example. Or if the HVAC was designed for office space, but the building is now used as manufacturing space, for example, the HVAC requirements will be different—depending upon what is being produced, and the municipality. So the company owners or school administrators must be reminded to assure their workers or parents that the workplace's/school's HVAC systems are compliant with current codes. This should also be reviewed for any apartment or condominium.

HVAC systems also should also be periodically cleaned. This includes the drip pans and ducting. These can build up with molds and other microorganisms, and infect their occupants. As we discussed earlier, cases have shown that extreme weather changes (from cold to warm or wet) can dramatically affect the HVAC system ducting in terms of mold and microorganisms—significantly infecting the building's occupants.

Flooring: Carpeting in workplaces and schools is particularly problematic. This is because they attract bacteria, molds, dander, allergens and other toxins quickly. Cleaning carpets is typically expensive and difficult. Wood, stone or concrete floors clean easier and can be disinfected more easily, as we've discussed.

Furniture: Chairs and sofas in the work place are susceptible to mold, toxin and allergen build-up as they age, and formaldehydes when newer. Therefore, they need to be periodically cleaned or replaced. Wooden furniture or furniture with cleanable surfaces and moisture barriers are preferred.

Windows: From an individual perspective, sitting or working close to an openable window is suggested in any workplace or school classroom. Any time there is an offensive odor or concern about indoor air quality, the window should be opened and left open until the risk has subsided. Hotel rooms can also be checked for openable windows before they are reserved. A closed-in room with a dirty HVAC system can significantly harm the integrity of our mucosal membranes.

Fans: Fans are a valuable and inexpensive addition to any room. These can help blow offensive air out the door or window, for example. Fans, in fact, are better strategies than air conditioning, because they do not artificially cool the body down—as we've discussed. In the opinion of this author, every workplace and school should be equipped with fans.

Air purifiers: Small air purifiers can significant help a person working in a workplace with questionable air. There are several purifiers that can be placed on the desk. These can significantly help remove particulates, mold and allergens from our immediate breathing airspace.

Regular Cleaning: This is a requisite for any workplace, school or apartment building. Common areas should be cleaned at least weekly. Floors and walls should be sanitized. Good natural cleaners include vinegar, lemon, borax and baking soda. Chlorine or rubbing alcohol can be used sparingly to disinfect. Furniture requires regular dusting and sanitization, and HVAC systems and ducts require regular cleaning.

Strengthened Immunity: No matter how clean we get our workplaces and schools, there will always be lots of toxins our mucosal membranes are exposed to. While these strategies can help remove toxin exposure, we still need to maintain strong mucosal membranes and strong immunity and tolerance.

Conclusion

We have proven, through the application and review of hundreds of scientific studies and rigorous clinical applications, that our mucosal membrane health is critical to our body's ability to avoid disease and remain healthy as long as possible.

We have shown the mechanisms, content and regions of the mucosal membranes, and have illustrated how defective membranes cause some of the most devastating disease conditions.

Furthermore, we have elaborated on how important probiotics are to the health of our mucosal membranes, and showed what elements can harm them along with harming our mucosal membranes in general.

And finally, we have shown that there are many things we can do to increase our mucosal health, and turn around defective mucosal membranes with simple, inexpensive and tasteful strategies.

Increasing our mucosal health is the future of medicine. By increasing the health of the barrier that keeps out invading microorganisms, allergens, toxins and other foreigners, we can avoid many illnesses, and keep the body healthy despite a growing risk of infection and toxic exposure in our modern world.

References and Bibliography

Abdureyim S, Amat N, Umar A, Upur H, Berke B, Moore N. Anti-inflammatory, immunomodulatory, and heme oxygenase-1 inhibitory activities of ravan napas, a formulation of uighur traditional medicine, in a rat model of allergic asthma. *Evid Based Complement Alternat Med.* 2011;2011. pii: 725926.

Aberg N, Hesselmar B, Aberg B, Eriksson B. Increase of asthma, allergic rhinitis and eczema in Swedish schoolchildren between 1979 and 1991. *Clin Exp Allergy.* 1995;25:815-819.

Adel-Patient K, Ah-Leung S, Creminon C, Nouaille S, Chatel JM, Langella P, Wal JM. Oral administration of recombinant Lactococcus lactis expressing bovine beta-lactoglobulin partially prevents mice from sensitization. *Clin Exp Allergy.* 2005 Apr;35(4):539-46.

Agache I, Ciobanu C. Risk factors and asthma phenotypes in children and adults with seasonal allergic rhinitis. *Phys Sportsmed.* 2010 Dec;38(4):81-6.

Agarwal SK, Singh SS, Verma S. Antifungal principle of sesquiterpene lactones from Anamirta cocculus. *Indian Drugs.* 1999;36:754-5.

Aggarwal BB, Harikumar KB. Potential therapeutic effects of curcumin, the anti-inflammatory agent, against neurodegenerative, cardiovascular, pulmonary, metabolic, autoimmune and neoplastic diseases. *Int J Biochem Cell Biol.* 2009 Jan;41(1):40-59.

Aggarwal BB, Sung B. Pharmacological basis for the role of curcumin in chronic diseases: an age-old spice with modern targets. *Trends Pharmacol Sci.* 2009 Feb;30(2):85-94.

Agostoni C, Fiocchi A, Riva E, Terracciano L, Sarratud T, Martelli A, Lodi F, D'Auria E, Zuccotti G, Giovannini M. Growth of infants with IgE-mediated cow's milk allergy fed different formulas in the complementary feeding period. *Pediatr Allergy Immunol.* 2007 Nov;18(7):599-606.

Aho K, Koskenvuo M, Tuominen J, Kaprio J. Occurrence of rheumatoid arthritis in a nationwide series of twins. *J Rheumatol.* 1986 Oct;13(5):899-902.

Akinbami LJ, Moorman JE, Garbe PL, Sondik EJ. Status of childhood asthma in the United States, 1980-2007. *Pediatrics.* 2009;123:S131-45.

Alemán A, Sastre J, Quirce S, de las Heras M, Carnés J, Fernández-Caldas E, Pastor C, Blázquez AB, Vivanco F, Cuesta-Herranz J. Allergy to kiwi: a double-blind, placebo-controlled food challenge study in patients from a birch-free area. *J Allergy Clin Immunol.* 2004 Mar;113(3):543-50.

Alexander DD, Cabana MD. Partially hydrolyzed 100% whey protein infant formula and reduced risk of atopic dermatitis: a meta-analysis. *J Pediatr Gastroenterol Nutr.* 2010 Apr;50(4):422-30.

Alexandrakis M, Letourneau R, Kempuraj D, Kandere-Grzybowska K, Huang M, Christodoulou S, Boucher W, Seretakis D, Theoharides TC. Flavones inhibit proliferation and increase mediator content in human leukemic mast cells (HMC-1). *Eur J Haematol.* 2003 Dec;71(6):448-54.

Al-Harrasi A, Al-Saidi S. Phytochemical analysis of the essential oil from botanically certified oleogum resin of Boswellia sacra (Omani Luban). *Molecules.* 2008 Sep 16;13(9):2181-9.

Almqvist C, Garden F, Xuan W, Mihrshahi S, Leeder SR, Oddy W, Webb K, Marks GB; CAPS team. Omega-3 and omega-6 fatty acid exposure from early life does not affect atopy and asthma at age 5 years. *J Allergy Clin Immunol.* 2007 Jun;119(6):1438-44.

Amato R, Pinelli M, Monticelli A, Miele G, Cocozza S. Schizophrenia and Vitamin D Related Genes Could Have Been Subject to Latitude-driven Adaptation. *BMC Evol Biol.* 2010 Nov 11;10(1):351.

American Conference of Governmental Industrial Hygienists. *Threshold limit values for chemical substances and physical agents in the work environment.* Cincinnati, OH: ACGIH, 1986.

American Dietetic Association; Dietitians of Canada. Position of the American Dietetic Association and Dietitians of Canada: vegetarian diets. *Can J Diet Pract Res.* 2003 Summer;64(2):62-81.

Ammon HP. Boswellic acids (components of frankincense) as the active principle in treatment of chronic inflammatory diseases. *Wien Med Wochenschr.* 2002;152(15-16):373-8.

Ammon HP. Boswellic acids in chronic inflammatory diseases. *Planta Med.* 2006 Oct;72(12):1100-16.

Anand P, Thomas SG, Kunnumakkara AB, Sundaram C, Harikumar KB, Sung B, Tharakan ST, Misra K, Priyadarsini IK, Rajasekharan KN, Aggarwal BB. Biological activities of curcumin and its analogues (Congeners) made by man and Mother Nature. *Biochem Pharmacol.* 2008 Dec 1;76(11):1590-611.

Anderson JL, May HT, Horne BD, Bair TL, Hall NL, Carlquist JF, Lappé DL, Muhlestein JB; Intermountain Heart Collaborative (IHC) Study Group. Relation of vitamin D deficiency to cardiovascular risk factors, disease status, and incident events in a general healthcare population. *Am J Cardiol.* 2010 Oct 1;106(7):963-8.

Anderson M., Grissom C. Increasing the Heavy Atom Effect of Xenon by Adsorption to Zeolites: Photolysis of 2,3-Diazabicyclo[2.2.2]oct-2-ene. *J. Am. Chem. Soc.* 1996;118:9552-9556.

Anderson RC, Anderson JH. Acute respiratory effects of diaper emissions. *Arch Environ Health.* 1999 Sep-Oct;54(5):353-8.
Anderson RC, Anderson JH. Acute toxic effects of fragrance products. *Arch Environ Health.* 1998 Mar-Apr;53(2):138-46.
Anderson RC, Anderson JH. Respiratory toxicity in mice exposed to mattress covers. *Arch Environ Health.* 1999 May-Jun;54(3):202-9.
Anderson RC, Anderson JH. Respiratory toxicity of fabric softener emissions. *J Toxicol Environ Health.* 2000 May 26;60(2):121-36.
Anderson RC, Anderson JH. Respiratory toxicity of mattress emissions in mice. *Arch Environ Health.* 2000 Jan-Feb;55(1):38-43.
Anderson RC, Anderson JH. Sensory irritation and multiple chemical sensitivity. *Toxicol Ind Health.* 1999 Apr-Jun;15(3-4):339-45.
Anderson RC, Anderson JH. Toxic effects of air freshener emissions. *Arch Environ Health.* 1997 Nov-Dec;52(6):433-41.
Anderson SD, Charlton B, Weiler JM, Nichols S, Spector SL, Pearlman DS; A305 Study Group. Comparison of mannitol and methacholine to predict exercise-induced bronchoconstriction and a clinical diagnosis of asthma. *Respir Res.* 2009 Jan 23;10:4.
Andoh T, Zhang Q, Yamamoto T, Tayama M, Hattori M, Tanaka K, Kuraishi Y. Inhibitory Effects of the Methanol Extract of Ganoderma lucidum on Mosquito Allergy-Induced Itch-Associated Responses in Mice. *J Pharmacol Sci.* 2010 Oct 8.
André C, André F, Colin L. Effect of allergen ingestion challenge with and without cromoglycate cover on intestinal permeability in atopic dermatitis, urticaria and other symptoms of food allergy. *Allergy.* 1989;44 Suppl 9:47-51.
André C. Food allergy. Objective diagnosis and test of therapeutic efficacy by measuring intestinal permeability. *Presse Med.* 1986 Jan 25;15(3):105-8.
Andre F, Andre C, Feknous M, Colin L, Cavagna S. Digestive permeability to different-sized molecules and to sodium cromoglycate in food allergy. *Allergy Proc.* 1991 Sep-Oct;12(5):293-8.
Anim-Nyame N, Sooranna SR, Johnson MR, Gamble J, Steer PJ. Garlic supplementation increases peripheral blood flow: a role for interleukin-6? *J Nutr Biochem.* 2004 Jan;15(1):30-6.
Annweiler C, Schott AM, Berrut G, Chauviré V, Le Gall D, Inzitari M, Beauchet O. Vitamin D and ageing: neurological issues. *Neuropsychobiology.* 2010 Aug;62(3):139-50.
Antczak A, Nowak D, Shariati B, Król M, Piasecka G, Kurmanowska Z. Increased hydrogen peroxide and thiobarbituric acid-reactive products in expired breath condensate of asthmatic patients. *Eur Respir J.* 1997 Jun;10(6):1235-41.
Aoki T, Usuda Y, Miyakoshi H, Tamura K, Herberman RB. Low natural killer syndrome: clinical and immunologic features. *Nat Immun Cell Growth Regul.* 1987;6(3):116-28.
Apáti P, Houghton PJ, Kite G, Steventon GB, Kéry A. In-vitro effect of flavonoids from Solidago canadensis extract on glutathione S-transferase. *J Pharm Pharmacol.* 2006 Feb;58(2):251-6.
APHA (American Public Health Association). Opposition to the Use of Hormone Growth Promoters in Beef and Dairy Cattle Production. Policy Date: 11/10/2009. Policy Number: 20098. http://www.apha.org/advocacy/policy/id=1379. Accessed Nov. 24, 2010.
Araki K, Shinozaki T, Irie Y, Miyazawa Y. Trial of oral administration of Bifidobacterium breve for the prevention of rotavirus infections. *Kansenshogaku Zasshi.* 1999 Apr;73(4):305-10.
Araujo AC, Aprile LR, Dantas RO, Terra-Filho J, Vianna EO. Bronchial responsiveness during esophageal acid infusion. *Lung.* 2008 Mar-Apr;186(2):123-8. 2008 Feb 23.
Arbes SJ Jr, Gergen PJ, Vaughn B, Zeldin DC. Asthma cases attributable to atopy: results from the Third National Health and Nutrition Examination Survey. *J Allergy Clin Immunol.* 2007 Nov;120(5):1139-45. 2007 Sep 24.
Argento A, Tiraferri E, Marzaloni M. Oral anticoagulants and medicinal plants. An emerging interaction. *Ann Ital Med Int.* 2000 Apr-Jun;15(2):139-43.
Arif AA, DelcIos GL, Colmer-Hamood J. Association between asthma, asthma symptoms and C-reactive protein in US adults: data from the National Health and Nutrition Examination Survey, 1999-2002. *Respirology.* 2007 Sep;12(5):675-82. .
Arif AA, Shah SM. Association between personal exposure to volatile organic compounds and asthma among US adult population. *Int Arch Occup Environ Health.* 2007 Aug;80(8):711-9.
Arshad SH, Bateman B, Sadeghnejad A, Gant C, Matthews SM. Prevention of allergic disease during childhood by allergen avoidance: the Isle of Wight prevention study. *J Allergy Clin Immunol.* 2007 Feb;119(2):307-13.
Arslanoglu S, Moro GE, Schmitt J, Tandoi L, Rizzardi S, Boehm G. Early dietary intervention with a mixture of prebiotic oligosaccharides reduces the incidence of allergic manifestations and infections during the first two years of life. *J Nutr.* 2008 Jun;138(6):1091-5.
Arslanoglu S, Moro GE, Schmitt J, Tandoi L, Rizzardi S, Boehm G. Early dietary intervention with a mixture of prebiotic oligosaccharides reduces the incidence of allergic manifestations and infections during the first two years of life. *J Nutr.* 2008 Jun;138(6):1091-5.
Arterburn LM, Oken HA, Bailey Hall E, Hamersley J, Kuratko CN, Hoffman JP. Algal-oil capsules and cooked salmon: nutritionally equivalent sources of docosahexaenoic acid. *J Am Diet Assoc.* 2008 Jul;108(7):1204-9.
Arterburn LM, Oken HA, Hoffman JP, Bailey-Hall E, Chung G, Rom D, Hamersley J, McCarthy D. Bioequivalence of Docosahexaenoic acid from different algal oils in capsules and in a DHA-fortified food. *Lipids.* 2007 Nov;42(11):1011-24.

REFERENCES AND BIBLIOGRAPHY

Arvaniti F, Priftis KN, Panagiotakos DB. Dietary habits and asthma: a review. *Allergy Asthma Proc.* 2010 Mar;31(2):e1-10.

Asero R, Antonicelli L, Arena A, Bommarito L, Caruso G, Colombo G, Crivellaro M, De Carli M, Della Torre E, Della Torre F, Heffler E, Lodi Rizzini F, Longo G, Manzotti G, Marcotulli M, Melchiorre A, Minale P, Morandi P, Moreni P, Moschella A, Murzilli F, Nebiolo F, Poppa M, Randazzo S, Rossi G, Senna GE. Causes of food-induced anaphylaxis in Italian adults: a multi-centre study. *Int Arch Allergy Immunol.* 2009;150(3):271-7.

Asero R, Mistrello G, Roncarolo D, Amato S, Caldironi G, Barocci F, van Ree R. Immunological cross-reactivity between lipid transfer proteins from botanically unrelated plant-derived foods: a clinical study. *Allergy.* 2002 Oct;57(10):900-6.

Ashrafi K, Chang FY, Watts JL, Fraser AG, Kamath RS, Ahringer J, Ruvkun G. Genome-wide RNAi analysis of Caenorhabditis elegans fat regulatory genes. *Nature.* 2003 Jan 16;421(6920):268-72.

Atkinson W, Harris J, Mills P, Moffat S, White C, Lynch O, Jones M, Cullinan P, Newman Taylor AJ. Domestic aeroallergen exposures among infants in an English town. *Eur Respir J.* 1999 Mar;13(3):583-9.

Atsumi T, Tonosaki K. Smelling lavender and rosemary increases free radical scavenging activity and decreases cortisol level in saliva. *Psychiatry Res.* 2007 Feb 28;150(1):89-96.

Bacopoulou F, Veltsista A, Vassi I, Gika A, Lekea V, Priftis K, Bakoula C. Can we be optimistic about asthma in childhood? A Greek cohort study. *J Asthma.* 2009 Mar;46(2):171-4.

Badar VA, Thawani VR, Wakode PT, Shrivastava MP, Gharpure KJ, Hingorani LL, Khiyani RM. Efficacy of Tinospora cordifolia in allergic rhinitis. *J Ethnopharmacol.* 2005 Jan 15;96(3):445-9.

Bae GS, Kim MS, Jung WS, Seo SW, Yun SW, Kim SG, Park RK, Kim EC, Song HJ, Park SJ. Inhibition of lipopolysaccharide-induced inflammatory responses by piperine. *Eur J Pharmacol.* 2010 Sep 10;642(1-3):154-62.

Bafadhel M, Singapuri A, Terry S, Hargadon B, Monteiro W, Green RH, Bradding PH, Wardlaw AJ, Pavord ID, Brightling CE. Body mass and fat mass in refractory asthma: an observational 1 year follow-up study. *J Allergy.* 2010;2010:251758. 2010 Dec 1.

Baker SM. *Detoxification and Healing.* Chicago: Contemporary Books, 2004.

Bakkeheim E, Mowinckel P, Carlsen KH, Håland G, Carlsen KC. Paracetamol in early infancy: the risk of childhood allergy and asthma. Acta Paediatr. 2011 Jan;100(1):90-6.

Balch P, Balch J. *Prescription for Nutritional Healing.* New York: Avery, 2000.

Ballentine R. *Diet & Nutrition: A holistic approach.* Honesdale, PA: Himalayan Int., 1978.

Ballentine R. *Radical Healing.* New York: Harmony Books, 1999.

Ballmer-Weber BK, Holzhauser T, Scibilia J, Mittag D, Zisa G, Ortolani C, Oesterballe M, Poulsen LK, Vieths S, Bindslev-Jensen C. Clinical characteristics of soybean allergy in Europe: a double-blind, placebo-controlled food challenge study. *J Allergy Clin Immunol.* 2007 Jun;119(6):1489-96.

Ballmer-Weber BK, Vieths S, Lüttkopf D, Heuschmann P, Wüthrich B. Celery allergy confirmed by double-blind, placebo-controlled food challenge: a clinical study in 32 subjects with a history of adverse reactions to celery root. *J Allergy Clin Immunol.* 2000 Aug;106(2):373-8.

Banno N, Akihisa T, Yasukawa K, Tokuda H, Tabata K, Nakamura Y, Nishimura R, Kimura Y, Suzuki T. Anti-inflammatory activities of the triterpene acids from the resin of Boswellia carteri. *J Ethnopharmacol.* 2006 Sep 19;107(2):249-53.

Bant A, Kruszewski J. Increased sensitization prevalence to common inhalant and food allergens in young adult Polish males. *Ann Agric Environ Med.* 2008 Jun;15(1):21-7.

Barnes M, Cullinan P, Athanasaki P, MacNeill S, Hole AM, Harris J, Kalogeraki S, Chatzinikolaou M, Drakonakis N, Bibaki-Liakou V, Newman Taylor AJ, Bibakis I. Crete: does farming explain urban and rural differences in atopy? *Clin Exp Allergy.* 2001 Dec;31(12):1822-8.

Barnetson RS, Drummond H, Ferguson A. Precipitins to dietary proteins in atopic eczema. *Br J Dermatol.* 1983 Dec;109(6):653-5.

Barnett AG, Williams GM, Schwartz J, Neller AH, Best TL, Petroeschevsky AL, Simpson RW. Air pollution and child respiratory health: a case-crossover study in Australia and New Zealand. *Am J Respir Crit Care Med.* 2005 Jun 1;171(11):1272-8.

Barrager E, Veltmann JR Jr, Schauss AG, Schiller RN. A multicentered, open-label trial on the safety and efficacy of methylsulfonylmethane in the treatment of seasonal allergic rhinitis. *J Altern Complement Med.* 2002 Apr;8(2):167-73.

Barros R, Moreira A, Fonseca J, de Oliveira JF, Delgado L, Castel-Branco MG, Haahtela T, Lopes C, Moreira P. Adherence to the Mediterranean diet and fresh fruit intake are associated with improved asthma control. *Allergy.* 2008 Jul;63(7):917-23.

Basu A, Devaraj S, Jialal I. Dietary factors that promote or retard inflammation. *Arterioscler Thromb Vasc Biol.* 2006 May;26(5):995-1001.

Bateman B, Warner JO, Hutchinson E, Dean T, Rowlandson P, Gant C, Grundy J, Fitzgerald T, Stevenson J. The effects of a double blind, placebo controlled, artificial food colourings and benzoate preservative challenge on hyperactivity in a general population sample of preschool children. *Arch Dis Child.* 2004 Jun;89(6):506-11.

Bates DW, Cullen DJ, Laird N, Petersen LA, Small SD, Servi D, Laffel G, Sweitzer BJ, Shea BF, Hallisey R, et al. Incidence of adverse drug events and potential adverse drug events. Implications for prevention. ADE Prevention Study Group. *JAMA*. 1995 Jul 5;274(1):29-34.

Batista R, Martins I, Jeno P, Ricardo CP, Oliveira MM. A proteomic study to identify soya allergens—the human response to transgenic versus non-transgenic soya samples. *Int Arch Allergy Immunol*. 2007;144(1):29-38.

Batmanghelidj F. Neurotransmitter histamine: an alternative view point, *Science in Medicine Simplified*. Falls Church, VA: Foundation for the Simple in Medicine, 1990.

Batmanghelidj F. Pain: a need for paradigm change. *Anticancer Res*. 1987 Sep-Oct;7(5B):971-89.

Batmanghelidj F. *Your Body's Many Cries for Water*. 2nd Ed. Vienna, VA: Global Health, 1997.

Beasley R, Clayton T, Crane J, von Mutius E, Lai CK, Montefort S, Stewart A; ISAAC Phase Three Study Group. Association between paracetamol use in infancy and childhood, and risk of asthma, rhinoconjunctivitis, and eczema in children aged 6-7 years: analysis from Phase Three of the ISAAC programme. *Lancet*. 2008 Sep. 20;372(9643):1039-48.

Beaulieu A, Fessele K. Agent Orange: management of patients exposed in Vietnam. *Clin J Oncol Nurs*. 2003 May-Jun;7(3):320-3.

Becker KG, Simon RM, Bailey-Wilson JE, Freidlin B, Biddison WE, McFarland HF, Trent JM. Clustering of non-major histocompatibility complex susceptibility candidate loci in human autoimmune diseases. *Proc Natl Acad Sci U S A*. 1998 Aug 18;95(17):9979-84.

Beddoe AF. *Biologic Ionization as Applied to Human Nutrition*. Warsaw: Wendell Whitman, 2002.

Beecher GR. Phytonutrients' role in metabolism: effects on resistance to degenerative processes. *Nutr Rev*. 1999 Sep;57(9 Pt 2):S3-6.

Belcaro G, Cesarone MR, Errichi S, Zulli C, Errichi BM, Vinciguerra G, Ledda A, Di Renzo A, Stuard S, Dugall M, Pellegrini L, Gizzi G, Ippolito E, Ricci A, Cacchio M, Cipollone G, Ruffini I, Fano F, Hosoi M, Rohdewald P. Variations in C-reactive protein, plasma free radicals and fibrinogen values in patients with osteoarthritis treated with Pycnogenol. *Redox Rep*. 2008;13(6):271-6.

Bell IR, Baldwin CM, Schwartz GE, Illness from low levels of environmental chemicals: relevance to chronic fatigue syndrome and fibromyalgia. *Am J Med*. 1998;105 (suppl 3A).:74-82. S.

Bell SJ, Potter PC. Milk whey-specific immune complexes in allergic and non-allergic subjects. *Allergy*. 1988 Oct;43(7):497-503.

Ben, X.M., Zhou, X.Y., Zhao, W.H., Yu, W.L., Pan, W., Zhang, W.L., Wu, S.M., Van Beusekom, C.M., Schaafsma, A. (2004) Supplementation of milk formula with galactooligosaccharides improves intestinal micro-flora and fermentation in term infants. *Chin Med J*. 117(6):927-931, 2004.

Benard A, Desreumeaux P, Huglo D, Hoorelbeke A, Tonnel AB, Wallaert B. Increased intestinal permeability in bronchial asthma. *J Allergy Clin Immunol*. 1996 Jun;97(6):1173-8.

Bengmark S. Curcumin, an atoxic antioxidant and natural NFkappaB, cyclooxygenase-2, lipooxygenase, and inducible nitric oxide synthase inhibitor: a shield against acute and chronic diseases. *JPEN J Parenter Enteral Nutr*. 2006 Jan-Feb;30(1):45-51.

Bengmark S. Immunonutrition: role of biosurfactants, fiber, and probiotic bacteria. *Nutrition*. 1998 Jul-Aug;14(7-8):585-94.

Benlounes N, Dupont C, Candalh C, Blaton MA, Darmon N, Desjeux JF, Heyman M. The threshold for immune cell reactivity to milk antigens decreases in cow's milk allergy with intestinal symptoms. *J Allergy Clin Immunol*. 1996 Oct;98(4):781-9.

Bennett WD, Zeman KL, Jarabek AM. Nasal contribution to breathing and fine particle deposition in children versus adults. *J Toxicol Environ Health A*. 2008;71(3):227-37.

Ben-Shoshan M, Harrington DW, Soller L, Fragapane J, Joseph L, St Pierre Y, Godefroy SB, Elliot SJ, Clarke AE. A population-based study on peanut, tree nut, fish, shellfish, and sesame allergy prevalence in Canada. *J Allergy Clin Immunol*. 2010 Jun;125(6):1327-35.

Ben-Shoshan M, Kagan R, Primeau MN, Alizadehfar R, Turnbull E, Harada L, Dufresne C, Allen M, Joseph L, St Pierre Y, Clarke A. Establishing the diagnosis of peanut allergy in children never exposed to peanut or with an uncertain history: a cross-Canada study. *Pediatr Allergy Immunol*. 2010 Sep;21(6):920-6.

Bensky D, Gable A, Kaptchuk T (transl.). *Chinese Herbal Medicine Materia Medica*. Seattle: Eastland Press, 1986.

Bergner P. *The Healing Power of Garlic*. Prima Publishing, Rocklin CA 1996.

Berin MC, Yang PC, Ciok L, Waserman S, Perdue MH. Role for IL-4 in macromolecular transport across human intestinal epithelium. *Am J Physiol*. 1999 May;276(5 Pt 1):C1046-52.

Berkow R., (Ed.) *The Merck Manual of Diagnosis and Therapy*. 16th Edition. Rahway, N.J.: Merck Research Labs, 1992.

Bernstein DI, Epstein T, Murphy-Berendts K, Liss GM. Surveillance of systemic reactions to subcutaneous immunotherapy injections: year 1 outcomes of the ACAAI and AAAAI collaborative study. *Ann Allergy Asthma Immunol*. 2010 Jun;104(6):530-5..

Berseth CL, Mitmesser SH, Ziegler EE, Marunycz JD, Vanderhoof J. Tolerance of a standard intact protein formula versus a partially hydrolyzed formula in healthy, term infants. *Nutr J*. 2009 Jun 19;8:27.

Berteau O and Mulloy B. 2003. Sulfated fucans, fresh perspectives: structures, functions, and biological properties of sulfated fucans and an overview of enzymes active toward this class of polysaccharide. *Glycobiology*. Jun;13(6):29R-40R.

REFERENCES AND BIBLIOGRAPHY

Beyer K, Morrow E, Li XM, Bardina L, Bannon GA, Burks AW, Sampson HA. Effects of cooking methods on peanut allergenicity. *J Allergy Clin Immunol.* 2001;107:1077-81.

Bielory BP, Perez VL, Bielory L. Treatment of seasonal allergic conjunctivitis with ophthalmic corticosteroids: in search of the perfect ocular corticosteroids in the treatment of allergic conjunctivitis. *Curr Opin Allergy Clin Immunol.* 2010 Oct;10(5):469-77.

Bielory L, Lupoli K. Herbal interventions in asthma and allergy. *J Asthma.* 1999;36:1-65.

Bielory L, Russin J, Zuckerman GB. Clinical efficacy, mechanisms of action, and adverse effects of complementary and alternative medicine therapies for asthma. *Allergy Asthma Proc.* 2004;25:283-91.

Bielory L. Complementary and alternative interventions in asthma, allergy, and immunology. *Ann Allergy Asthma Immunol.* 2004 Aug;93(2 Suppl 1):S45-54.

Bindslev-Jensen C, Skov PS, Roggen EL, Hvass P, Brinch DS. Investigation on possible allergenicity of 19 different commercial enzymes used in the food industry. *Food Chem Toxicol.* 2006 Nov;44(11):1909-15.

Birch EE, Khoury JC, Berseth CL, Castañeda YS, Couch JM, Bean J, Tamer R, Harris CL, Mitmesser SH, Scalabrin DM. The impact of early nutrition on incidence of allergic manifestations and common respiratory illnesses in children. *J Pediatr.* 2010 Jun;156(6):902-6, 906.e1. 2010 Mar 15.

Bisgaard H, Loland L, Holst KK, Pipper CB. Prenatal determinants of neonatal lung function in high-risk newborns. *J Allergy Clin Immunol.* 2009 Mar;123(3):651-7, 657.e1-4. 2009 Jan 18.

Bisset N.. *Herbal Drugs and Phytopharmaceuticals.* Stuttgart: CRC, 1994.

Bjarnason I, MacPherson A, Hollander D. Intestinal permeability: an overview. *Gastroenterology.* 1995 May;108(5):1566-81.

Blackhall K, Appleton S, Cates FJ. Ionisers for chronic asthma. *Cochrane Database Syst Rev* 2003;(3):CD002986.

Blood AJ, Zatorre RJ, Bermudez P, Evans AC. Emotional responses to pleasant and unpleasant music correlate with activity in paralimbic brain regions. *Nat Neurosci.* 1999;2:382-7.

Blumenthal M (ed.) *The Complete German Commission E Monographs.* Boston: Amer Botan Council, 1998.

Blumenthal M, Brinckmann J, Goldberg A (eds). *Herbal Medicine: Expanded Commission E Monographs.* Newton, MA: Integrative Med., 2000.

Boccafogli A, Vicentini L, Camerani A, Cogliati P, D'Ambrosi A, Scolozzi R. Adverse food reactions in patients with grass pollen allergic respiratory disease. *Ann Allergy.* 1994 Oct;73(4):301-8.

Bode C, Bode JC. Effect of alcohol consumption on the gut. *Best Pract Res Clin Gastroenterol.* 2003 Aug;17(4):575-92.

Bodinier M, Legoux MA, Pineau F, Triballeau S, Segain JP, Brossard C, Denery-Papini S. Intestinal translocation capabilities of wheat allergens using the Caco-2 cell line. *J Agric Food Chem.* 2007 May 30;55(11):4576-83.

Boehm, G., Lidestri, M., Casetta, P., Jelinek, J., Negretti, F., Stahl, B., Martini, A. (2002) Supplementation of a bovine milk formula with an oligosaccharide mixture increases counts of faecal bifidobacteria in preterm infants. *Arch Dis Child Fetal Neonatal Ed.* 86: F178-F181

Bolhaar ST, Tiemessen MM, Zuidmeer L, van Leeuwen A, Hoffmann-Sommergruber K, Bruijnzeel-Koomen CA, Taams LS, Knol EF, van Hoffen E, van Ree R, Knulst AC. Efficacy of birch-pollen immunotherapy on cross-reactive food allergy confirmed by skin tests and double-blind food challenges. *Clin Exp Allergy.* 2004 May;34(5):761-9.

Bolleddula J, Goldfarb J, Wang R, Sampson H, Li XM. Synergistic Modulation Of Eotaxin And Il-4 Secretion By Constituents Of An Anti-asthma Herbal Formula (ASHMI) In Vitro. *J Allergy Clin Immunol.* 2007;119:S172.

Bonfils P, Halimi P, Malinvaud D. Adrenal suppression and osteoporosis after treatment of nasal polyposis. *Acta Otolaryngol.* 2006 Dec;126(11):1195-200.

Bongaerts GP, Severijnen RS. Preventive and curative effects of probiotics in atopic patients. *Med Hypotheses.* 2005;64(6):1089-92.

Bongartz D, Hesse A. Selective extraction of quercetrin in vegetable drugs and urine by off-line coupling of boronic acid affinity chromatography and high-performance liquid chromatography. *J Chromatogr B Biomed Appl.* 1995 Nov 17;673(2):223-30.

Bonsignore MR, La Grutta S, Cibella F, Scichilone N, Cuttitta G, Interrante A, Marchese M, Veca M, Virzi' M, Bonanno A, Profita M, Morici G. Effects of exercise training and montelukast in children with mild asthma. *Med Sci Sports Exerc.* 2008 Mar;40(3):405-12.

Borchers AT, Hackman RM, Keen CL, Stern JS, Gershwin ME. Complementary medicine: a review of immunomodulatory effects of Chinese herbal medicines. *Am J Clin Nutr.* 1997 Dec;66(6):1303-12.

Borchert VE, Czyborra P, Fetscher C, Goepel M, Michel MC. Extracts from Rhois aromatica and Solidaginis virgaurea inhibit rat and human bladder contraction. *Naunyn Schmiedebergs Arch Pharmacol.* 2004 Mar;369(3):281-6.

Böttcher MF, Jenmalm MC, Voor T, Julge K, Holt PG, Björkstén B. Cytokine responses to allergens during the first 2 years of life in Estonian and Swedish children. *Clin Exp Allergy.* 2006 May;36(5):619-28.

Bottema RW, Kerkhof M, Reijmerink NE, Thijs C, Smit HA, van Schayck CP, Brunekreef B, van Oosterhout AJ, Postma DS, Koppelman GH. Gene-gene interaction in regulatory T-cell function in atopy and asthma development in childhood. *J Allergy Clin Immunol.* 2010 Aug;126(2):338-46, 346.e1-10.

Bouchez-Mahiout I, Pecquet C, Kerre S, Snégaroff J, Raison-Peyron N, Laurière M. High molecular weight entities in industrial wheat protein hydrolysates are immunoreactive with IgE from allergic patients. *J Agric Food Chem.* 2010 Apr 14;58(7):4207-15.

Bougault V, Turmel J, Boulet LP. Bronchial challenges and respiratory symptoms in elite swimmers and winter sport athletes: Airway hyperresponsiveness in asthma: its measurement and clinical significance. *Chest.* 2010 Aug;138(2 Suppl):31S-37S. 2010 Apr 2.

Boyce JA, Assa'ad A, Burks AW, Jones SM, Sampson HA, Wood RA, Plaut M, Cooper SF, Fenton MJ, Arshad SH, Bahna SL, Beck LA, Byrd-Bredbenner C, Camargo CA Jr, Eichenfield L, Furuta GT, Hanifin JM, Jones C, Kraft M, Levy BD, Lieberman P, Luccioli S, McCall KM, Schneider LC, Simon RA, Simons FE, Teach SJ, Yawn BP, Schwaninger JM. Guidelines for the diagnosis and management of food allergy in the United States: report of the NIAID-sponsored expert panel. *J Allergy Clin Immunol.* 2010 Dec;126(6 Suppl):S1-58.

Bråbäck L, Kjellman NI, Sandin A, Björkstén B. Atopy among schoolchildren in northern and southern Sweden in relation to pet ownership and early life events. *Pediatr Allergy Immunol.* 2001 Feb;12(1):4-10.

Bradette-Hébert ME, Legault J, Lavoie S, Pichette A. A new labdane diterpene from the flowers of Solidago canadensis. *Chem Pharm Bull.* 2008 Jan;56(1):82-4.

Brandtzaeg P. The mucosal immune system and its integration with the mammary glands. *J Pediatr.* 2010 Feb;156(2 Suppl):S8-15.

Brehm JM, Schuemann B, Fuhlbrigge AL, Hollis BW, Strunk RC, Zeiger RS, Weiss ST, Litonjua AA; Childhood Asthma Management Program Research Group. Serum vitamin D levels and severe asthma exacerbations in the Childhood Asthma Management Program study. *J Allergy Clin Immunol.* 2010 Jul;126(1):52-8.e5. 2010 Jun 9.

Brighenti F, Valtueña S, Pellegrini N, Ardigò D, Del Rio D, Salvatore S, Piatti P, Serafini M, Zavaroni I. Total antioxidant capacity of the diet is inversely and independently related to plasma concentration of high-sensitivity C-reactive protein in adult Italian subjects. *Br J Nutr.* 2005 May;93(5):619-25.

Brodtkorb TH, Zetterström O, Tinghög G. Cost-effectiveness of clean air administered to the breathing zone in allergic asthma. *Clin Respir J.* 2010 Apr;4(2):104-10.

Brody J. *Jane Brody's Nutrition Book.* New York: WW Norton, 1981.

Broekhuizen BD, Sachs AP, Hoes AW, Moons KG, van den Berg JW, Dalinghaus WH, Lammers E, Verheij TJ. Undetected chronic obstructive pulmonary disease and asthma in people over 50 years with persistent cough. *Br J Gen Pract.* 2010 Jul;60(576):489-94.

Brostoff J, Gamlin L, Brostoff J. *Food Allergies and Food Intolerance: The Complete Guide to Their Identification and Treatment.* Rochester, VT: Healing Arts, 2000.

Brownstein D. *Salt: Your Way to Health.* West Bloomfield, MI: Medical Alternatives, 2006.

Brown-Whitehorn TF, Spergel JM. The link between allergies and eosinophilic esophagitis: implications for management strategies. *Expert Rev Clin Immunol.* 2010 Jan;6(1):101-9.

Bruce S, Nyberg F, Melén E, James A, Pulkkinen V, Orsmark-Pietras C, Bergström A, Dahlén B, Wickman M, von Mutius E, Doekes G, Lauener R, Riedler J, Eder W, van Hage M, Pershagen G, Scheynius A, Kere J. The protective effect of farm animal exposure on childhood allergy is modified by NPSR1 polymorphisms. *J Med Genet.* 2009 Mar;46(3):159-67. 2008 Feb 19.

Bruneton J. *Pharmacognosy, Phytochemistry, Medicinal Plants.* Paris: Lavoisier, 1995.

Bruton A, Lewith GT. The Buteyko breathing technique for asthma: a review. *Complement Ther Med.* 2005 Mar;13(1):41-6. 2005 Apr 18.

Bruton A, Thomas M. The role of breathing training in asthma management. *Curr Opin Allergy Clin Immunol.* 2011 Feb;11(1):53-7.

Bublin M, Pfister M, Radauer C, Oberhuber C, Bulley S, Dewitt AM, Lidholm J, Reese G, Vieths S, Breiteneder H, Hoffmann-Sommergruber K, Ballmer-Weber BK. Component-resolved diagnosis of kiwifruit allergy with purified natural and recombinant kiwifruit allergens. *J Allergy Clin Immunol.* 2010 Mar;125(3):687-94, 694.e1.

Buchanan TW, Lutz K, Mirzazade S, Specht K, Shah NJ, Zilles K, et al. Recognition of emotional prosody and verbal components of spoken language: an fMRI study. *Cogn Brain Res.* 2000;9:227-38.

Bucher X, Pichler WJ, Dahinden CA, Helbling A. Effect of tree pollen specific, subcutaneous immunotherapy on the oral allergy syndrome to apple and hazelnut. *Allergy.* 2004 Dec;59(12):1272-6.

Budzianowski J. Coumarins, caffeoyltartaric acids and their artifactual methyl esters from Taraxacum officinale leaves. *Planta Med.* 1997 Jun;63(3):288.

REFERENCES AND BIBLIOGRAPHY

Bueso AK, Berntsen S, Mowinckel P, Andersen LF, Lødrup Carlsen KC, Carlsen KH. Dietary intake in adolescents with asthma - potential for improvement. *Pediatr Allergy Immunol.* 2010 Oct 20. doi: 10.1111/j.1399-3038.2010.01013.x.

Bundy R, Walker AF, Middleton RW, Booth J. Turmeric extract may improve irritable bowel syndrome symptomology in otherwise healthy adults: a pilot study. *J Altern Complement Med.* 2004 Dec;10(6):1015-8.

Burdge GC, Jones AE, Wootton SA. Eicosapentaenoic and docosapentaenoic acids are the principal products of alpha-linolenic acid metabolism in young men. *B J Nutr.* 2002 Oct;88(4):355-63.

Buret AG. How stress induces intestinal hypersensitivity. *Am J Pathol.* 2006 Jan;168(1):3-5.

Burgess CD, Bremner P, Thomson CD, Crane J, Siebers RW, Beasley R. Nebulized beta 2-adrenoceptor agonists do not affect plasma selenium or glutathione peroxidase activity in patients with asthma. *Int J Clin Pharmacol Ther.* 1994 Jun;32(6):290-2.

Burks W, Jones SM, Berseth CL, Harris C, Sampson HA, Scalabrin DM. Hypoallergenicity and effects on growth and tolerance of a new amino acid-based formula with docosahexaenoic acid and arachidonic acid. *J Pediatr.* 2008 Aug;153(2):266-71.

Burney PG, Luczynska C, Chinn S, Jarvis D. The European Community Respiratory Health Survey. *Eur Respir J.* 1994;7: 954-960.

Burr ML, Butland BK, King S, Vaughan-Williams E. Changes in asthma prevalence: two surveys 15 years apart. *Arch Dis Child.* 1989;64:1452-1456.

Busse PJ, Wen MC, Huang CK, Srivastava K, Zhang TF, Schofield B, Sampson HA, Li XM. Therapeutic effects of the Chinese herbal formula, MSSM-03d, on persistent airway hyperreactivity and airway remodeling. *J Allergy Clin Immunol.* 2004;113:S220.

Byrne AM, Malka-Rais J, Burks AW, Fleischer DM. How do we know when peanut and tree nut allergy have resolved, and how do we keep it resolved? *Clin Exp Allergy.* 2010 Sep;40(9):1303-11.

Cabanillas B, Pedrosa MM, Rodríguez J, González A, Muzquiz M, Cuadrado C, Crespo JF, Burbano C. Effects of enzymatic hydrolysis on lentil allergenicity. *Mol Nutr Food Res.* 2010 Mar 19.

Caglar E, Kavaloglu SC, Kuscu OO, Sandalli N, Holgerson PL, Twetman S. Effect of chewing gums containing xylitol or probiotic bacteria on salivary mutans streptococci and lactobacilli. *Clin Oral Investig.* 2007 Dec;11(4):425-9.

Caglar E, Kuscu OO, Cildir SK, Kuvvetli SS, Sandalli N. A probiotic lozenge administered medical device and its effect on salivary mutans streptococci and lactobacilli. *Int J Paediatr Dent.* 2008 Jan;18(1):35-9.

Caglar E, Kuscu OO, Selvi Kuvvetli S, Kavaloglu Cildir S, Sandalli N, Twetman S. Short-term effect of ice-cream containing *Bifidobacterium lactis* Bb-12 on the number of salivary mutans streptococci and lactobacilli. *Acta Odontol Scand.* 2008 Jun;66(3):154-8.

Calder PC. Dietary modification of inflammation with lipids. *Proc Nutr Soc.* 2002 Aug;61(3):345-58.

Camargo CA Jr, Ingham T, Wickens K, Thadhani R, Silvers KM, Epton MJ, Town GI, Pattemore PK, Espinola JA, Crane J; New Zealand Asthma and Allergy Cohort Study Group. Cord-blood 25-hydroxyvitamin D levels and risk of respiratory infection, wheezing, and asthma. *Pediatrics.* 2011 Jan;127(1):e180-7.

Caminiti L, Passalacqua G, Barberi S, Vita D, Barberio G, De Luca R, Pajno GB. A new protocol for specific oral tolerance induction in children with IgE-mediated cow's milk allergy. *Allergy Asthma Proc.* 2009 Jul-Aug;30(4):443-8.

Campbell TC, Campbell TM. *The China Study.* Dallas, TX: Benbella Books, 2006.

Canali R, Comitato R, Schonlau F, Virgili F. The anti-inflammatory pharmacology of Pycnogenol in humans involves COX-2 and 5-LOX mRNA expression in leukocytes. *Int Immunopharmacol.* 2009 Sep;9(10):1145-9.

Canonica GW, Passalacqua G. Noninjection routes for immunotherapy. *J Allergy Clin Immunol.* 2003 Mar;111(3):437-48; quiz 449.

Cantani A, Micera M. Natural history of cow's milk allergy. An eight-year follow-up study in 115 atopic children. *Eur Rev Med Pharmacol Sci.* 2004 Jul-Aug;8(4):153-64.

Cantani A, Micera M. The prick by prick test is safe and reliable in 58 children with atopic dermatitis and food allergy. *Eur Rev Med Pharmacol Sci.* 2006 May-Jun;10(3):115-20.

Cao G, Alessio HM, Cutler RG. Oxygen-radical absorbance capacity assay for antioxidants. *Free Radic Biol Med.* 1993 Mar;14(3):303-11.

Cao G, Shukitt-Hale B, Bickford PC, Joseph JA, McEwen J, Prior RL. Hyperoxia-induced changes in antioxidant capacity and the effect of dietary antioxidants. *J Appl Physiol.* 1999 Jun;86(6):1817-22.

Caramia G. The essential fatty acids omega-6 and omega-3: from their discovery to their use in therapy. *Minerva Pediatr.* 2008 Apr;60(2):219-33.

Carey DG, Aase KA, Pliego GJ. The acute effect of cold air exercise in determination of exercise-induced bronchospasm in apparently healthy athletes. J Strength Cond Res. 2010 Aug;24(8):2172-8.

Carroccio A, Cavataio F, Montalto G, D'Amico D, Alabrese L, Iacono G. Intolerance to hydrolysed cow's milk proteins in infants: clinical characteristics and dietary treatment. *Clin Exp Allergy.* 2000 Nov;30(11):1597-603.

Carroll D. *The Complete Book of Natural Medicines.* New York: Summit, 1980.

Caruso M, Frasca G, Di Giuseppe PL, Pennisi A, Tringali G, Bonina FP. Effects of a new nutraceutical ingredient on allergen-induced sulphidoleukotrienes production and CD63 expression in allergic subjects. *Int Immunopharmacol.* 2008 Dec 20;8(13-14):1781-6.

Casale TB, Amin BV. Allergic rhinitis/asthma interrelationship. *Clin Rev Allergy Immunol.* 2001;21:27-49.

Cats A, Kuipers EJ, Bosschaert MA, Pot RG, Vandenbroucke-Grauls CM, Kusters JG. Effect of frequent consumption of a Lactobacillus casei-containing milk drink in Helicobacter pylori-colonized subjects. *Aliment Pharmacol Ther.* 2003 Feb;17(3):429-35.

Caughey AB, Nicholson JM, Cheng YW, Lyell DJ, Washington AE. Induction of labor and Cesarean delivery by gestational age. *Am J Obstet Gynecol.* 2006 Sep;195(3):700-5.

Celakovská J, Vaněcková J, Ettlerová K, Ettler K, Bukac J. The role of atopy patch test in diagnosis of food allergy in atopic eczema/dermatitis syndrom in patients over 14 years of age. *Acta Medica (Hradec Kralove).* 2010;53(2):101-8.

Celikel S, Karakaya G, Yurtsever N, Sorkun K, Kalyoncu AF. Bee and bee products allergy in Turkish beekeepers: determination of risk factors for systemic reactions. *Allergol Immunopathol (Madr).* 2006 Sep-Oct;34(5):180-4.

Centers for Disease Control and Prevention (CDC). Obesity prevalence among low-income, preschool-aged children - United States, 1998-2008. *MMWR Morb Mortal Wkly Rep.* 2009 Jul 24;58(28):769-73.

Centers for Disease Control and Prevention (CDC). Vital signs: nonsmokers' exposure to secondhand smoke - United States, 1999-2008. *MMWR Morb Mortal Wkly Rep.* 2010 Sep 10;59(35):1141-6.

Centre for Molecular, Environmental, Genetic and Analytic Epidemiology, School of Population Health, The UniverGumowski P, Lech B, Chaves I, Girard JP. Chronic asthma and rhinitis due to Candida albicans, epidermophyton, and trichophyton. *Ann Allergy.* 1987 Jul;59(1):48-51.

Cereijido M, Contreras RG, Flores-Benítez D, Flores-Maldonado C, Larre I, Ruiz A, Shoshani L. New diseases derived or associated with the tight junction. *Arch Med Res.* 2007 Jul;38(5):465-78.

Chafen JJ, Newberry SJ, Riedl MA, Bravata DM, Maglione M, Suttorp MJ, Sundaram V, Paige NM, Towfigh A, Hulley BJ, Shekelle PG. Diagnosing and managing common food allergies: a systematic review. *JAMA.* 2010 May 12;303(18):1848-56.

Chahine BG, Bahna SL. The role of the gut mucosal immunity in the development of tolerance versus development of allergy to food. *Curr Opin Allergy Clin Immunol.* 2010 Aug;10(4):394-9.

Chaitow L, Trenev N. *Probiotics.* New York: Thorsons, 1990.

Chaitow L. *Conquer Pain the Natural Way.* San Francisco: Chronicle Books, 2002.

Chakürski I, Matev M, Koïchev A, Angelova I, Stefanov G. Treatment of chronic colitis with an herbal combination of Taraxacum officinale, Hipericum perforatum, Melissa officinaliss, Calendula officinalis and Foeniculum vulgare. *Vutr Boles.* 1981;20(6):51-4.

Chan CK, Kuo ML, Shen JJ, See LC, Chang HH, Huang JL. Ding Chuan Tang, a Chinese herb decoction, could improve airway hyperresponsiveness in stabilized asthmatic children: a randomized, double-blind clinical trial. *Pediatr Allergy Immunol.* 2006;17:316-22.

Chandra RK. Prospective studies of the effect of breast feeding on incidence of infection and allergy. *Acta Paediatr Scand.* 1979 Sep;68(5):691-4.

Chaney M, Ross M. *Nutrition.* New York: Houghton Mifflin, 1971.

Chang HT, Tseng LJ, Hung TJ, Kao BT, Lin WY, Fan TC, Chang MD, Pai TW. Inhibition of the interactions between eosinophil cationic protein and airway epithelial cells by traditional Chinese herbs. *BMC Syst Biol.* 2010 Sep 13;4 Suppl 2:S8.

Chang TT, Huang CC, Hsu CH. Clinical evaluation of the Chinese herbal medicine formula STA-1 in the treatment of allergic asthma. *Phytother Res.* 2006;20:342-7.

Chang TT, Huang CC, Hsu CH. Inhibition of mite-induced immunoglobulin E synthesis, airway inflammation, and hyperreactivity by herbal medicine STA-1. *Immunopharmacol Immunotoxicol.* 2006;28:683-95.

Chao A, Thun MJ, Connell CJ, McCullough ML, Jacobs EJ, Flanders WD, Rodriguez C, Sinha R, Calle EE. Meat consumption and risk of colorectal cancer. *JAMA.* 2005 Jan 12;293(2):172-82.

Characterization and quantitation of Antioxidant Constituents of Sweet Pepper (Capsicum annuum - Cayenne). *J Agric Food Chem.* 2004 Jun 16;52(12):3861-9.

Chatzi L, Apostolaki G, Bibakis I, Skypala I, Bibaki-Liakou V, Tzanakis N, Kogevinas M, Cullinan P. Protective effect of fruits, vegetables and the Mediterranean diet on asthma and allergies among children in Crete. *Thorax.* 2007 Aug;62(8):677-83.

Chatzi L, Torrent M, Romieu I, Garcia-Esteban R, Ferrer C, Vioque J, Kogevinas M, Sunyer J. Mediterranean diet in pregnancy is protective for wheeze and atopy in childhood. *Thorax.* 2008 Jun;63(6):507-13.

Chaves TC, de Andrade e Silva TS, Monteiro SA, Watanabe PC, Oliveira AS, Grossi DB. Craniocervical posture and hyoid bone position in children with mild and moderate asthma and mouth breathing. *Int J Pediatr Otorhinolaryngol.* 2010 Sep;74(9):1021-7.

Chehade M, Aceves SS. Food allergy and eosinophilic esophagitis. *Curr Opin Allergy Clin Immunol.* 2010 Jun;10(3):231-7.

REFERENCES AND BIBLIOGRAPHY

Chellini E, Talassi F, Corbo G, Berti G, De Sario M, Rusconi F, Piffer S, Caranci N, Petronio MG, Sestini P, Dell'Orco V, Bonci E, Armenio L, La Grutta S; Gruppo Collaborativo SIDRIA-2. Environmental, social and demographic characteristics of children and adolescents, resident in different Italian areas. *Epidemiol Prev.* 2005 Mar-Apr;29(2 Suppl):14-23.

Chen HJ, Shih CK, Hsu HY, Chiang W. Mast cell-dependent allergic responses are inhibited by ethanolic extract of adlay (Coix lachryma-jobi L. var. ma-yuen Stapf) testa. *J Agric Food Chem.* 2010 Feb 24;58(4):2596-601.

Chen JX, Ji B, Lu ZL, Hu LS. Effects of chai hu (radix burpleuri) containing formulation on plasma beta-endorphin, epinephrine and dopamine on patients. *Am J Chin Med.* 2005;33(5):737-45.

Chen Y, Blaser MJ. Helicobacter pylori colonization is inversely associated with childhood asthma. *J Infect Dis.* 2008 Aug 15;198(4):553-60.

Chen Y, Blaser MJ. Inverse associations of Helicobacter pylori with asthma and allergy. *Arch Intern Med.* 2007 Apr 23;167(8):821-7.

Cheney G, Waxler SH, Miller IJ. Vitamin U therapy of peptic ulcer; experience at San Quentin Prison. *Calif Med.* 1956 Jan;84(1):39-42.

Chevallier A. *Encyclopedia of Medicinal Plants.* New York, NY: DK Publishing; 1996.

Chevrier MR, Ryan AE, Lee DY, Zhongze M, Wu-Yan Z, Via CS. Boswellia carterii extract inhibits TH1 cytokines and promotes TH2 cytokines in vitro. *Clin Diagn Lab Immunol.* 2005 May;12(5):575-80.

Chilton FH, Rudel LL, Parks JS, Arm JP, Seeds MC. Mechanisms by which botanical lipids affect inflammatory disorders. *Am J Clin Nutr.* 2008 Feb;87(2):498S-503S.

Chilton FH, Tucker L. *Win the War Within.* New York: Rodale, 2006.

Chin A Paw MJ, de Jong N, Pallast EG, Kloek GC, Schouten EG, Kok FJ. Immunity in frail elderly: a randomized controlled trial of exercise and enriched foods. *Med Sci Sports Exerc.* 2000 Dec;32(12):2005-11.

Choi BW, Yoo KH, Jeong JW, Yoon HJ, Kim SH, Park YM, Kim WK, Oh JW, Rha YH, Pyun BY, Chang SI, Moon HB, Kim YY, Cho SH. Easy diagnosis of asthma: computer-assisted, symptom-based diagnosis. *J Korean Med Sci.* 2007 Oct;22(5):832-8.

Choi SY, Sohn JH, Lee YW, Lee EK, Hong CS, Park JW. Characterization of buckwheat 19-kD allergen and its application for diagnosing clinical reactivity. *Int Arch Allergy Immunol.* 2007;144(4):267-74.

Choi SZ, Choi SU, Lee KR. Phytochemical constituents of the aerial parts from Solidago virga-aurea var. gigantea. *Arch Pharm Res.* 2004 Feb;27(2):164-8.

Chong Neto HJ, Rosário NA; Grupo EISL Curitiba (Estudio Internacional de Sibilancias en Lactantes). Risk factors for wheezing in the first year of life. *J Pediatr.* 2008 Nov-Dec;84(6):495-502.

Chopra RN, Nayar SL, Chopra IC, eds. *Glossary of Indian Medicinal plants.* New Delhi: CSIR, 1956.

Choudhry S, Seibold MA, Borrell LN, Tang H, Serebrisky D, Chapela R, Rodriguez-Santana JR, Avila PC, Ziv E, Rodriguez-Cintron W, Risch NJ, Burchard EG. Dissecting complex diseases in complex populations: asthma in latino americans. *Proc Am Thorac Soc.* 2007 Jul;4(3):226-33.

Christopher JR. *School of Natural Healing.* Springville UT: Christopher Publ, 1976.

Chu YF, Liu RH. Cranberries inhibit LDL oxidation and induce LDL receptor expression in hepatocytes. *Life Sci.* 2005;77(15):1892-1901. 27.

Chung SY, Butts CL, Maleki SJ, Champagne ET Linking peanut allergenicity to the processes of maturation, curing, and roasting. *J Agric Food Chem.* 2003;51: 4273-4277.

Cibella F, Cuttitta G. Nocturnal asthma and gastroesophageal reflux. *Am J Med.* 2001 Dec 3;111 Suppl 8A:31S-36S.

Cingi C, Demirbas D, Songu M. Allergic rhinitis caused by food allergies. *Eur Arch Otorhinolaryngol.* 2010 Sep;267(9):1327-35.

Cisneros C, García-Río F, Romera D, Villasante C, Girón R, Ancochea J. Bronchial reactivity indices are determinants of health-related quality of life in patients with stable asthma. *Thorax.* 2010 Sep;65(9):795-800.

Clark S, Bock SA, Gaeta TJ, Brenner BE, Cydulka RK, Camargo CA; Multicenter Airway Research Collaboration-8 Investigators. Multicenter study of emergency department visits for food allergies. *J Allergy Clin Immunol.* 2004 Feb;113(2):347-52.

Clement YN, Williams AF, Aranda D, Chase R, Watson N, Mohammed R, Stubbs O, Williamson D. Medicinal herb use among asthmatic patients attending a specialty care facility in Trinidad. *BMC Complement Altern Med.* 2005 Feb 15;5:3.

Cobo Sanz JM, Mateos JA, Muñoz Conejo A. Effect of *Lactobacillus casei* on the incidence of infectious conditions in children. *Nutr Hosp.* 2006 Jul-Aug;21(4):547-51.

Codispoti CD, Levin L, LeMasters GK, Ryan P, Reponen T, Villareal M, Burkle J, Stanforth S, Lockey JE, Khurana Hershey GK, Bernstein DI. Breast-feeding, aeroallergen sensitization, and environmental exposures during infancy are determinants of childhood allergic rhinitis. *J Allergy Clin Immunol.* 2010 May;125(5):1054-1060.e1.

Cohen A, Goldberg M, Levy B, Leshno M, Katz Y. Sesame food allergy and sensitization in children: the natural history and long-term follow-up. *Pediatr Allergy Immunol.* 2007 May;18(3):217-23.

Cohen RT, Raby BA, Van Steen K, Fuhlbrigge AL, Celedón JC, Rosner BA, Strunk RC, Zeiger RS, Weiss ST; Childhood Asthma Management Program Research Group. In utero smoke exposure and impaired response to inhaled corticosteroids in children with asthma. *J Allergy Clin Immunol.* 2010 Sep;126(3):491-7. 2010 Jul 31.;.

Collipp PJ, Goldzier S 3rd, Weiss N, Soleymani Y, Snyder R. Pyridoxine treatment of childhood bronchial asthma. *Ann Allergy.* 1975 Aug;35(2):93-7.

Conquer JA, Holub BJ. Dietary docosahexaenoic acid as a source of eicosapentaenoic acid in vegetarians and omnivores. *Lipids.* 1997 Mar;32(3):341-5.

Cooper GS, Miller FW, Germolec DR: Occupational exposures and autoimmune diseases. *Int Immunopharm* 2002, 2:303-313.

Cooper K. *The Aerobics Program for Total Well-Being.* New York: Evans, 1980.

Corbe C, Boissin JP, Siou A. Light vision and chorioretinal circulation. Study of the effect of procyanidolic oligomers (Endotelon). *J Fr Ophtalmol.* 1988;11(5):453-60.

Corbo GM, Forastiere F, De Sario M, Brunetti L, Bonci E, Bugiani M, Chellini E, La Grutta S, Migliore E, Pistelli R, Rusconi F, Russo A, Simoni M, Talassi F, Galassi C; Sidria-2 Collaborative Group. Wheeze and asthma in children: associations with body mass index, sports, television viewing, and diet. *Epidemiology.* 2008 Sep;19(5):747-55.

Cory S, Ussery-Hall A, Griffin-Blake S, Easton A, Vigeant J, Balluz L, Garvin W, Greenlund K; Centers for Disease Control and Prevention (CDC). Prevalence of selected risk behaviors and chronic diseases and conditions-steps communities, United States, 2006-2007. *MMWR Surveill Summ.* 2010 Sep 24;59(8):1-37.

Courtney R, Cohen M. Investigating the claims of Konstantin Buteyko, M.D., Ph.D.: the relationship of breath holding time to end tidal CO_2 and other proposed measures of dysfunctional breathing. *J Altern Complement Med.* 2008 Mar;14(2):115-23.

Couzy F, Kastenmayer P, Vigo M, Clough J, Munoz-Box R, Barclay DV. Calcium bioavailability from a calcium- and sulfate-rich mineral water, compared with milk, in young adult women. *Am J Clin Nutr.* 1995 Dec;62(6):1239-44.

Covar R, Gleason M, Macomber B, Stewart L, Szefler P, Engelhardt K, Murphy J, Liu A, Wood S, DeMichele S, Gelfand EW, Szefler SJ. Impact of a novel nutritional formula on asthma control and biomarkers of allergic airway inflammation in children. *Clin Exp Allergy.* 2010 Aug;40(8):1163-74. 2010 Jun 7.

Crane J, Ellis I, Siebers R, Grimmet D, Lewis S, Fitzharris P. A pilot study of the effect of mechanical ventilation and heat exchange on house-dust mites and Der p 1 in New Zealand homes. *Allergy.* 1998 Aug;53(8):755-62.

Crescente M, Jessen G, Momi S, Höltje HD, Gresele P, Cerletti C, de Gaetano G. Interactions of gallic acid, resveratrol, quercetin and aspirin at the platelet cyclooxygenase-1 level. Functional and modelling studies. *Thromb Haemost.* 2009 Aug;102(2):336-46.

Crinnion WJ. Toxic effects of the easily avoidable phthalates and parabens. *Altern Med Rev.* 2010 Sep;15(3):190-6.

Cserhati E. Current view on the etiology of childhood bronchial asthma. *Orv Hetil.* 2000;141:759-760.

Cuesta-Herranz J, Barber D, Blanco C, Cistero-Bahíma A, Crespo JF, Fernández-Rivas M, Fernández-Sánchez J, Florido JF, Ibáñez MD, Rodríguez R, Salcedo G, Garcia BE, Lombardero M, Quiralte J, Rodriguez J, Sánchez-Monge R, Vereda A, Villalba M, Alonso Díaz de Durana MD, Basagaña M, Carrillo T, Fernández-Nieto M, Tabar AI. Differences among Pollen-Allergic Patients with and without Plant Food Allergy. *Int Arch Allergy Immunol.* 2010 Apr 23;153(2):182-192.

Cummings M. *Human Heredity: Principles and Issues.* St. Paul, MN: West, 1988.

Custovic A, Simpson BM, Simpson A, Kissen P, Woodcock A; NAC Manchester Asthma and Allergy Study Group. Effect of environmental manipulation in pregnancy and early life on respiratory symptoms and atopy during first year of life: a randomised trial. *Lancet.* 2001 Jul 21;358(9277):188-93.

Dallinga JW, Robroeks CM, van Berkel JJ, Moonen EJ, Godschalk RW, Jöbsis Q, Dompeling E, Wouters EF, van Schooten FJ. Volatile organic compounds in exhaled breath as a diagnostic tool for asthma in children. Clin Exp Allergy. 2010 Jan;40(1):68-76.

D'Anneo RW, Bruno ME, Falagiani P. Sublingual allergoid immunotherapy: a new 4-day induction phase in patients allergic to house dust mites. *Int J Immunopathol Pharmacol.* 2010 Apr-Jun;23(2):553-60.

D'Auria E, Sala M, Lodi F, Radaelli G, Riva E, Giovannini M. Nutritional value of a rice-hydrolysate formula in infants with cows' milk protein allergy: a randomized pilot study. *J Int Med Res.* 2003 May-Jun;31(3):215-22.

Davidson T. *Rhinology: The Collected Writings of Maurice H. Cottle, M.D.* San Diego, CA: American Rhinologic Society, 1987.

Davies G. *Timetables of Medicine.* New York: Black Dog & Leventhal, 2000.

Davin JC, Forget P, Mahieu PR. Increased intestinal permeability to (51 Cr) EDTA is correlated with IgA immune complex-plasma levels in children with IgA-associated nephropathies. *Acta Paediatr Scand.* 1988 Jan;77(1):118-24.

de Boissieu D, Dupont C, Badoual J. Allergy to nondairy proteins in mother's milk as assessed by intestinal permeability tests. *Allergy.* 1994 Dec;49(10):882-4.

de Boissieu D, Matarazzo P, Rocchiccioli F, Dupont C. Multiple food allergy: a possible diagnosis in breastfed infants. *Acta Paediatr.* 1997 Oct;86(10):1042-6.

De Lucca AJ, Bland JM, Vigo CB, Cushion M, Selitrennikoff CP, Peter J, Walsh TJ. CAY-I, a fungicidal saponin from Capsicum sp. fruit. *Med Mycol.* 2002 Apr;40(2):131-7.

REFERENCES AND BIBLIOGRAPHY

de Martino M, Novembre E, Galli L, de Marco A, Botarelli P, Marano E, Vierucci A. Allergy to different fish species in cod-allergic children: in vivo and in vitro studies. *J Allergy Clin Immunol.* 1990;86:909-914.

De Smet PA. Herbal remedies. *N Engl J Med.* 2002;347:2046-2056.

Dean C. *Death by Modern Medicine.* Belleville, ON: Matrix Verite-Media, 2005.

Debley JS, Carter ER, Redding GJ. Prevalence and impact of gastroesophageal reflux in adolescents with asthma: a population-based study. *Pediatr Pulmonol.* 2006 May;41(5):475-81.

Dehlink E, Yen E, Leichtner AM, Hait EJ, Fiebiger E. First evidence of a possible association between gastric acid suppression during pregnancy and childhood asthma: a population-based register study. *Clin Exp Allergy.* 2009 Feb;39(2):246-53. 2008 Dec 9.

del Giudice MM, Leonardi S, Maiello N, Brunese FP. Food allergy and probiotics in childhood. *J Clin Gastroenterol.* 2010 Sep;44 Suppl 1:S22-5.

Delacourt C. Bronchial changes in untreated asthma. *Arch Pediatr.* 2004 Jun;11 Suppl 2:71s-73s.

Del-Rio-Navarro B, Berber A, Blandón-Vijil V, Ramírez-Aguilar M, Romieu I, Ramírez-Chanona N, Heras-Acevedo S, Serrano-Sierra A, Barraza-Villareal A, Baeza-Bacab M, Sienra-Monge JJ. Identification of asthma risk factors in Mexico City in an International Study of Asthma and Allergy in Childhood survey. *Allergy Asthma Proc.* 2006 Jul-Aug;27(4):325-33.

Dengate S, Ruben A. Controlled trial of cumulative behavioural effects of a common bread preservative. *J Paediatr Child Health.* 2002 Aug;38(4):373-6.

Dente FL, Bacci E, Bartoli ML, Cianchetti S, Costa F, Di Franco A, Malagrinò L, Vagaggini B, Paggiaro P. Effects of oral prednisone on sputum eosinophils and cytokines in patients with severe refractory asthma. *Ann Allergy Asthma Immunol.* 2010 Jun;104(6):464-70.

Derebery MJ, Berliner KI. Allergy and its relation to Meniere's disease. *Otolaryngol Clin North Am.* 2010 Oct;43(5):1047-58.

Desjeux JF, Heyman M. Milk proteins, cytokines and intestinal epithelial functions in children. *Acta Paediatr Jpn.* 1994 Oct;36(5):592-6.

DesRoches A, Infante-Rivard C, Paradis L, Paradis J, Haddad E. Peanut allergy: is maternal transmission of antigens during pregnancy and breastfeeding a risk factor? *J Investig Allergol Clin Immunol.* 2010;20(4):289-94.

Deutsche Gesellschaft für Ernährung. Drink distilled water? *Med. Mo. Pharm.* 1993;16:146.

Devaraj TL. *Speaking of Ayurvedic Remedies for Common Diseases.* New Delhi: Sterling, 1985.

Devirgiliis C, Zalewski PD, Perozzi G, Murgia C. Zinc fluxes and zinc transporter genes in chronic diseases. *Mutat Res.* 2007 Sep 1;622(1-2):84-93. 2007 Feb 17.

Dharmage SC, Erbas B, Jarvis D, Wjst M, Raherison C, Norbäck D, Heinrich J, Sunyer J, Svanes C. Do childhood respiratory infections continue to influence adult respiratory morbidity? *Eur Respir J.* 2009 Feb;33(2):237-44.

Di Gioacchino M, Cavallucci E, Di Stefano F, Paolini F, Ramondo S, Di Sciascio MB, Ciuffreda S, Riccioni G, Della Vecchia R, Romano A, Boscolo P. Effect of natural allergen exposure on non-specific bronchial reactivity in asthmatic farmers. *Sci Total Environ.* 2001 Apr 10;270(1-3):43-8.

Di Gioacchino M, Cavallucci E, Di Stefano F, Verna N, Ramondo S, Ciuffreda S, Riccioni G, Boscolo P. Influence of total IgE and seasonal increase of eosinophil cationic protein on bronchial hyperreactivity in asthmatic grass-sensitized farmers. *Allergy.* 2000 Nov;55(11):1030-4.

Di Marco F, Santus P, Centanni S. Anxiety and depression in asthma. *Curr Opin Pulm Med.* 2011 Jan;17(1):39-44.

Dierksen KP, Moore CJ, Inglis M, Wescombe PA, Tagg JR. The effect of ingestion of milk supplemented with salivaricin A-producing Streptococcus salivarius on the bacteriocin-like inhibitory activity of streptococcal populations on the tongue. *FEMS Microbiol Ecol.* 2007 Mar;59(3):584-91.

Diğrak M, Ilçim A, Hakki Alma M. Antimicrobial activities of several parts of Pinus brutia, Juniperus oxycedrus, Abies cilicia, Cedrus libani and Pinus nigra. *Phytother Res.* 1999 Nov;13(7):584-7.

DiMango E, Holbrook JT, Simpson E, Reibman J, Richter J, Narula S, Prusakowski N, Mastronarde JG, Wise RA; American Lung Association Asthma Clinical Research Centers. Effects of asymptomatic proximal and distal gastroesophageal reflux on asthma severity. *Am J Respir Crit Care Med.* 2009 Nov 1;180(9):809-16. 2009 Aug 6.

Din FV, Theodoratou E, Farrington SM, Tenesa A, Barnetson RA, Cetnarskyj R, Stark L, Porteous ME, Campbell H, Dunlop MG. Effect of aspirin and NSAIDs on risk and survival from colorectal cancer. *Gut.* 2010 Dec;59(12):1670-9.

Diop L, Guillou S, Durand H. Probiotic food supplement reduces stress-induced gastrointestinal symptoms in volunteers: a double-blind, placebo-controlled, randomized trial. *Nutr Res.* 2008 Jan;28(1):1-5.

Dixon AE, Kaminsky DA, Holbrook JT, Wise RA, Shade DM, Irvin CG. Allergic rhinitis and sinusitis in asthma: differential effects on symptoms and pulmonary function. *Chest.* 2006 Aug;130(2):429-35.

Dona A, Arvanitoyannis IS. Health risks of genetically modified foods. *Crit Rev Food Sci Nutr.* 2009 Feb;49(2):164-75.

Donato F, Monarca S, Premi S., and Gelatti, U. Drinking water hardness and chronic degenerative diseases. Part III. Tumors, urolithiasis, fetal malformations, deterioration of the cognitive function in the aged and atopic eczema. *Ann. Ig.* 2003;15:57-70.

Dooley, M.A. and Hogan S.L. Environmental epidemiology and risk factors for autoimmune disease. *Curr Opin Rheum.* 2003;15(2):99-103.
D'Orazio N, Ficoneri C, Riccioni G, Conti P, Theoharides TC, Bollea MR. Conjugated linoleic acid: a functional food? *Int J Immunopathol Pharmacol.* 2003 Sep-Dec;16(3):215-20.
dos Santos LH, Ribeiro IO, Sánchez PG, Hetzel JL, Felicetti JC, Cardoso PF. Evaluation of pantoprazol treatment response of patients with asthma and gastroesophageal reflux: a randomized prospective double-blind placebo-controlled study. *J Bras Pneumol.* 2007 Apr;33(2):119-27.
Dotolo Institute. *The Study of Colon Hydrotherapy.* Pinellas Park, FL: Dotolo, 2003.
Dove MS, Dockery DW, Connolly GN. Smoke-free air laws and asthma prevalence, symptoms, and severity among nonsmoking youth. *Pediatrics.* 2011 Jan;127(1):102-9. 2010 Dec 13.
Dowd JB, Zajacova A, Aiello A. Early origins of health disparities: burden of infection, health, and socioeconomic status in U.S. children. *Soc Sci Med.* 2009 Feb;68(4):699-707. 2009 Jan 17.
Ducrotté P. Irritable bowel syndrome: from the gut to the brain-gut. *Gastroenterol Clin Biol.* 2009 Aug-Sep;33(8-9):703-12.
Duke J. *CRC Handbook of Medicinal Herbs.* Boca Raton: CRC; 1989.
Duke J. *The Green Pharmacy.* New York: St. Martins, 1997.
Dunstan JA, Roper J, Mitoulas L, Hartmann PE, Simmer K, Prescott SL. The effect of supplementation with fish oil during pregnancy on breast milk immunoglobulin A, soluble CD14, cytokine levels and fatty acid composition. *Clin Exp Allergy.* 2004 Aug;34(8):1237-42.
Duong M, Subbarao P, Adelroth E, Obminski G, Strinich T, Inman M, Pedersen S, O'Byrne PM. Sputum eosinophils and the response of exercise-induced bronchoconstriction to corticosteroid in asthma. *Chest.* 2008 Feb;133(2):404-11. 2007 Dec 10.
Dupont C, Barau E, Molkhou P, Raynaud F, Barbet JP, Dehennin L. Food-induced alterations of intestinal permeability in children with cow's milk-sensitive enteropathy and atopic dermatitis. *J Pediatr Gastroenterol Nutr.* 1989 May;8(4):459-65.
Dupont C, Barau E, Molkhou P. Intestinal permeability disorders in children. *Allerg Immunol.* 1991 Mar;23(3):95-103.
Dupont C, Soulaines P, Lapillonne A, Donne N, Kalach N, Benhamou P. Atopy patch test for early diagnosis of cow's milk allergy in preterm infants. *J Pediatr Gastroenterol Nutr.* 2010 Apr;50(4):463-4.
Dupuy P, Cassé M, André F, Dhivert-Donnadieu H, Pinton J, Hernandez-Pion C. Low-salt water reduces intestinal permeability in atopic patients. *Dermatology.* 1999;198(2):153-5.
Duran-Tauleria E, Vignati G, Guedan MJ, Petersson CJ. The utility of specific immunoglobulin E measurements in primary care. *Allergy.* 2004 Aug;59 Suppl 78:35-41.
D'Urbano LE, Pellegrino K, Artesani MC, Donnanno S, Luciano R, Riccardi C, Tozzi AE, Ravà L, De Benedetti F, Cavagni G. Performance of a component-based allergen-microarray in the diagnosis of cow's milk and hen's egg allergy. *Clin Exp Allergy.* 2010 Jul 13.
Duwiejua M, Zeitlin IJ, Waterman PG, Chapman J, Mhango GJ, Provan GJ. Anti-inflammatory activity of resins from some species of the plant family Burseraceae. *Planta Med.* 1993 Feb;59(1):12-6.
Dykewicz MS, Lemmon JK, Keaney DL. Comparison of the Multi-Test II and Skintestor Omni allergy skin test devices. *Ann Allergy Asthma Immunol.* 2007 Jun;98(6):559-62.
Eastham EJ, Walker WA. Effect of cow's milk on the gastrointestinal tract: a persistent dilemma for the pediatrician. *Pediatrics.* 1977 Oct;60(4):477-81.
Eaton KK, Howard M, Howard JM. Gut permeability measured by polyethylene glycol absorption in abnormal gut fermentation as compared with food intolerance. *J R Soc Med.* 1995 Feb;88(2):63-6.
Ebers GC, Kukay K, Bulman DE, Sadovnick AD, Rice G, Anderson C, Armstrong H, Cousin K, Bell RB, Hader W, Paty DW, Hashimoto S, Oger J, Duquette P, Warren S, Gray T, O'Connor P, Nath A, Auty A, Metz L, Francis G, Paulseth JE, Murray TJ, Pryse-Phillips W, Nelson R, Freedman M, Brunet D, Bouchard JP, Hinds D, Risch N. A full genome search in multiple sclerosis. *Nat Genet.* 1996 Aug;13(4):472-6.
Eccles R. Menthol and related cooling compounds. *J Pharm Pharmacol.* 1994 Aug;46(8):618-30.
ECRHS (2002) The European Community Respiratory Health Survey II. *Eur Respir J.* 20: 1071-1079.
Edgecombe K, Latter S, Peters S, Roberts G. Health experiences of adolescents with uncontrolled severe asthma. *Arch Dis Child.* 2010 Dec;95(12):985-91. 2010 Jul 30.
Edgell PG. The psychology of asthma. *Can Med Assoc J.* 1952 Aug;67(2):121-5.
Egashira Y, Nagano H. A multicenter clinical trial of TJ-96 in patients with steroid-dependent bronchial asthma. A comparison of groups allocated by the envelope method. *Ann N Y Acad Sci.* 1993 Jun 23;685:580-3.
Ege MJ, Frei R, Bieli C, Schram-Bijkerk D, Waser M, Benz MR, Weiss G, Nyberg F, van Hage M, Pershagen G, Brunekreef B, Riedler J, Lauener R, Braun-Fahrländer C, von Mutius E; PARSIFAL Study team. Not all farming environments protect against the development of asthma and wheeze in children. *J Allergy Clin Immunol.* 2007 May;119(5):1140-7.

REFERENCES AND BIBLIOGRAPHY

Ege MJ, Herzum I, Büchele G, Krauss-Etschmann S, Lauener RP, Roponen M, Hyvärinen A, Vuitton DA, Riedler J, Brunekreef B, Dalphin JC, Braun-Fahrländer C, Pekkanen J, Renz H, von Mutius E; Protection Against Allergy Study in Rural Environments (PASTURE) Study group. Prenatal exposure to a farm environment modifies atopic sensitization at birth. *J Allergy Clin Immunol*. 2008 Aug;122(2):407-12, 412.e1-4.

Eggermont E. Cow's milk protein allergy. *Tijdschr Kindergeneeskd*. 1981 Feb;49(1):16-20.

Ehling S, Hengel M, and Shibamoto T. Formation of acrylamide from lipids. *Adv Exp Med Biol* 2005, 561:223-233.

Ehnert B, Lau-Schadendorf S, Weber A, Buettner P, Schou C, Wahn U. Reducing domestic exposure to dust mite allergen reduces bronchial hyperreactivity in sensitive children with asthma. *J Allergy Clin Immunol*. 1992 Jul;90(1):135-8.

Ehren J, Morón B, Martin E, Bethune MT, Gray GM, Khosla C. A food-grade enzyme preparation with modest gluten detoxification properties. *PLoS One*. 2009 Jul 21;4(7):e6313.

Eijkemans M, Mommers M, de Vries SI, van Buuren S, Stafleu A, Bakker I, Thijs C. Asthmatic symptoms, physical activity, and overweight in young children: a cohort study. *Pediatrics*. 2008 Mar;121(3):e666-72.

Eldridge MW, Peden DB. Allergen provocation augments endotoxin-induced nasal inflammation in subjects with atopic asthma. *J Allergy Clin Immunol*. 2000 Mar;105(3):475-81.

el-Ghazaly M, Khayyal MT, Okpanyi SN, Arens-Corell M. Study of the anti-inflammatory activity of Populus tremula, Solidago virgaurea and Fraxinus excelsior. *Arzneimittelforschung*. 1992 Mar;42(3):333-6.

Ellingwood F. *American Materia Medica, Therapeutics and Pharmacognosy*. Portland: Eclectic Medical Publ., 1983.

Elliott RB, Harris DP, Hill JP, Bibby NJ, Wasmuth HE. Type I (insulin-dependent) diabetes mellitus and cow milk: casein variant consumption. *Diabetologia*. 1999 Mar;42(3):292-6.

Elwood PC. Epidemiology and trace elements. *Clin Endocrinol Metab*. 1985 Aug;14(3):617-28.

Emmanouil E, Manios Y, Grammatikaki E, Kondaki K, Oikonomou E, Papadopoulos N, Vassilopoulou E. Association of nutrient intake and wheeze or asthma in a Greek pre-school population. *Pediatr Allergy Immunol*. 2010 Feb;21(1 Pt 1):90-5. 2009 Sep 9.

Engler RJ. Alternative and complementary medicine: a source of improved therapies for asthma? A challenge for redefining the specialty? *J Allergy Clin Immunol*. 2000;106:627-9.

Environmental Working Group. *Human Toxome Project*. 2007. http://www.ewg.org/sites/humantoxome/. Accessed: 2007 Sep.

EPA. *A Brief Guide to Mold, Moisture and Your Home*. Environmental Protection Agency, Office of Air and Radiation/Indoor Environments Division. EPA 2002;402-K-02-003.

Epstein GN, Halper JP, Barrett EA, Birdsall C, McGee M, Baron KP, Lowenstein S. A pilot study of mind-body changes in adults with asthma who practice mental imagery. *Altern Ther Health Med*. 2004 Jul-Aug;10(4):66-71.

Erkkola M, Kaila M, Nwaru BI, Kronberg-Kippilä C, Ahonen S, Nevalainen J, Veijola R, Pekkanen J, Ilonen J, Simell O, Knip M, Virtanen SM. Maternal vitamin D intake during pregnancy is inversely associated with asthma and allergic rhinitis in 5-year-old children. *Clin Exp Allergy*. 2009 Jun;39(6):875-82.

Ernst E. Frankincense: systematic review. *BMJ*. 2008 Dec 17;337:a2813.

Erwin EA, James HR, Gutekunst HM, Russo JM, Kelleher KJ, Platts-Mills TA. Serum IgE measurement and detection of food allergy in pediatric patients with eosinophilic esophagitis. *Ann Allergy Asthma Immunol*. 2010 Jun;104(6):496-502.

EuroPrevall. *WP 1.1 Birth Cohort Update*. 1st Quarter 2006. Berlin, Germany: Charité University Medical Centre.

Evans P, Forte D, Jacobs C, Fredhoi C, Aitchison E, Hucklebridge F, Clow A. Cortisol secretory activity in older people in relation to positive and negative well-being. *Psychoneuroendocrinology*. 2007 Aug 7

Everhart JE. *Digestive Diseases in the United States*. Darby, PA: Diane Pub, 1994.

FAAN. *Public Comment on 2005 Food Safety Survey: Docket No. 2004N-0516 (2005 FSS)*. Fairfax, VA: Food Allergy & Anaphylaxis Network.

Fairchild SS, Shannon K, Kwan E, Mishell RI. T cell-derived glucosteroid response-modifying factor (GRMFT): a unique lymphokine made by normal T lymphocytes and a T cell hybridoma. *J Immunol*. 1984 Feb;132(2):821-7.

Fajac I, Frossard N. Neuropeptides of the nasal innervation and allergic rhinitis. *Rev Mal Respir*. 1994;11(4):357-67.

Fälth-Magnusson K, Kjellman NI, Magnusson KE, Sundqvist T. Intestinal permeability in healthy and allergic children before and after sodium-cromoglycate treatment assessed with different-sized polyethyleneglycols (PEG 400 and PEG 1000). *Clin Allergy*. 1984 May;14(3):277-86.

Fälth-Magnusson K, Kjellman NI, Odelram H, Sundqvist T, Magnusson KE. Gastrointestinal permeability in children with cow's milk allergy: effect of milk challenge and sodium cromoglycate as assessed with polyethyleneglycols (PEG 400 and PEG 1000). *Clin Allergy*. 1986 Nov;16(6):543-51.

Fan AY, Lao L, Zhang RX, Zhou AN, Wang LB, Moudgil KD, Lee DY, Ma ZZ, Zhang WY, Berman BM. Effects of an acetone extract of Boswellia carterii Birdw. (Burseraceae) gum resin on adjuvant-induced arthritis in lewis rats. *J Ethnopharmacol*. 2005 Oct 3;101(1-3):104-9.

Fanaro S, Marten B, Bagna R, Vigi V, Fabris C, Peña-Quintana, Argüelles F, Scholz-Ahrens KE, Sawatzki G, Zelenka R, Schrezenmeir J, de Vrese M and Bertino E. Galacto-oligosaccharides are bifidogenic and safe at weaning: A double-blind Randomized Multicenter study. *J Pediatr Gastroent Nutr.* 2009 48; 82-88

Fang SP, Tanaka T, Tago F, Okamoto T, Kojima S. Immunomodulatory effects of gyokuheifusan on INF-gamma/IL-4 (Th1/Th2) balance in ovalbumin (OVA)-induced asthma model mice. *Biol Pharm Bull.* 2005;28:829-33.

FAO/WHO Expert Committee. *Fats and Oils in Human Nutrition.* Food and Nutrition Paper. 1994;(57).

Fawell J, Nieuwenhuijsen MJ. Contaminants in drinking water. *Br Med Bull.* 2003;68:199-208.

Fecka I. Qualitative and quantitative determination of hydrolysable tannins and other polyphenols in herbal products from meadowsweet and dog rose. *Phytochem Anal.* 2009 May;20(3):177-90.

Felley CP, Corthésy-Theulaz I, Rivero JL, Sipponen P, Kaufmann M, Bauerfeind P, Wiesel PH, Brassart D, Pfeifer A, Blum AL, Michetti P. Favourable effect of an acidified milk (LC-1) on Helicobacter pylori gastritis in man. *Eur J Gastroenterol Hepatol.* 2001 Jan;13(1):25-9.

Fernández-Rivas M, Garrido Fernández S, Nadal JA, Díaz de Durana MD, García BE, González-Mancebo E, Martín S, Barber D, Rico P, Tabar AI. Randomized double-blind, placebo-controlled trial of sublingual immunotherapy with a Pru p 3 quantified peach extract. *Allergy.* 2009 Jun;64(6):876-83.

Fernández-Rivas M, González-Mancebo E, Rodríguez-Pérez R, Benito C, Sánchez-Monge R, Salcedo G, Alonso MD, Rosado A, Tejedor MA, Vila C, Casas ML. Clinically relevant peach allergy is related to peach lipid transfer protein, Pru p 3, in the Spanish population. *J Allergy Clin Immunol.* 2003 Oct;112(4):789-95.

Ferrari M, Benini L, Brotto E, Locatelli F, De Iorio F, Bonella F, Tacchella N, Corradini C, Lo Cascio V, Vantini I. Omeprazole reduces the response to capsaicin but not to methacholine in asthmatic patients with proximal reflux. *Scand J Gastroenterol.* 2007 Mar;42(3):299-307.

Ferrier L, Berard F, Debrauwer L, Chabo C, Langella P, Bueno L, Fioramonti J. Impairment of the intestinal barrier by ethanol involves enteric microflora and mast cell activation in rodents. *Am J Pathol.* 2006 Apr;168(4):1148-54.

Field RW, Krewski D, Lubin JH, Zielinski JM, Alavanja M, Catalan VS, Klotz JB, Létourneau EG, Lynch CF, Lyon JL, Sandler DP, Schoenberg JB, Steck DJ, Stolwijk JA, Weinberg C, Wilcox HB. An overview of the North American residential radon and lung cancer case-control studies. *J Toxicol Environ Health A.* 2006 Apr;69(7):599-631.

Field T, Henteleff T, Hernandez-Reif M, Martinez E, Mavunda K, Kuhn C, Schanberg S. Children with asthma have improved pulmonary functions after massage therapy. *J Pediatr.* 1998 May;132(5):854-8.

Finkelman FD, Boyce JA, Vercelli D, Rothenberg ME. Key advances in mechanisms of asthma, allergy, and immunology in 2009. *J Allergy Clin Immunol.* 2010 Feb;125(2):312-8.

Fiocchi A, Restani P, Bernardo L, Martelli A, Ballabio C, D'Auria E, Riva E. Tolerance of heat-treated kiwi by children with kiwifruit allergy. *Pediatr Allergy Immunol.* 2004 Oct;15(5):454-8.

Fiocchi A, Travaini M, D'Auria E, Banderali G, Bernardo L, Riva E. Tolerance to a rice hydrolysate formula in children allergic to cow's milk and soy. *Clin Exp Allergy.* 2003 Nov;33(11):1576-80.

Fiocchi, A; Restani, P; Riva, E; Qualizza, R; Bruni, P; Restelli, AR; Galli, CL. Meat allergy: I. Specific IgE to BSA and OSA in atopic, beef sensitive children. *J Am Coll Nutr.* 1995 14: 239-244.

Fjeld T, Veiersted B, Sandvik L, Riise G, Levy F. The Effect of Indoor Foliage Plants on Health and Discomfort Symptoms among Office Workers. *Ind Built Environ.* 1998 July;7(4): 204-209.

Flandrin, J, Montanari M. (eds.). *Food: A Culinary History from Antiquity to the Present.* New York: Penguin Books, 1999.

Fleischer DM, Conover-Walker MK, Christie L, Burks AW, Wood RA. Peanut allergy: recurrence and its management. *J Allergy Clin Immunol.* 2004 Nov;114(5):1195-201.

Flinterman AE, van Hoffen E, den Hartog Jager CF, Koppelman S, Pasmans SG, Hoekstra MO, Bruijnzeel-Koomen CA, Knulst AC, Knol EF. Children with peanut allergy recognize predominantly Ara h2 and Ara h6, which remains stable over time. *Clin Exp Allergy.* 2007 Aug;37(8):1221-8.

Foliaki S, Annesi-Maesano I, Tuuau-Potoi N, Waqatakirewa L, Cheng S, Douwes J, Pearce N. Risk factors for symptoms of childhood asthma, allergic rhinoconjunctivitis and eczema in the Pacific: an ISAAC Phase III study. *Int J Tuberc Lung Dis.* 2008 Jul;12(7):799-806.

Forbes EE, Groschwitz K, Abonia JP, Brandt EB, Cohen E, Blanchard C, Ahrens R, Seidu L, McKenzie A, Strait R, Finkelman FD, Foster PS, Matthaei KI, Rothenberg ME, Hogan SP. IL-9- and mast cell-mediated intestinal permeability predisposes to oral antigen hypersensitivity. *J Exp Med.* 2008 Apr 14;205(4):897-913.

Forestier C, Guelon D, Cluytens V, Gillart T, Sirot J, De Champs C. Oral probiotic and prevention of Pseudomonas aeruginosa infections: a randomized, double-blind, placebo-controlled pilot study in intensive care unit patients. *Crit Care.* 2008;12(3):R69.

Forget-Dubois N, Boivin M, Dionne G, Pierce T, Tremblay RE, Pérusse D. A longitudinal twin study of the genetic and environmental etiology of maternal hostile-reactive behavior during infancy and toddlerhood. *Infant Behav Dev.* 2007

REFERENCES AND BIBLIOGRAPHY

Foster S, Hobbs C. *Medicinal Plants and Herbs.* Boston: Houghton Mifflin, 2002.

Fox RD, *Algoculture.* Doctorate Dissertation, 1983 Jul.

Francavilla R, Lionetti E, Castellaneta SP, Magistà AM, Maurogiovanni G, Bucci N, De Canio A, Indrio F, Cavallo L, Ierardi E, Miniello VL. Inhibition of Helicobacter pylori infection in humans by Lactobacillus reuteri ATCC 55730 and effect on eradication therapy: a pilot study. *Helicobacter.* 2008 Apr;13(2):127-34.

Francis H, Fletcher G, Anthony C, Pickering C, Oldham L, Hadley E, Custovic A, Niven R. Clinical effects of air filters in homes of asthmatic adults sensitized and exposed to pet allergens. *Clin Exp Allergy.* 2003 Jan;33(1):101-5.

Frank PI, Morris JA, Hazell ML, Linehan MF, Frank TL. Long term prognosis in preschool children with wheeze: longitudinal postal questionnaire study 1993-2004. *BMJ.* 2008 Jun 21;336(7658):1423-6. 2008 Jun 16.

Frawley D, Lad V. *The Yoga of Herbs.* Sante Fe: Lotus Press, 1986.

Freedman BJ. A dietary free from additives in the management of allergic disease. *Clin Allergy.* 1977 Sep;7(5):417-21.

Fremont S, Moneret-Vautrin DA, Franck P, Morisset M, Croizier A, Codreanu F, Kanny G. Prospective study of sensitization and food allergy to flaxseed in 1317 subjects. *Eur Ann Allergy Clin Immunol.* 2010 Jun;42(3):103-11.

Frias J, Song YS, Martínez-Villaluenga C, González de Mejia E, Vidal-Valverde C. Immunoreactivity and amino acid content of fermented soybean products. *J Agric Food Chem.* 2008 Jan 9;56(1):99-105.

Friedman LS, Harvard Health Publ. Ed. *Controlling GERD and Chronic Heartburn.* Boston: Harvard Health, 2008.

Frumkin H. Beyond toxicity: human health and the natural environment. *Am J Prev Med.* 2001;20(3):234-40.

Fu G, Zhong Y, Li C, Li Y, Lin X, Liao B, Tsang EW, Wu K, Huang S. Epigenetic regulation of peanut allergen gene Ara h 3 in developing embryos. *Planta.* 2010 Apr;231(5):1049-60.

Fu JX. Measurement of MEFV in 66 cases of asthma in the convalescent stage and after treatment with Chinese herbs. *Zhong Xi Yi Jie He Za Zhi.* 1989 Nov;9(11):658-9, 644.

Fujii T, Ohtsuka Y, Lee T, Kudo T, Shoji H, Sato H, Nagata S, Shimizu T, Yamashiro Y. Bifidobacterium breve enhances transforming growth factor beta1 signaling by regulating Smad7 expression in preterm in-fants. *J Pediatr Gastroenterol Nutr.* 2006 Jul;43(1):83-8.

Furuhjelm C, Warstedt K, Larsson J, Fredriksson M, Böttcher MF, Fälth-Magnusson K, Duchén K. Fish oil supplementation in pregnancy and lactation may decrease the risk of infant allergy. *Acta Paediatr.* 2009 Sep;98(9):1461-7.

Gabory A, Attig L, Junien C. Sexual dimorphism in environmental epigenetic programming. *Mol Cell Endocrinol.* 2009 May 25;304(1-2):8-18. 2009 Mar 9.

Gamboa PM, Cáceres O, Antepara I, Sánchez-Monge R, Ahrazem O, Salcedo G, Barber D, Lombardero M, Sanz ML. Two different profiles of peach allergy in the north of Spain. *Allergy.* 2007 Apr;62(4):408-14.

Gao X, Wang W, Wei S, Li W. Review of pharmacological effects of Glycyrrhiza radix and its bioactive compounds. *Zhongguo Zhong Yao Za Zhi.* 2009 Nov;34(21):2695-700.

Garavello W, Somigliana E, Acaia B, Gaini L, Pignataro L, Gaini RM. Nasal lavage in pregnant women with seasonal allergic rhinitis: a randomized study. *Int Arch Allergy Immunol.* 2010;151(2):137-41. 2009 Sep 15. 19752567.

Garcia Gomez LJ, Sanchez-Muniz FJ. Review: cardiovascular effect of garlic (Allium sativum). *Arch Latinoam Nutr.* 2000 Sep;50(3):219-29.

García-Compeán D, González MV, Galindo G, Mar DA, Treviño JL, Martínez R, Bosques F, Maldonado H. Prevalence of gastroesophageal reflux disease in patients with extraesophageal symptoms referred from otolaryngology, allergy, and cardiology practices: a prospective study. *Dig Dis.* 2000;18(3):178-82.

Garcia-Marcos L, Canflanca IM, Garrido JB, Varela AL, Garcia-Hernandez G, Guillen Grima F, Gonzalez-Diaz C, Carvajal-Urueña I, Arnedo-Pena A, Busquets-Monge RM, Morales Suarez-Varela M, Blanco-Quiros A. Relationship of asthma and rhinoconjunctivitis with obesity, exercise and Mediterranean diet in Spanish schoolchildren. *Thorax.* 2007 Jun;62(6):503-8.

Gardner ML. Gastrointestinal absorption of intact proteins. Annu Rev Nutr. 1988;8:329-50.

Gary WK, Fanny WS, David SC. Factors associated with difference in prevalence of asthma in children from three cities in China: multicentre epidemiological survey. *BMJ.* 2004;329:1-4.

Garzi A, Messina M, Frati F, Carfagna L, Zagordo L, Belcastro M, Parmiani S, Sensi L, Marcucci F. An extensively hydrolysed cow's milk formula improves clinical symptoms of gastroesophageal reflux and reduces the gastric emptying time in infants. *Allergol Immunopathol (Madr).* 2002 Jan-Feb;30(1):36-41.

Gazdik F, Horvathova M, Gazdikova K, Jahnova E. The influence of selenium supplementation on the immunity of corticoid-dependent asthmatics. *Bratisl Lek Listy.* 2002;103(1):17-21.

Gazdik F, Kadrabova J, Gazdikova K. Decreased consumption of corticosteroids after selenium supplementation in corticoid-dependent asthmatics. *Bratisl Lek Listy.* 2002;103(1):22-5.

Geha RS, Beiser A, Ren C, Patterson R, Greenberger PA, Grammer LC, Ditto AM, Harris KE, Shaughnessy MA, Yarnold PR, Corren J, Saxon A. Multicenter, double-blind, placebo-controlled, multiple-challenge evaluation of reported reactions to monosodium glutamate. *J Allergy Clin Immunol.* 2000 Nov;106(5):973-80.

Gerez IF, Shek LP, Chng HH, Lee BW. Diagnostic tests for food allergy. *Singapore* Med J. 2010 Jan;51(1):4-9.

Gergen PJ, Arbes SJ Jr, Calatroni A, Mitchell HE, Zeldin DC. Total IgE levels and asthma prevalence in the US population: results from the National Health and Nutrition Examination Survey 2005-2006. *J Allergy Clin Immunol.* 2009 Sep;124(3):447-53. 2009 Aug 3.

Ghadioungui P. (transl.) *The Ebers Papyrus.* Academy of Scientific Research. Cairo, 1987.

Giampietro PG, Kjellman NI, Oldaeus G, Wouters-Wesseling W, Businco L. Hypoallergenicity of an extensively hydrolyzed whey formula. *Pediatr Allergy Immunol.* 2001 Apr;12(2):83-6.

Gibbons E. *Stalking the Healthful Herbs.* New York: David McKay, 1966.

Gibson RA. Docosa-hexaenoic acid (DHA) accumulation is regulated by the polyunsaturated fat content of the diet: Is it synthesis or is it incorporation? *Asia Pac J Clin Nutr.* 2004;13(Suppl):S78.

Gilbert CR, Arum SM, Smith CM. Vitamin D deficiency and chronic lung disease. *Can Respir J.* 2009 May-Jun;16(3):75-80.

Gill HS, Rutherfurd KJ, Cross ML, Gopal PK. Enhancement of immunity in the elderly by dietary supplementation with the probiotic Bifidobacterium lactis HN019. *Am J Clin Nutr.* 2001 Dec;74(6):833-9.

Gillman A, Douglass JA. What do asthmatics have to fear from food and additive allergy? *Clin Exp Allergy.* 2010 Sep;40(9):1295-302.

Ginde AA, Mansbach JM, Camargo CA Jr. Association between serum 25-hydroxyvitamin D level and upper respiratory tract infection in the Third National Health and Nutrition Examination Survey. *Arch Intern Med.* 2009 Feb 23;169(4):384-90.

Glück U, Gebbers J. Ingested probiotics reduce nasal colonization with pathogenic bacteria (Staphylococcus aureus, Streptococcus pneumoniae, and b-hemolytic streptococci. *Am J. Clin. Nutr.* 2003;77:517-520.

Goedsche K, Förster M, Kroegel C, Uhlemann C. Repeated cold water stimulations (hydrotherapy according to Kneipp) in patients with COPD. *Forsch Komplementmed.* 2007 Jun;14(3):158-66.

Goel V, Dolan RJ. The functional anatomy of humor: segregating cognitive and affective components. *Nat Neurosci.* 2001;4:237-8.

Gohil K, Packer L. Bioflavonoid-Rich Botanical Extracts Show Antioxidant and Gene Regulatory Activity. *Ann N Y Acad Sci.* 2002:957:70-7.

Goldin BR, Adlercreutz H, Dwyer JT, Swenson L, Warram JH, Gorbach SL. Effect of diet on excretion of estrogens in pre- and postmenopausal women. *Cancer Res.* 1981 Sep;41(9 Pt 2):3771-3.

Goldin BR, Adlercreutz H, Gorbach SL, Warram JH, Dwyer JT, Swenson L, Woods MN. Estrogen excretion patterns and plasma levels in vegetarian and omnivorous women. *N Engl J Med.* 1982 Dec 16;307(25):1542-7.

Goldin BR, Swenson L, Dwyer J, Sexton M, Gorbach SL. Effect of diet and Lactobacillus acidophilus supplements on human fecal bacterial enzymes. *J Natl Cancer Inst.* 1980 Feb;64(2):255-61.

Goldstein JL, Aisenberg J, Zakko SF, Berger MF, Dodge WE. Endoscopic ulcer rates in healthy subjects associated with use of aspirin (81 mg q.d.) alone or coadministered with celecoxib or naproxen: a randomized, 1-week trial. *Dig Dis Sci.* 2008 Mar;53(3):647-56.

Golub E. *The Limits of Medicine.* New York: Times Books, 1994.

Gonzales M, Malcoe LH, Myers OB, Espinoza J. Risk factors for asthma and cough among Hispanic children in the southwestern United States of America, 2003-2004. *Rev Panam Salud Publica.* 2007 May;21(5):274-81.

González Alvarez R, Arruzazabala ML. Current views of the mechanism of action of prophylactic antiallergic drugs. *Allergol Immunopathol (Madr).* 1981 Nov-Dec;9(6):501-8.

González J, Fernández M, García Fragoso L. Exclusive breastfeeding reduces asthma in a group of children from the Caguas municipality of Puerto Rico. *Bol Asoc Med P R.* 2010 Jan-Mar;102(1):10-2.

González Morales JE, Leal de Hernández L, González Spencer D. Asthma associated with gastroesophageal reflux. *Rev Alerg Mex.* 1998 Jan-Feb;45(1):16-21.

González-Pérez A, Aponte Z, Vidaurre CF, Rodríguez LA. Anaphylaxis epidemiology in patients with and patients without asthma: a United Kingdom database review. *J Allergy Clin Immunol.* 2010 May;125(5):1098-1104.e1.

González-Sánchez R, Trujillo X, Trujillo-Hernández B, Vásquez C, Huerta M, Elizalde A. Forskolin versus sodium cromoglycate for prevention of asthma attacks: a single-blinded clinical trial. *J Int Med Res.* 2006 Mar-Apr;34(2):200-7.

Gordon BR. Patch testing for allergies. *Curr Opin Otolaryngol Head Neck Surg.* 2010 Jun;18(3):191-4.

Gore KV, Rao AK, Guruswamy MN. Physiological studies with Tylophora asthmatica in bronchial asthma. *Indian J Med Res.* 1980 Jan;71:144-8.

Goren AI, Hellmann S. Changes prevalence of asthma among schoolchildren in Israel. *Eur Respir J.* 1997;10:2279-2284.

Gotteland M, Poliak L, Cruchet S, Brunser O. Effect of regular ingestion of Saccharomyces boulardii plus inulin or Lactobacillus acidophilus LB in children colonized by Helicobacter pylori. *Acta Paediatr.* 2005 Dec;94(12):1747-51.

Govindan S, Viswanathan S, Vijayasekaran V, Alagappan R. A pilot study on the clinical efficacy of Solanum xanthocarpum and Solanum trilobatum in bronchial asthma. *J Ethnopharmacol.* 1999 Aug;66(2):205-10.

REFERENCES AND BIBLIOGRAPHY

Govindan S, Viswanathan S, Vijayasekaran V, Alagappan R. Further studies on the clinical efficacy of Solanum xanthocarpum and Solanum trilobatum in bronchial asthma. *Phytother Res.* 2004 Oct;18(10):805-9.

Grant WB, Holick MF. Benefits and requirements of vitamin D for optimal health: a review. *Altern Med Rev.* 2005 Jun;10(2):94-111.

Grant WB. Hypothesis—ultraviolet-B irradiance and vitamin D reduce the risk of viral infections and thus their sequelae, including autoimmune diseases and some cancers. *Photochem Photobiol.* 2008 Mar-Apr;84(2):356-65. 2008 Jan 7.

Gray H. *Anatomy, Descriptive and Surgical.* 15th Edition. New York: Random House, 1977.

Gray-Davison F. *Ayurvedic Healing.* New York: Keats, 2002.

Greskevitch M, Kullman G, Bang KM, Mazurek JM. Respiratory disease in agricultural workers: mortality and morbidity statistics. J Agromedicine. 2007;12(3):5-10.

Griffith HW. *Healing Herbs: The Essential Guide.* Tucson: Fisher Books, 2000.

Grimm T, Chovanová Z, Muchová J, Sumegová K, Liptáková A, Duracková Z, Högger P. Inhibition of NF-kappaB activation and MMP-9 secretion by plasma of human volunteers after ingestion of maritime pine bark extract (Pycnogenol). J Inflamm (Lond). 2006 Jan 27;3:1.

Grimm T, Schäfer A, Högger P. Antioxidant activity and inhibition of matrix metalloproteinases by metabolites of maritime pine bark extract (pycnogenol). *Free Radic Biol Med.* 2004 Mar 15;36(6):811-22.

Grimm T, Skrabala R, Chovanová Z, Muchová J, Sumegová K, Liptáková A, Duracková Z, Högger P. Single and multiple dose pharmacokinetics of maritime pine bark extract (pycnogenol) after oral administration to healthy volunteers. *BMC Clin Pharmacol.* 2006 Aug 3;6:4.

Gropper SS, Smith JL, Groff JL. *Advanced nutrition and human metabolism.* Belmonth, CA: Wadsworth Publ, 2008.

Groschwitz KR, Ahrens R, Osterfeld H, Gurish MF, Han X, Abrink M, Finkelman FD, Pejler G, Hogan SP. Mast cells regulate homeostatic intestinal epithelial migration and barrier function by a chymase/Mcpt4-dependent mechanism. *Proc Natl Acad Sci U S A.* 2009 Dec 29;106(52):22381-6.

Grosser BI, Monti-Bloch L, Jennings-White C, Berliner DL. Behavioral and electrophysiological effects of androstadienone, a human pheromone. *Psychoneuroendocrinology.* 2000 Apr;25(3):289-99.

Grzanna R, Lindmark L, Frondoza CG. Ginger—an herbal medicinal product with broad anti-inflammatory actions. *J Med Food.* 2005 Summer;8(2):125-32.

Guandalini S. The influence of gluten: weaning recommendations for healthy children and children at risk for celiac disease. *Nestle Nutr Workshop Ser Pediatr Program.* 2007;60:139-51; discussion 151-5.

Guerin M, Huntley ME, Olaizola M. Haematococcus astaxanthin: applications for human health and nutrition. *Trends Biotechnol.* 2003 May;21(5):210-6.

Guinot P, Brambilla C, Duchier J, Braquet P, Bonvoisin B, Cournot A. Effect of BN 52063, a specific PAF-acether antagonist, on bronchial provocation test to allergens in asthmatic patients. A preliminary study. *Prostaglandins.* 1987 Nov;34(5):723-31.

Gundermann KJ, Müller J. Phytodolor—effects and efficacy of a herbal medicine. *Wien Med Wochenschr.* 2007;157(13-14):343-7.

Gupta I, Gupta V, Parihar A, Gupta S, Lüdtke R, Safayhi H, Ammon HP. Effects of Boswellia serrata gum resin in patients with bronchial asthma: results of a double-blind, placebo-controlled, 6-week clinical study. *Eur J Med Res.* 1998 Nov 17;3(11):511-4.

Gupta R, Sheikh A, Strachan DP, Anderson HR (2006) Time trends in allergic disorders in the UK. *Thorax,* published online. doi: 10.1136/thx.2004.038844.

Gupta S, George P, Gupta V, Tandon VR, Sundaram KR. Tylophora indica in bronchial asthma—a double blind study. *Indian J Med Res.* 1979 Jun;69:981-9.

Gutmanis J. *Hawaiian Herbal Medicine.* Waipahu, HI: Island Heritage, 2001.

Haggag EG, Abou-Moustafa MA, Boucher W, Theoharides TC. The effect of a herbal water-extract on histamine release from mast cells and on allergic asthma. *J Herb Pharmacother.* 2003;3(4):41-54.

Haines JL, Ter-Minassian M, Bazyk A, Gusella JF, Kim DJ, Terwedow H, Pericak-Vance MA, Rimmler JB, Haynes CS, Roses AD, Lee A, Shaner B, Menold M, Seboun E, Fitoussi RP, Gartioux C, Reyes C, Ribierre F, Gyapay G, Weissenbach J, Hauser SL, Goodkin DE, Lincoln R, Usuku K, Oksenberg JR, et al. A complete genomic screen for multiple sclerosis underscores a role for the major histocompatability complex. The Multiple Sclerosis Genetics Group. *Nat Genet.* 1996 Aug;13(4):469-71..

Halász A, Cserháti E. The prognosis of bronchial asthma in childhood in Hungary: a long-term follow-up. *J Asthma.* 2002 Dec;39(8):693-9.

Halken S, Hansen KS, Jacobsen HP, Estmann A, Faelling AE, Hansen LG, Kier SR, Lassen K, Lintrup M, Mortensen S, Ibsen KK, Osterballe O, Høst A. Comparison of a partially hydrolyzed infant formula with two extensively hydrolyzed formulas for allergy prevention: a prospective, randomized study. *Pediatr Allergy Immunol.* 2000 Aug;11(3):149-61.

Halpern GM, Miller AH. *Medicinal Mushrooms: Ancient Remedies for Modern Ailments.* New York: M. Evans, 2002.

Hamasaki Y, Kobayashi I, Hayasaki R, Zaitu M, Muro E, Yamamoto S, Ichimaru T, Miyazaki S. The Chinese herbal medicine, shinpi-to, inhibits IgE-mediated leukotriene synthesis in rat basophilic leukemia-2H3 cells. *J Ethnopharmacol.* 1997 Apr;56(2):123-31.

Hamelmann E, Beyer K, Gruber C, Lau S, Matricardi PM, Nickel R, Niggemann B, Wahn U. Primary prevention of allergy: avoiding risk or providing protection? *Clin Exp Allergy.* 2008 Feb;38(2):233-45.

Hamilton RG. Clinical laboratory assessment of immediate-type hypersensitivity. *J Allergy Clin Immunol.* 2010 Feb;125(2 Suppl 2):S284-96.

Hammond BG, Mayhew DA, Kier LD, Mast RW, Sander WJ. Safety assessment of DHA-rich microalgae from Schizochytrium sp. *Regul Toxicol Pharmacol.* 2002 Apr;35(2 Pt 1):255-65.

Han ER, Choi IS, Kim HK, Kang YW, Park JG, Lim JR, Seo JH, Choi JH. Inhaled corticosteroid-related tooth problems in asthmatics. *J Asthma.* 2009 Mar;46(2):160-4.

Han SN, Leka LS, Lichtenstein AH, Ausman LM, Meydani SN. Effect of a therapeutic lifestyle change diet on immune functions of moderately hypercholesterolemic humans. *J Lipid Res.* 2003 Dec;44(12):2304-10.

Hansen KS, Ballmer-Weber BK, Lüttkopf D, Skov PS, Wüthrich B, Bindslev-Jensen C, Vieths S, Poulsen LK. Roasted hazelnuts—allergenic activity evaluated by double-blind, placebo-controlled food challenge. *Allergy.* 2003 Feb;58(2):132-8.

Hansen KS, Ballmer-Weber BK, Sastre J, Lidholm J, Andersson K, Oberhofer H, Lluch-Bernal M, Ostling J, Mattsson L, Schocker F, Vieths S, Poulsen LK. Component-resolved in vitro diagnosis of hazelnut allergy in Europe. *J Allergy Clin Immunol.* 2009 May;123(5):1134-41, 1141.e1-3.

Hansen KS, Khinchi MS, Skov PS, Bindslev-Jensen C, Poulsen LK, Malling HJ. Food allergy to apple and specific immunotherapy with birch pollen. *Mol Nutr Food Res.* 2004 Nov;48(6):441-8.

Haranath PS, Shyamalakumari S. Experimental study on mode of action of Tylophora asthmatica in bronchial asthma. *Indian J Med Res.* 1975 May;63(5):661-70.

Harrington JJ, Lee-Chiong T Jr. Sleep and older patients. *Clin Chest Med.* 2007 Dec;28(4):673-84, v.

Hartz C, Lauer I, Del Mar San Miguel Moncin M, Cistero-Bahima A, Foetisch K, Lidholm J, Vieths S, Scheurer S. Comparison of IgE-Binding Capacity, Cross-Reactivity and Biological Potency of Allergenic Non-Specific Lipid Transfer Proteins from Peach, Cherry and Hazelnut. *Int Arch Allergy Immunol.* 2010 Jun 17;153(4):335-346.

Harvald B, Hauge M: Hereditary factors elucidated by twin studies. In *Genetics and the Epidemiology of Chronic Disease.* Edited by Neel JV, Shaw MV, Schull WJ. Washington, DC: Dept Health, Education and Welfare, 1965:64-76.

Hassan AM. Selenium status in patients with aspirin-induced asthma. *Ann Clin Biochem.* 2008 Sep;45(Pt 5):508-12.

Hasselmark L, Malmgren R, Zetterström O, Unge G. Selenium supplementation in intrinsic asthma. *Allergy.* 1993 Jan;48(1):30-6.

Hata K, Ishikawa K, Hori K, Konishi T. Differentiation-inducing activity of lupeol, a lupane-type triterpene from Chinese dandelion root (Hokouei-kon), on a mouse melanoma cell line. *Biol Pharm Bull.* 2000 Aug;23(8):962-7.

Hattori K, Sasai M, Yamamoto A, Taniuchi S, Kojima T, Kobayashi Y, Iwamoto H, Yaeshima T, Hayasawa H. Intestinal flora of infants with cow milk hypersensitivity fed on casein-hydrolyzed formula supplemented raffinose. *Arerugi.* 2000 Dec;49(12):1146-55.

Heaney LG, Brightling CE, Menzies-Gow A, Stevenson M, Niven RM; British Thoracic Society Difficult Asthma Network. Refractory asthma in the UK: cross-sectional findings from a UK multicentre registry. *Thorax.* 2010 Sep;65(9):787-94.

Heaney RP, Dowell MS. Absorbability of the calcium in a high-calcium mineral water. *Osteoporos Int.* 1994 Nov;4(6):323-4.

Heap GA, van Heel DA. Genetics and pathogenesis of coeliac disease. *Semin Immunol.* May 13 2009.

Hemmer W, Focke M, Marzban G, Swoboda I, Jarisch R, Laimer M. Identification of Bet v 1-related allergens in fig and other Moraceae fruits. *Clin Exp Allergy.* 2010 Apr;40(4):679-87.

Hendel B, Ferreira P. *Water & Salt: The Essence of Life.* Gaithersburg: Natural Resources, 2003.

Herbert V. Vitamin B12: Plant sources, requirements, and assay. *Am J Clin Nutr.* 1988;48:852-858.

Herman PM, Drost LM. Evaluating the clinical relevance of food sensitivity tests: a single subject experiment. *Altern Med Rev.* 2004 Jun;9(2):198-207.

Herzog AM, Black KA, Fountaine DJ, Knotts TR. Reflection and attentional recovery as two distinctive benefits of restorative environments. *J Environ Psychol.* 1997;17:165-70.

Hess-Kosa K. *Indoor Air Quality: Sampling Methodologies.* Boca Rataon: CRC Press, 2002.

Heyman M, Grasset E, Ducroc R, Desjeux JF. Antigen absorption by the jejunal epithelium of children with cow's milk allergy. *Pediatr Res.* 1988 Aug;24(2):197-202.

Hide DW, Matthews S, Tariq S, Arshad SH. Allergen avoidance in infancy and allergy at 4 years of age. *Allergy.* 1996 Feb;51(2):89-93.

Hijazi Z, Molla AM, Al-Habashi H, Muawad WM, Molla AM, Sharma PN. Intestinal permeability is increased in bronchial asthma. *Arch Dis Child.* 2004 Mar;89(3):227-9.

REFERENCES AND BIBLIOGRAPHY

Hill J, Micklewright A, Lewis S, Britton J. Investigation of the effect of short-term change in dietary magnesium intake in asthma. *Eur Respir J.* 1997 Oct;10(10):2225-9.

Hirose Y, Murosaki S, Yamamoto Y, Yoshikai Y, Tsuru T. Daily intake of heat-killed Lactobacillus plantarum L-137 augments acquired immunity in healthy adults. *J Nutr.* 2006 Dec;136(12):3069-73.

Hobbs C. *Medicinal Mushrooms.* Summertown, TN: Botanica Press, 2003.

Hobbs C. *Stress & Natural Healing.* Loveland, CO: Interweave Press, 1997.

Hoffmann D. *Holistic Herbal.* London: Thorsons, 2002.

Hofmann D, Hecker M, Völp A. Efficacy of dry extract of ivy leaves in children with bronchial asthma-a review of randomized controlled trials. *Phytomedicine.* 2003 Mar;10(2-3):213-20.

Höiby AS, Strand V, Robinson DS, Sager A, Rak S. Efficacy, safety, and immunological effects of a 2-year immunotherapy with Depigoid birch pollen extract: a randomized, double-blind, placebo-controlled study. *Clin Exp Allergy.* 2010 Jul;40(7):1062-70.

Holick MF. Sunlight and vitamin D for bone health and prevention of autoimmune diseases, cancers, and cardiovascular disease. *Am J Clin Nutr.* 2004 Dec;80(6 Suppl):1678S-88S.

Holick MF. The vitamin D deficiency pandemic and consequences for nonskeletal health: mechanisms of action. *Mol Aspects Med.* 2008 Dec;29(6):361-8

Holick MF. Vitamin D status: measurement, interpretation, and clinical application. *Ann Epidemiol.* 2009 Feb;19(2):73-8.

Holladay, S.D. Prenatal Immunotoxicant Exposure and Postnatal Autoimmune Disease. *Environ Health Perspect.* 1999; 107(suppl 5):687-691.

Holt GA. Food & Drug Interactions. Chicago: Precept Press, 1998, 83.

Homma M, Oka K, Niitsuma T, Itoh H. A novel 11 beta-hydroxysteroid dehydrogenase inhibitor contained in saiboku-to, a herbal remedy for steroid-dependent bronchial asthma. *J Pharm Pharmacol.* 1994 Apr;46(4):305-9.

Hönscheid A, Rink L, Haase H. T-lymphocytes: a target for stimulatory and inhibitory effects of zinc ions. *Endocr Metab Immune Disord Drug Targets.* 2009 Jun;9(2):132-44.

Hooper R, Calvert J, Thompson RL, Deetlefs ME, Burney P. Urban/rural differences in diet and atopy in South Africa. *Allergy.* 2008 Apr;63(4):425-31.

Hope BE, Massey DG, Fournier-Massey G. Hawaiian materia medica for asthma. *Hawaii Med J.* 1993 Jun;52(6):160-6.

Horak E, Morass B, Ulmer H. Association between environmental tobacco smoke exposure and wheezing disorders in Austrian preschool children. *Swiss Med Wkly.* 2007 Nov 3;137(43-44):608-13.

Horrobin DF. Effects of evening primrose oil in rheumatoid arthritis. *Ann Rheum Dis.* 1989 Nov;48(11):965-6.

Hospers IC, de Vries-Vrolijk K, Brand PL. Double-blind, placebo-controlled cow's milk challenge in children with alleged cow's milk allergies, performed in a general hospital: diagnosis rejected in two-thirds of the children. *Ned Tijdschr Geneeskd.* 2006 Jun 10;150(23):1292-7.

Hosseini S, Pishnamazi S, Sadrzadeh SM, Farid F, Farid R, Watson RR. Pycnogenol((R)) in the Management of Asthma. *J Med Food.* 2001 Winter;4(4):201-209.

Hougee S, Vriesema AJ, Wijering SC, Knippels LM, Folkerts G, Nijkamp FP, Knol J, Garssen J. Oral treatment with probiotics reduces allergic symptoms in ovalbumin-sensitized mice: a bacterial strain comparative study. *Int Arch Allergy Immunol.* 2010;151(2):107-17. 2009 Sep 15.

Houle CR, Leo HL, Clark NM. A developmental, community, and psychosocial approach to food allergies in children. *Curr Allergy Asthma Rep.* 2010 Sep;10(5):381-6.

Houssen ME, Ragab A, Mesbah A, El-Samanoudy AZ, Othman G, Moustafa AF, Badria FA. Natural anti-inflammatory products and leukotriene inhibitors as complementary therapy for bronchial asthma. *Clin Biochem.* 2010 Jul;43(10-11):887-90.

Hsieh KH. Evaluation of efficacy of traditional Chinese medicines in the treatment of childhood bronchial asthma: clinical trial, immunological tests and animal study. Taiwan Asthma Study Group. *Pediatr Allergy Immunol.* 1996 Aug;7(3):130-40.

Hsu CH, Lu CM, Chang TT. Efficacy and safety of modified Mai-Men-Dong-Tang for treatment of allergic asthma. *Pediatr Allergy Immunol.* 2005;16:76-81.

Hu C, Kitts DD. Antioxidant, prooxidant, and cytotoxic activities of solvent-fractionated dandelion (Taraxacum officinale) flower extracts in vitro. *J Agric Food Chem.* 2003 Jan 1;51(1):301-10.

Hu C, Kitts DD. Dandelion (Taraxacum officinale) flower extract suppresses both reactive oxygen species and nitric oxide and prevents lipid oxidation in vitro. *Phytomedicine.* 2005 Aug;12(8):588-97.

Hu C, Kitts DD. Luteolin and luteolin-7-O-glucoside from dandelion flower suppress iNOS and COX-2 in RAW264.7 cells. *Mol Cell Biochem.* 2004 Oct;265(1-2):107-13.

Huang D, Ou B, Prior RL. The chemistry behind antioxidant capacity assays. *J Agric Food Chem.* 2005 Mar 23;53(6):1841-56.

Huang M, Wang W, Wei S. Investigation on medicinal plant resources of Glycyrrhiza uralensis in China and chemical assessment of its underground part. *Zhongguo Zhong Yao Za Zhi.* 2010 Apr;35(8):947-52.

Huntley A, Ernst E: Herbal medicines for asthma: a systematic review. *Thorax.* 2000, 55:925-929.
Hur YM, Rushton JP. Genetic and environmental contributions to prosocial behaviour in 2- to 9-year-old South Korean twins. *Biol Lett.* 2007 Dec 22;3(6):664-6.
Husby S. Dietary antigens: uptake and humoral immunity in man. *APMIS Suppl.* 1988;1:1-40.
Hyndman SJ, Vickers LM, Htut T, Maunder JW, Peock A, Higenbottam TW. A randomized trial of dehumidification in the control of house dust mite. Clin Exp Allergy. 2000 Aug;30(8):1172-80.
Ibero M, Boné J, Martín B, Martínez J. Evaluation of an extensively hydrolysed casein formula (Damira 2000) in children with allergy to cow's milk proteins. *Allergol Immunopathol (Madr).* 2010 Mar-Apr;38(2):60-8.
Inbar O, Dotan R, Dlin RA, Neuman I, Bar-Or O. Breathing dry or humid air and exercise-induced asthma during swimming. *Eur J Appl Physiol Occup Physiol.* 1980;44(1):43-50.
Indrio F, Ladisa G, Mautone A, Montagna O. Effect of a fermented formula on thymus size and stool pH in healthy term infants. *Pediatr Res.* 2007 Jul;62(1):98-100.
Innis SM, Hansen JW. Plasma fatty acid responses, metabolic effects, and safety of microalgal and fungal oils rich in arachidonic and docosahexaenoic acids in adults. *Am J Clin Nutr.* 1996 Aug;64(2):159-67.
Ionescu JG. New insights in the pathogenesis of atopic disease. *J Med Life.* 2009 Apr-Jun;2(2):146-54.
Iribarren C, Tolstykh IV, Miller MK, Eisner MD. Asthma and the prospective risk of anaphylactic shock and other allergy diagnoses in a large integrated health care delivery system. *Ann Allergy Asthma Immunol.* 2010 May;104(5):371-7.
ISAAC. The International Study of Asthma and Allergies in Childhood (ISAAC) Steering Committee. Worldwide variation in prevalence of symptoms of asthma, allergic rhinoconjunctivitis, and atopic eczema: ISAAC. *Lancet.* 1998;351:1225-1232.
Ishida Y, Nakamura F, Kanzato H, Sawada D, Hirata H, Nishimura A, Kajimoto O, Fujiwara S. Clinical effects of *Lactobacillus acidophilus* strain L-92 on perennial allergic rhinitis: a double-blind, placebo-controlled study. *J Dairy Sci.* 2005 Feb;88(2):527-33.
Ishtiaq M, Hanif W, Khan MA, Ashraf M, Butt AM. An ethnomedicinal survey and documentation of important medicinal folklore food phytonims of flora of Samahni valley, (Azad Kashmir) Pakistan. *Pak J Biol Sci.* 2007 Jul 1;10(13):2241-56.
Ivory K, Chambers SJ, Pin C, Prieto E, Arqués JL, Nicoletti C. Oral delivery of *Lactobacillus casei* Shirota modifies allergen-induced immune responses in allergic rhinitis. *Clin Exp Allergy.* 2008 Aug;38(8):1282-9.
Izbicki G, Chavko R, Banauch GI, Weiden MD, Berger KI, Aldrich TK, Hall C, Kelly KJ, Prezant DJ. World trade center "sarcoid-like" granulomatous pulmonary disease in New York City fire department rescue workers. *Chest.* 2007 May;131(5):1414-23.
Izquierdo JL, Martín A, de Lucas P, Rodríguez-González-Moro JM, Almonacid C, Paravisini A. Misdiagnosis of patients receiving inhaled therapies in primary care. *Int J Chron Obstruct Pulmon Dis.* 2010 Aug 9;5:241-9.
Izumi K, Aihara M, Ikezawa Z. Effects of non steroidal antiinflammatory drugs (NSAIDs) on immediate-type food allergy analysis of Japanese cases from 1998 to 2009. *Arerugi.* 2009 Dec;58(12):1629-39.
Jaber R. Respiratory and allergic diseases: from upper respiratory tract infections to asthma. *Prim Care.* 2002 Jun;29(2):231-61.
Jackson DJ, Lemanske RF Jr. The role of respiratory virus infections in childhood asthma inception. *Immunol Allergy Clin North Am.* 2010 Nov;30(4):513-22, vi.
Jacobs DE, Wilson J, Dixon SL, Smith J, Evens A. The relationship of housing and population health: a 30-year retrospective analysis. *Environ Health Perspect.* 2009 Apr;117(4):597-604. 2008 Dec 16.
Jagetia GC, Aggarwal BB. "Spicing up" of the immune system by curcumin. *J Clin Immunol.* 2007 Jan;27(1):19-35.
Jagetia GC, Nayak V, Vidyasagar MS. Evaluation of the antineoplastic activity of guduchi (Tinospora cordifolia) in cultured HeLa cells. *Cancer Lett.* 1998 May 15;127(1-2):71-82.
Jagetia GC, Rao SK. Evaluation of Cytotoxic Effects of Dichloromethane Extract of Guduchi (Tinospora cordifolia Miers ex Hook F & THOMS) on Cultured HeLa Cells. *Evid Based Complement Alternat Med.* 2006 Jun;3(2):267-72.
Jahnova E, Horvathova M, Gazdik F, Weissova S. Effects of selenium supplementation on expression of adhesion molecules in corticoid-dependent asthmatics. *Bratisl Lek Listy.* 2002;103(1):12-4.
Jaiswal M, Prajapati PK, Patgiri BJ Ravishankar B. A Comparative Pharmaco - Clinical Study on Anti-Asthmatic Effect of Shirisharishta Prepared by Bark, Sapwood and Heartwood of Albizia Lebbeck. *J Res Ayurv.* 2006;27(3):67-74.
Jaiswal M, Prajapati PK, Patgiri, BJ, Ravishankar, B. Clinical Study on Anti-Asthmatic Effect of Shirisharishta Prepared by Bark, Sapwood and Heartwood of Albizia Lebbeck. *Pharmaco.* 2006 27(3): 67-74
Janson C, Anto J, Burney P, Chinn S, de Marco R, Heinrich J, Jarvis D, Kuenzli N, Leynaert B, Luczynska C, Neukirch F, Svanes C, Sunyer J, Wjst M; European Community Respiratory Health Survey II. The European Community Respiratory Health Survey: what are the main results so far? European Community Respiratory Health Survey II. *Eur Respir J.* 2001 Sep;18(3):598-611.
Jarocka-Cyrta E, Baniukiewicz A, Wasilewska J, Pawlak J, Kaczmarski M. Focal villous atrophy of the duodenum in children who have outgrown cow's milk allergy. Chromoendoscopy and magnification endoscopy evaluation. *Med Wieku Rozwoj.* 2007 Apr-Jun;11(2 Pt 1):123-7.

REFERENCES AND BIBLIOGRAPHY

Jayaprakasam B, Doddaga S, Wang R, Holmes D, Goldfarb J, Li XM. Licorice flavonoids inhibit eotaxin-1 secretion by human fetal lung fibroblasts in vitro. *J Agric Food Chem.* 2009 Feb 11;57(3):820-5.

Jennings S, Prescott SL. Early dietary exposures and feeding practices: role in pathogenesis and prevention of allergic disease? *Postgrad Med J.* 2010 Feb;86(1012):94-9.

Jensen B. *Foods that Heal.* Garden City Park, NY: Avery Publ, 1988, 1993.

Jensen B. *Nature Has a Remedy.* Los Angeles: Keats, 2001.

Jeon HJ, Kang HJ, Jung HJ, Kang YS, Lim CJ, Kim YM, Park EH. Anti-inflammatory activity of Taraxacum officinale. *J Ethnopharmacol.* 2008 Jan 4;115(1):82-8.

Johansson G, Holmén A, Persson L, Högstedt B, Wassén C, Ottova L, Gustafsson JA. Long-term effects of a change from a mixed diet to a lacto-vegetarian diet on human urinary and faecal mutagenic activity. *Mutagenesis.* 1998 Mar;13(2):167-71.

Johansson G, Holmén A, Persson L, Högstedt B, Wassén C, Ottova L, Gustafsson JA. Dietary influence on some proposed risk factors for colon cancer: fecal and urinary mutagenic activity and the activity of some intestinal bacterial enzymes. *Cancer Detect Prev.* 1997;21(3):258-66.

Johansson G, Holmén A, Persson L, Högstedt R, Wassén C, Ottova L, Gustafsson JA. The effect of a shift from a mixed diet to a lacto-vegetarian diet on human urinary and fecal mutagenic activity. *Carcinogenesis.* 1992 Feb;13(2):153-7.

Johansson G, Ravald N. Comparison of some salivary variables between vegetarians and omnivores. *Eur J Oral Sci.* 1995 Apr;103(2 (Pt 1)):95-8.

Johari H. *Ayurvedic Massage: Traditional Indian Techniques for Balancing Body and Mind.* Rochester, VT: Healing Arts, 1996.

Johnson LM. Gitksan medicinal plants—cultural choice and efficacy. *J Ethnobiol Ethnomed.* 2006 Jun 21;2:29.

Jones MA, Silman AJ, Whiting S, et al. Occurrence of rheumatoid arthritis is not increased in the first degree relatives of a population based inception cohort of inflammatory polyarthritis. *Ann Rheum Dis.* 1996;55(2): 89-93.

José RJ, Roberts J, Bakerly ND. The effectiveness of a social marketing model on case-finding for COPD in a deprived inner city population. *Prim Care Respir J.* 2010 Jun;19(2):104-8.

Joseph SP, Borrell LN, Shapiro A. Self-reported lifetime asthma and nativity status in U.S. children and adolescents: results from the National Health and Nutrition Examination Survey 1999-2004. *J Health Care Poor Underserved.* 2010 May;21(2 Suppl):125-39.

Juergens UR, Dethlefsen U, Steinkamp G, Gillissen A, Repges R, Vetter H. Anti-inflammatory activity of 1.8-cineol (eucalyptol) in bronchial asthma: a double-blind placebo-controlled trial. *Respir Med.* 2003 Mar;97(3):250-6.

Julkunen-Tiitto R. A chemotaxonomic survey of phenolics in leaves of northern Salicaceae species. Phytochemistry. 1986;25(3):663-667.

Jung HA, Yokozawa T, Kim BW, Jung JH, Choi JS. Selective inhibition of prenylated flavonoids from Sophora flavescens against BACE1 and cholinesterases. *Am J Chin Med.* 2010;38(2):415-29.

Jurenka JS. Anti-inflammatory properties of curcumin, a major constituent of Curcuma longa: a review of preclinical and clinical research. *Altern Med Rev.* 2009 Feb;14(2):141-153.

Juvonen R, Bloigu A, Peitso A, Silvennoinen-Kassinen S, Saikku P, Leinonen M, Hassi J, Harju T. Training improves physical fitness and decreases CRP also in asthmatic conscripts. *J Asthma.* 2008 Apr;45(3):237-42.

Kähkönen MP, Hopia AI, Vuorela HJ, Rauha JP, Pihlaja K, Kujala TS, Heinonen M. Antioxidant activity of plant extracts containing phenolic compounds. *J Agric Food Chem.* 1999 Oct;47(10):3954-62.

Kaila M, Vanto T, Valovirta E, Koivikko A, Juntunen-Backman K. Diagnosis of food allergy in Finland: survey of pediatric practices. *Pediatr Allergy Immunol.* 2000 Nov;11(4):246-9.

Kalach N, Benhamou PH, Campeotto F, Dupont Ch. Anemia impairs small intestinal absorption measured by intestinal permeability in children. *Eur Ann Allergy Clin Immunol.* 2007 Jan;39(1):20-2.

Kaliner M, Shelhamer JH, Borson B, Nadel J, Patow C, Marom Z. Human respiratory mucus. *Am Rev Respir Dis.* 1986 Sep;134(3):612-21.

Kalliomäki M, Salminen S, Arvilommi H, Kero P, Koskinen P, Isolauri E. Probiotics in primary prevention of atopic disease: a randomised placebo-controlled trial. *Lancet.* 2001 Apr 7;357(9262):1076-9.

Kamdar T, Bryce PJ. Immunotherapy in food allergy. Immunotherapy. 2010 May;2(3):329-38.

Kang SK, Kim JK, Ahn SH, Oh JE, Kim JH, Lim DH, Son BK. Relationship between silent gastroesophageal reflux and food sensitization in infants and young children with recurrent wheezing. *J Korean Med Sci.* 2010 Mar;25(3):425-8.

Kanny G, Grignon G, Dauca M, Guedenet JC, Moneret-Vautrin DA. Ultrastructural changes in the duodenal mucosa induced by ingested histamine in patients with chronic urticaria. *Allergy.* 1996 Dec;51(12):935-9.

Kapil A, Sharma S. Immunopotentiating compounds from Tinospora cordifolia. *J Ethnopharmacol.* 1997 Oct;58(2):89-95.

Kaplan C. Indoor air pollution from unprocessed solid fuels in developing countries. *Rev Environ Health.* 2010 Jul-Sep;25(3):221-42.

Kaplan M, Mutlu EA, Benson M, Fields JZ, Banan A, Keshavarzian A. Use of herbal preparations in the treatment of oxidant-mediated inflammatory disorders. *Complement Ther Med.* 2007 Sep;15(3):207-16. 2006 Aug 21.
Kaplan R. The nature of the view from home: psychological benefits. *Environ Behav.* 2001;33(4):507-42.
Kaplan R. Wilderness perception and psychological benefits: an analysis of a continuing program. *Leisure Sci.* 1984;6(3):271-90.
Karkoulias K, Patouchas D, Alahiotis S, Tsiamita M, Vrodakis K, Spiropoulos K. Specific sensitization in wheat flour and contributing factors in traditional bakers. *Eur Rev Med Pharmacol Sci.* 2007 May-Jun;11(3):141-8.
Karpińska J, Mikołuć B, Motkowski R, Piotrowska-Jastrzebska J. HPLC method for simultaneous determination of retinol, alpha-tocopherol and coenzyme Q10 in human plasma. *J Pharm Biomed Anal.* 2006 Sep 18;42(2):232-6.
Kashiwada Y, Takanaka K, Tsukada H, Miwa Y, Taga T, Tanaka S, Ikeshiro Y. Sesquiterpene glucosides from anti-leukotriene B4 release fraction of Taraxacum officinale. *J Asian Nat Prod Res.* 2001;3(3):191-7.
Katial RK, Strand M, Prasertsuntarasai T, Leung R, Zheng W, Alam R. The effect of aspirin desensitization on novel biomarkers in aspirin-exacerbated respiratory diseases. *J Allergy Clin Immunol.* 2010 Oct;126(4):738-44. 2010 Aug 21.
Kattan JD, Srivastava KD, Sampson HA, Li XM. Pharmacologic and Immunologic Effects of Individual Herbs of Food Allergy Herbal Formula 2 in a Murine Model of Peanut Allergy. *J Allergy Clin Immunol.* 2006;117(2):S34.
Kattan JD, Srivastava KD, Zou ZM, Goldfarb J, Sampson HA, Li XM. Pharmacological and immunological effects of individual herbs in the Food Allergy Herbal Formula-2 (FAHF-2) on peanut allergy. *Phytother Res.* 2008 May;22(5):651-9.
Katz DL, Cushman D, Reynolds J, Njike V, Treu JA, Walker J, Smith E, Katz C. Putting physical activity where it fits in the school day: preliminary results of the ABC (Activity Bursts in the Classroom) for fitness program. *Prev Chronic Dis.* 2010 Jul;7(4):A82. 2010 Jun 15.
Katz Y, Rajuan N, Goldberg MR, Eisenberg E, Heyman E, Cohen A, Leshno M. Early exposure to cow's milk protein is protective against IgE-mediated cow's milk protein allergy. *J Allergy Clin Immunol.* 2010 Jul;126(1):77-82.e1.
Kazaks AG, Uriu-Adams JY, Albertson TE, Shenoy SF, Stern JS. Effect of oral magnesium supplementation on measures of airway resistance and subjective assessment of asthma control and quality of life in men and women with mild to moderate asthma: a randomized placebo controlled trial. *J Asthma.* 2010 Feb;47(1):83-92.
Kazansky DB. MHC restriction and allogeneic immune responses. *J Immunotoxicol.* 2008 Oct;5(4):369-84.
Kazłowska K, Hsu T, Hou CC, Yang WC, Tsai GJ. Anti-inflammatory properties of phenolic compounds and crude extract from Porphyra dentata. *J Ethnopharmacol.* 2010 Mar 2;128(1):123-30.
Keita AV, Söderholm JD. The intestinal barrier and its regulation by neuroimmune factors. *Neurogastroenterol Motil.* 2010 Jul;22(7):718-33.
Kekkonen RA, Lummela N, Karjalainen H, Latvala S, Tynkkynen S, Jarvenpaa S, Kautiainen H, Julkunen I, Vapaatalo H, Korpela R. Probiotic intervention has strain-specific anti-inflammatory effects in healthy adults. *World J Gastroenterol.* 2008 Apr 7;14(13):2029-36.
Kekkonen RA, Sysi-Aho M, Seppanen-Laakso T, Julkunen I, Vapaatalo H, Oresic M, Korpela R. Effect of probiotic *Lactobacillus rhamnosus* GG intervention on global serum lipidomic profiles in healthy adults. *World J Gastroenterol.* 2008 May 28;14(20):3188-94.
Kekkonen RA, Vasankari TJ, Vuorimaa T, Haahtela T, Julkunen I, Korpela R. The effect of probiotics on respiratory infections and gastrointestinal symptoms during training in marathon runners. *Int J Sport Nutr Exerc Metab.* 2007 Aug;17(4):352-63.
Kelder P. *Ancient Secret of the Fountain of Youth.* New York: Doubleday, 1998.
Kelly HW, Van Natta ML, Covar RA, Tonascia J, Green RP, Strunk RC; CAMP Research Group. Effect of long-term corticosteroid use on bone mineral density in children: a prospective longitudinal assessment in the childhood Asthma Management Program (CAMP) study. *Pediatrics.* 2008 Jul;122(1):e53-61.
Kelly-Pieper K, Patil SP, Busse P, Yang N, Sampson H, Li XM, Wisnivesky JP, Kattan M. Safety and tolerability of an antiasthma herbal Formula (ASHMI) in adult subjects with asthma: a randomized, double-blinded, placebo-controlled, dose-escalation phase I study. *J Altern Complement Med.* 2009 Jul;15(7):735-43.
Kenia P, Houghton T, Beardsmore C. Does inhaling menthol affect nasal patency or cough? *Pediatr Pulmonol.* 2008 Jun;43(6):532-7.
Keogh JB, Grieger JA, Noakes M, Clifton PM. Flow-Mediated Dilatation Is Impaired by a High-Saturated Fat Diet but Not by a High-Carbohydrate Diet. *Arterioscler Thromb Vasc Biol.* 2005 Mar 17
Kerckhoffs DA, Brouns F, Hornstra G, Mensink RP. Effects on the human serum lipoprotein profile of beta-glucan, soy protein and isoflavones, plant sterols and stanols, garlic and tocotrienols. *J Nutr.* 2002 Sep;132(9):2494-505.
Kerkhof M, Postma DS, Brunekreef B, Reijmerink NE, Wijga AH, de Jongste JC, Gehring U, Koppelman GH. Toll-like receptor 2 and 4 genes influence susceptibility to adverse effects of traffic-related air pollution on childhood asthma. *Thorax.* 2010 Aug;65(8):690-7.
Key T, Appleby P, Davey G, Allen N, Spencer E, Travis R. Mortality in British vegetarians: review and preliminary results from EPIC-Oxford. *Amer. Jour. Clin. Nutr. Suppl.* 2003;78(3): 533S-538S.

REFERENCES AND BIBLIOGRAPHY

Kiefte-de Jong JC, Escher JC, Arends LR, Jaddoe VW, Hofman A, Raat H, Moll HA. Infant nutritional factors and functional constipation in childhood: the Generation R study. *Am J Gastroenterol.* 2010 Apr;105(4):940-5.

Kim HM, Shin HY, Lim KH, Ryu ST, Shin TY, Chae HJ, Kim HR, Lyu YS, An NH, Lim KS. Taraxacum officinale inhibits tumor necrosis factor-alpha production from rat astrocytes. *Immunopharmacol Immunotoxicol.* 2000 Aug;22(3):519-30.

Kim JH, An S, Kim JE, Choi GS, Ye YM, Park HS. Beef-induced anaphylaxis confirmed by the basophil activation test. *Allergy Asthma Immunol Res.* 2010 Jul;2(3):206-8.

Kim JH, Ellwood PE, Asher MI. Diet and asthma: looking back, moving forward. *Respir Res.* 2009 Jun 12;10:49.

Kim JH, Lee SY, Kim HB, Jin HS, Yu JH, Kim BJ, Kim BS, Kang MJ, Jang SO, Hong SJ. TBXA2R gene polymorphism and responsiveness to leukotriene receptor antagonist in children with asthma. *Clin Exp Allergy.* 2008 Jan;38(1):51-9.

Kim JY, Kim DY, Lee YS, Lee BK, Lee KH, Ro JY. DA-9601, Artemisia asiatica herbal extract, ameliorates airway inflammation of allergic asthma in mice. *Mol Cells.* 2006;22:104-12.

Kim NI, Jo Y, Ahn SB, Son BK, Kim SH, Park YS, Kim SH, Ju JE. A case of eosinophilic esophagitis with food hypersensitivity. *J Neurogastroenterol Motil.* 2010 Jul;16(3):315-8.

Kim SJ, Jung JY, Kim HW, Park T. Anti-obesity effects of Juniperus chinensis extract are associated with increased AMP-activated protein kinase expression and phosphorylation in the visceral adipose tissue of rats. *Biol Pharm Bull.* 2008 Jul;31(7):1415-21.

Kim TE, Park SW, Noh G, Lee S. Comparison of skin prick test results between crude allergen extracts from foods and commercial allergen extracts in atopic dermatitis by double-blind placebo-controlled food challenge for milk, egg, and soybean. *Yonsei Med J.* 2002 Oct;43(5):613-20.

Kim YH, Kim KS, Han CS, Yang HC, Park SH, Ko KI, Lee SH, Kim KH, Lee NH, Kim JM, Son K. Inhibitory effects of natural plants of Jeju Island on elastase and MMP-1 expression. *Int J Cosmet Sci.* 2007 Dec;29(6):487-8.

Kimata H. Effect of viewing a humorous vs. nonhumorous film on bronchial responsiveness in patients with bronchial asthma. *Physiol Behav.* 2004 Jun;81(4):681-4.

Kimata M, Inagaki N, Nagai H. Effects of luteolin and other flavonoids on IgE-mediated allergic reactions. *Planta Med.* 2000 Feb;66(1):25-9.

Kimata M, Shichijo M, Miura T, Serizawa I, Inagaki N, Nagai H. Effects of luteolin, quercetin and baicalein on immunoglobulin E-mediated mediator release from human cultured mast cells. *Clin Exp Allergy.* 2000 Apr;30(4):501-8.

Kimmatkar N, Thawani V, Hingorani L, Khiyani R. Efficacy and tolerability of Boswellia serrata extract in treatment of osteoarthritis of knee—a randomized double blind placebo controlled trial. *Phytomedicine.* 2003 Jan;10(1):3-7.

Kinaciyan T, Jahn-Schmid B, Radakovics A, Zwölfer B, Schreiber C, Francis JN, Ebner C, Bohle B. Successful sublingual immunotherapy with birch pollen has limited effects on concomitant food allergy to apple and the immune response to the Bet v 1 homolog Mal d 1. *J Allergy Clin Immunol.* 2007 Apr;119(4):937-43.

Kinross JM, von Roon AC, Holmes E, Darzi A, Nicholson JK. The human gut microbiome: implications for future health care. *Curr Gastroenterol Rep.* 2008 Aug;10(4):396-403.

Kippelen P, Larsson J, Anderson SD, Brannan JD, Dahlén B, Dahlén SE. Effect of sodium cromoglycate on mast cell mediators during hyperpnea in athletes. *Med Sci Sports Exerc.* 2010 Oct;42(10):1853-60.

Kirjavainen PV, Salminen SJ, Isolauri E. Probiotic bacteria in the management of atopic disease: underscoring the importance of viability. *J Pediatr Gastroenterol Nutr.* 2003 Feb;36(2):223-7.

Kisiel W, Barszcz B. Further sesquiterpenoids and phenolics from Taraxacum officinale. *Fitoterapia.* 2000 Jun;71(3):269-73.

Kisiel W, Michalska K. Sesquiterpenoids and phenolics from Taraxacum hondoense. *Fitoterapia.* 2005 Sep;76(5):520-4.

Klein R, Landau MG. *Healing: The Body Betrayed.* Minneapolis: DCI:Chronimed, 1992.

Klein-Galczinsky C. Pharmacological and clinical effectiveness of a fixed phytogenic combination trembling poplar (Populus tremula), true goldenrod (Solidago virgaurea) and ash (Fraxinus excelsior) in mild to moderate rheumatic complaints. *Wien Med Wochenschr.* 1999;149(8-10):248-53.

Klemola T, Vanto T, Juntunen-Backman K, Kalimo K, Korpela R, Varjonen E. Allergy to soy formula and to extensively hydrolyzed whey formula in infants with cow's milk allergy: a prospective, randomized study with a follow-up to the age of 2 years. *J Pediatr.* 2002 Feb;140(2):219-24.

Kloss J. *Back to Eden.* Twin Oaks, WI: Lotus Press, 1939-1999.

Knutson TW, Bengtsson U, Dannaeus A, Ahlstedt S, Knutson L. Effects of luminal antigen on intestinal albumin and hyaluronan permeability and ion transport in atopic patients. *J Allergy Clin Immunol.* 1996 Jun;97(6):1225-32.

Ko J, Busse PJ, Shek L, Noone SA, Sampson HA, Li XM. Effect of Chinese Herbal Formulas on T Cell Responses in Patients with Peanut Allergy or Asthma. *J Allergy Clin Immunol.* 2005;115:S34.

Ko J, Lee JI, Munoz-Furlong A, Li XM, Sicherer SH. Use of complementary and alternative medicine by food-allergic patients. *Ann Allergy Asthma Immunol.* 2006;97:365-9.

Kobayashi I, Hamasaki Y, Sato R, Zaitu M, Muro E, Yamamoto S, Ichimaru T, Miyazaki S. Saiboku-To, a herbal extract mixture, selectively inhibits 5-lipoxygenase activity in leukotriene synthesis in rat basophilic leukemia-1 cells. *J Ethnopharmacol.* 1995 Aug 11;48(1):33-41.

Kokwaro JO. *Medicinal Plants of East Africa.* Nairobi: Univ of Neirobi Press, 2009.

Kong LF, Guo LH, Zheng XY. Effect of yiqi bushen huoxue herbs in treating children asthma and on levels of nitric oxide, endothelin-1 and serum endothelial cells. *Zhongguo Zhong Xi Yi Jie He Za Zhi.* 2001 Sep;21(9):667-9.

Koo HN, Hong SH, Song BK, Kim CH, Yoo YH, Kim HM. Taraxacum officinale induces cytotoxicity through TNF-alpha and IL-1alpha secretion in Hep G2 cells. *Life Sci.* 2004 Jan 16;74(9):1149-57.

Kootstra HS, Vlieg-Boerstra BJ, Dubois AE. Assessment of the reduced allergenic properties of the Santana apple. *Ann Allergy Asthma Immunol.* 2007 Dec;99(6):522-5.

Kotzampassi K, Giamarellos-Bourboulis EJ, Voudouris A, Kazamias P, Eleftheriadis E. Benefits of a synbiotic formula (Synbiotic 2000Forte) in critically Ill trauma patients: early results of a randomized controlled trial. *World J Surg.* 2006 Oct;30(10):1848-55.

Kovács T, Mette H, Per B, Kun L, Schmelczer M, Barta J, Jean-Claude D, Nagy J. Relationship between intestinal permeability and antibodies against food antigens in IgA nephropathy. *Orv Hetil.* 1996 Jan 14;137(2):65-9.

Kowalchik C, Hylton W (eds). *Rodale's Illustrated Encyclopedia of Herbs.* Emmaus, PA: 1987.

Kowalczyk E, Krzesiński P, Kura M, Niedworok J, Kowalski J, Błaszczyk J. Pharmacological effects of flavonoids from Scutellaria baicalensis. *Przegl Lek.* 2006;63(2):95-6.

Kozlowski LT, Mehta NY, Sweeney CT, Schwartz SS, Vogler GP, Jarvis MJ, West RJ. Filter ventilation and nicotine content of tobacco in cigarettes from Canada, the United Kingdom, and the United States. *Tob Control.* 1998 Winter;7(4):369-75.

Kreig M. *Black Market Medicine.* New York: Bantam, 1968.

Kremmyda LS, Vlachava M, Noakes PS, Diaper ND, Miles EA, Calder PC. Atopy Risk in Infants and Children in Relation to Early Exposure to Fish, Oily Fish, or Long-Chain Omega-3 Fatty Acids: A Systematic Review. *Clin Rev Allergy Immunol.* 2009 Dec 9.

Krogulska A, Dynowski J, Wasowska-Królikowska K. Bronchial reactivity in schoolchildren allergic to food. *Ann Allergy Asthma Immunol.* 2010 Jul;105(1):31-8.

Krogulska A, Wasowska-Królikowska K, Dynowski J. Evaluation of bronchial hyperreactivity in children with asthma undergoing food challenges. *Pol Merkur Lekarski.* 2007 Jul;23(133):30-5.

Krogulska A, Wasowska-Królikowska K, Polakowska E, Chrul S. Cytokine profile in children with asthma undergoing food challenges. *J Investig Allergol Clin Immunol.* 2009;19(1):43-8.

Krogulska A, Wasowska-Królikowska K, Polakowska E, Chrul S. Evaluation of receptor expression on immune system cells in the peripheral blood of asthmatic children undergoing food challenges. Int Arch Allergy Immunol. 2009;150(4):377-88. 2009 Jul 1.

Krogulska A, Wasowska-Królikowska K, Trzeźwińska B. Food challenges in children with asthma. *Pol Merkur Lekarski.* 2007 Jul;23(133):22-9.

Kroidl RF, Schwichtenberg U, Frank E. Bronchial asthma due to storage mite allergy. Pneumologie. 2007 Aug;61(8):525-30.

Krueger AP, Reed EJ. Biological impact of small air Ions. *Science.* 1976 Sep 24;193(4259):1209-13.

Krüger P, Kanzer J, Hummel J, Fricker G, Schubert-Zsilavecz M, Abdel-Tawab M. Permeation of Boswellia extract in the Caco-2 model and possible interactions of its constituents KBA and AKBA with OATP1B3 and MRP2. *Eur J Pharm Sci.* 2009 Feb 15;36(2-3):275-84.

Kuitunen M, Kukkonen K, Juntunen-Backman K, Korpela R, Poussa T, Tuure T, Haahtela T, Savilahti E. Probiotics prevent IgE-associated allergy until age 5 years in Cesarean-delivered children but not in the total cohort. *J Allergy Clin Immunol.* 2009 Feb;123(2):335-41.

Kuitunen M, Savilahti E, Sarnesto A. Human alpha-lactalbumin and bovine beta-lactoglobulin absorption in infants. *Allergy.* 1994 May;49(5):354-60.

Kuitunen M, Savilahti E. Mucosal IgA, mucosal cow's milk antibodies, serum cow's milk antibodies and gastrointestinal permeability in infants. *Pediatr Allergy Immunol.* 1995 Feb;6(1):30-5.

Kukkonen K, Kuitunen M, Haahtela T, Korpela R, Poussa T, Savilahti E. High intestinal IgA associates with reduced risk of IgE-associated allergic diseases. *Pediatr Allergy Immunol.* 2010 Feb;21(1 Pt 1):67-73.

Kukkonen K, Savilahti E, Haahtela T, Juntunen-Backman K, Korpela R, Poussa T, Tuure T, Kuitunen M. Probiotics and prebiotic galacto-oligosaccharides in the prevention of allergic diseases: a randomized, double-blind, placebo-controlled trial. *J Allergy Clin Immunol.* 2007 Jan;119(1):192-8.

Kulka M. The potential of natural products as effective treatments for allergic inflammation: implications for allergic rhinitis. *Curr Top Med Chem.* 2009;9(17):1611-24.

REFERENCES AND BIBLIOGRAPHY

Kull I, Bergström A, Lilja G, Pershagen G, Wickman M. Fish consumption during the first year of life and development of allergic diseases during childhood. *Allergy.* 2006 Aug;61(8):1009-15.

Kull I, Melen E, Alm J, Hallberg J, Svartengren M, van Hage M, Pershagen G, Wickman M, Bergström A. Breast-feeding in relation to asthma, lung function, and sensitization in young schoolchildren. *J Allergy Clin Immunol.* 2010 May;125(5):1013-9.

Kumar A, Panghal S, Mallapur SS, Kumar M, Ram V, Singh BK. Antiinflammatory Activity of Piper longum Fruit Oil. *Indian J Pharm Sci.* 2009 Jul;71(4):454-6.

Kumar A, Saluja AK, Shah UD, Mayavanshi AV. Pharmacological potential of Albizzia lebbeck: A Review. *Pharmacog.* 2007 Jan-May; 1(1) 171-174.

Kumar R, Singh BP, Srivastava P, Sridhara S, Arora N, Gaur SN. Relevance of serum IgE estimation in allergic bronchial asthma with special reference to food allergy. *Asian Pac J Allergy Immunol.* 2006 Dec;24(4):191-9.

Kummeling I, Mills EN, Clausen M, Dubakiene R, Pérez CF, Fernández-Rivas M, Knulst AC, Kowalski ML, Lidholm J, Le TM, Metzler C, Mustakov T, Popov T, Potts J, van Ree R, Sakellariou A, Töndury B, Tzannis K, Burney P. The EuroPrevall surveys on the prevalence of food allergies in children and adults: background and study methodology. *Allergy.* 2009 Oct;64(10):1493-7.

Kung HC, Hoyert DL, Xu J, Murphy SL. Deaths: Final Data for 2005. *National Vital Statistics Reports.* 2008;56(10). http://www.cdc.gov/nchs/data/ nvsr/nvsr56/nvsr56_10.pdf. Accessed: 2008 Jun.

Kunisawa J, Kiyono H. Aberrant interaction of the gut immune system with environmental factors in the development of food allergies. *Curr Allergy Asthma Rep.* 2010 May;10(3):215-21.

Kurth T, Barr RG, Gaziano JM, Buring JE. Randomised aspirin assignment and risk of adult-onset asthma in the Women's Health Study. *Thorax.* 2008 Jun;63(6):514-8. 2008 Mar 13.

Kusunoki T, Morimoto T, Nishikomori R, Yasumi T, Heike T, Mukaida K, Fujii T, Nakahata T. Breastfeeding and the prevalence of allergic diseases in schoolchildren: Does reverse causation matter? *Pediatr Allergy Immunol.* 2010 Feb;21(1 Pt 1):60-6.

Kuvaeva IB. Permeability of the gastrointestinal tract for macromolecules in health and disease. *Hum Physiol.* 1979 Mar-Apr;4(2):272-83.

Kuz'mina IaS, Vavilova NN. Kinesitherapy of patients with bronchial asthma and excessive body weight at the early stage of rehabilitation treatment. *Vopr Kurortol Fizioter Lech Fiz Kult.* 2009 Sep-Oct;(5):17-20.

Kuznetsova TA, Shevchenko NM, Zviagintseva TN, Besednova NN. Biological activity of fucoidans from brown algae and the prospects of their use in medicine]. *Antibiot Khimioter.* 2004;49(5):24-30.

Kvamme JM, Wilsgaard T, Florholmen J, Jacobsen BK. Body mass index and disease burden in elderly men and women: the Tromsø Study. *Eur J Epidemiol.* 2010 Mar;25(3):183-93. 2010 Jan 20.

Lad V. *Ayurveda: The Science of Self-Healing.* Twin Lakes, WI: Lotus Press.

Lamaison JL, Carnat A, Petitjean-Freytet C. Tannin content and inhibiting activity of elastase in Rosaceae. *Ann Pharm Fr.* 1990;48(6):335-40.

Laney AS, Cragin LA, Blevins LZ, Sumner AD, Cox-Ganser JM, Kreiss K, Moffatt SG, Lohff CJ. Sarcoidosis, asthma, and asthma-like symptoms among occupants of a historically water-damaged office building. *Indoor Air.* 2009 Feb;19(1):83-90.

Lang CJ, Hansen M, Roscioli E, Jones J, Murgia C, Leigh Ackland M, Zalewski P, Anderson G, Ruffin R. Dietary zinc mediates inflammation and protects against wasting and metabolic derangement caused by sustained cigarette smoke exposure in mice. *Biometals.* 2011 Feb;24(1):23-39. 2010 Aug 29.

Lange NE, Rifas-Shiman SL, Camargo CA Jr, Gold DR, Gillman MW, Litonjua AA. Maternal dietary pattern during pregnancy is not associated with recurrent wheeze in children. *J Allergy Clin Immunol.* 2010 Aug;126(2):250-5, 255.e1-4.

Lappe FM. *Diet for a Small Planet.* New York: Ballantine, 1971.

Larenas-Linnemann D, Matta JJ, Shah-Hosseini K, Michels A, Mösges R. Skin prick test evaluation of Dermatophagoides pteronyssinus diagnostic extracts from Europe, Mexico, and the United States. *Ann Allergy Asthma Immunol.* 2010 May;104(5):420-5.

Lau BH, Riesen SK, Truong KP, Lau EW, Rohdewald P, Barreta RA. Pycnogenol as an adjunct in the management of childhood asthma. *J Asthma.* 2004;41(8):825-32.

Laubereau B, Filipiak-Pittroff B, von Berg A, Grübl A, Reinhardt D, Wichmann HE, Koletzko S; GINI Study Group. Caesarean section and gastrointestinal symptoms, atopic dermatitis, and sensitisation during the first year of life. *Arch Dis Child.* 2004 Nov;89(11):993-7.

Laurière M, Pecquet C, Bouchez-Mahiout I, Snégaroff J, Bayrou O, Raison-Peyron N, Vigan M. Hydrolysed wheat proteins present in cosmetics can induce immediate hypersensitivities. *Contact Dermatitis.* 2006 May;54(5):283-9.

LaValle JB. *The Cox-2 Connection.* Rochester, VT: Healing Arts, 2001.

Lazarou J, Pomeranz BH, Corey PN. Incidence of adverse drug reactions in hospitalized patients: a meta-analysis of prospective studies. *JAMA.* 1998 Apr.

Lean G. US study links more than 200 diseases to pollution. *London Independent.* 2004 Nov 14.

Leander M, Cronqvist A, Janson C, Uddenfeldt M, Rask-Andersen A. Health-related quality of life predicts onset of asthma in a longitudinal population study. *Respir Med.* 2009 Feb;103(2):194-200.

Lecheler J, Pfannebecker B, Nguyen DT, Petzold U, Munzel U, Kremer HJ, Maus J. Prevention of exercise-induced asthma by a fixed combination of disodium cromoglycate plus reproterol compared with montelukast in young patients. *Arzneimittelforschung.* 2008;58(6):303-9.

Lee E, Haa K, Yook JM, Jin MH, Seo CS, Son KH, Kim HP, Bae KH, Kang SS, Son JK, Chang HW. Anti-asthmatic activity of an ethanol extract from Saururus chinensis. *Biol Pharm Bull.* 2006 Feb;29(2):211-5.

Lee JH, Noh J, Noh G, Kim HS, Mun SH, Choi WS, Cho S, Lee S. Allergen-specific B cell subset responses in cow's milk allergy of late eczematous reactions in atopic dermatitis. *Cell Immunol.* 2010;262(1):44-51.

Lee JY, Kim CJ. Determination of allergenic egg proteins in food by protein-, mass spectrometry-, and DNA-based methods. *J AOAC Int.* 2010 Mar-Apr;93(2):462-77.

Lee KH, Yeh MH, Kao ST, Hung CM, Chen BC, Liu CJ, Yeh CC. Xia-bai-san inhibits lipopolysaccharide-induced activation of intercellular adhesion molecule-1 and nuclear factor-kappa B in human lung cells. *J Ethnopharmacol.* 2009 Jul 30;124(3):530-8.

Lee YS, Kim SH, Jung SH, Kim JK, Pan CH, Lim SS. Aldose reductase inhibitory compounds from Glycyrrhiza uralensis. *Biol Pharm Bull.* 2010;33(5):917-21.

Lehmann B. The vitamin D3 pathway in human skin and its role for regulation of biological processes. *Photochem Photobiol.* 2005 Nov-Dec;81(6):1246-51.

Lehto M, Airaksinen L, Puustinen A, Tillander S, Hannula S, Nyman T, Toskala E, Alenius H, Lauerma A. Thaumatin-like protein and baker's respiratory allergy. *Ann Allergy Asthma Immunol.* 2010 Feb;104(2):139-46.

Leitzmann C. Vegetarian diets: what are the advantages? *Forum Nutr.* 2005;(57):147-56.

Leu YL, Shi LS, Damu AG. Chemical constituents of Taraxacum formosanum. Chem *Pharm Bull.* 2003 May;51(5):599-601.

Leu YL, Wang YL, Huang SC, Shi LS. Chemical constituents from roots of Taraxacum formosanum. *Chem Pharm Bull.* 2005 Jul;53(7):853-5.

Leung DY, Sampson HA, Yunginger JW, Burks AW Jr, Schneider LC, Wortel CH, Davis FM, Hyun JD, Shanahan WR Jr; Avon Longitudinal Study of Parents and Children Study Team. Effect of anti-IgE therapy in patients with peanut allergy. *N Engl J Med.* 2003 Mar 13;348(11):986-93.

Leung DY, Shanahan WR Jr, Li XM, Sampson HA. New approaches for the treatment of anaphylaxis. *Novartis Found Symp.* 2004;257:248-60; discussion 260-4, 276-85.

Lewerin C, Jacobsson S, Lindstedt G, Nilsson-Ehle H. Serum biomarkers for atrophic gastritis and antibodies against Helicobacter pylori in the elderly: Implications for vitamin B12, folic acid and iron status and response to oral vitamin therapy. *Scand J Gastroenterol.* 2008;43(9):1050-6.

Lewis SA, Grimshaw KE, Warner JO, Hourihane JO. The promiscuity of immunoglobulin E binding to peanut allergens, as determined by Western blotting, correlates with the severity of clinical symptoms. *Clin Exp Allergy.* 2005 Jun;35(6):767-73.

Lewis WH, Elvin-Lewis MPF. *Medical Botany: Plants Affecting Man's Health.* New York: Wiley, 1977.

Lewontin R. *The Genetic Basis of Evolutionary Change.* New York: Columbia Univ Press, 1974.

Leyel CF. *Culpeper's English Physician & Complete Herbal.* Hollywood, CA: Wilshire, 1971.

Leynadier F. Mast cells and basophils in asthma. Ann Biol Clin (Paris). 1989;47(6):351-6.

Li J, Sun B, Huang Y, Lin X, Zhao D, Tan G, Wu J, Zhao H, Cao L, Zhong N. A multicentre study assessing the prevalence of sensitizations in patients with asthma and/or rhinitis in China. *Allergy.* 2009;64:1083-1092.

Li MH, Zhang HL, Yang BY. Effects of ginkgo leaf concentrated oral liquor in treating asthma. *Zhongguo Zhong Xi Yi Jie He Za Zhi.* 1997 Apr;17(4):216-8. 5.

Li S, Li W, Wang Y, Asada Y, Koike K. Prenylflavonoids from Glycyrrhiza uralensis and their protein tyrosine phosphatase-1B inhibitory activities. *Bioorg Med Chem Lett.* 2010 Sep 15;20(18):5398-401.

Li XM, Huang CK, Zhang TF, Teper AA, Srivastava K, Schofield BH, Sampson HA. The chinese herbal medicine formula MSSM-002 suppresses allergic airway hyperreactivity and modulates TH1/TH2 responses in a murine model of allergic asthma. *J Allergy Clin Immunol.* 2000;106:660-8.

Li XM, Srivastava K. Traditional Chinese medicine for the therapy of allergic disorders. *Curr Opin Otolaryngol Head Neck Surg.* 2006 Jun;14(3):191-6.

Li XM, Zhang TF, Huang CK, Srivastava K, Teper AA, Zhang L, Schofield BH, Sampson HA. Food Allergy Herbal Formula-1 (FAHF-1) blocks peanut-induced anaphylaxis in a murine model. *J Allergy Clin Immunol.* 2001;108:639-46.

Li XM, Zhang TF, Sampson H, Zou ZM, Beyer K, Wen MC, Schofield B. The potential use of Chinese herbal medicines in treating allergic asthma. *Ann Allergy Asthma Immunol.* 2004;93:S35-S44.

Li XM. Beyond allergen avoidance: update on developing therapies for peanut allergy. *Curr Opin Allergy Clin Immunol.* 2005;5:287-92.

REFERENCES AND BIBLIOGRAPHY

Li YQ, Yuan W, Zhang SL. Clinical and experimental study of xiao er ke cuan ling oral liquid in the treatment of infantile bronchopneumonia. *Zhongguo Zhong Xi Yi Jie He Za Zhi*. 1992 Dec;12(12):719-21, 737, 708.

Lied GA, Lillestøl K, Valeur J, Berstad A. Intestinal B cell-activating factor: an indicator of non-IgE-mediated hypersensitivity reactions to food? *Aliment Pharmacol Ther*. 2010 Jul;32(1):66-73.

Lillestøl K, Berstad A, Lind R, Florvaag E, Arslan Lied G, Tangen T. Anxiety and depression in patients with self-reported food hypersensitivity. *Gen Hosp Psychiatry*. 2010 Jan-Feb;32(1):42-8.

Lima JA, Fischer GB, Sarria EE, Mattiello R, Solé D. Prevalence of and risk factors for wheezing in the first year of life. *J Bras Pneumol*. 2010 Oct;36(5):525-31. English, Portuguese.

Limb SL, Brown KC, Wood RA, Wise RA, Eggleston PA, Tonascia J, Hamilton RG, Adkinson NF Jr. Adult asthma severity in individuals with a history of childhood asthma. *J Allergy Clin Immunol*. 2005 Jan;115(1):61-6.

Lindahl O, Lindwall L, Spångberg A, Stenram A, Ockerman PA. Vegan regimen with reduced medication in the treatment of bronchial asthma. *J Asthma*. 1985;22(1):45-55.

Ling WH, Hänninen O. Shifting from a conventional diet to an uncooked vegan diet reversibly alters fecal hydrolytic activities in humans. J Nutr. 1992 Apr;122(4):924-30.

Lininger S, Gaby A, Austin S, Brown D, Wright J, Duncan A. *The Natural Pharmacy*. New York: Three Rivers, 1999.

Linsalata M, Russo F, Berloco P, Caruso ML, Matteo GD, Cifone MG, Simone CD, Ierardi E, Di Leo A. The influence of Lactobacillus brevis on ornithine decarboxylase activity and polyamine profiles in Helicobacter pylori-infected gastric mucosa. Helicobacter. 2004 Apr;9(2):165-72.

Lipski E. *Digestive Wellness*. Los Angeles, CA: Keats, 2000.

Liu AH, Jaramillo R, Sicherer SH, Wood RA, Bock SA, Burks AW, Massing M, Cohn RD, Zeldin DC. National prevalence and risk factors for food allergy and relationship to asthma: results from the National Health and Nutrition Examination Survey 2005-2006. *J Allergy Clin Immunol*. 2010 Oct;126(4):798-806.e13.

Liu GM, Cao MJ, Huang YY, Cai QF, Weng WY, Su WJ. Comparative study of in vitro digestibility of major allergen tropomyosin and other food proteins of Chinese mitten crab (Eriocheir sinensis). *J Sci Food Agric*. 2010 Aug 15;90(10):1614-20.

Liu HY, Giday Z, Moore BF. Possible pathogenetic mechanisms producing bovine milk protein inducible malabsorption: a hypothesis. *Ann Allergy*. 1977 Jul;39(1):1-7.

Liu JY, Hu JH, Zhu QG, Li FQ, Wang J, Sun HJ. Effect of matrine on the expression of substance P receptor and inflammatory cytokines production in human skin keratinocytes and fibroblasts. *Int Immunopharmacol*. 2007 Jun;7(6):816-23.

Liu T, Valdez R, Yoon PW, Crocker D, Moonesinghe R, Khoury MJ. The association between family history of asthma and the prevalence of asthma among US adults: National Health and Nutrition Examination Survey, 1999-2004. *Genet Med*. 2009 May;11(5):323-8.

Liu X, Beaty TH, Deindl P, Huang SK, Lau S, Sommerfeld C, Fallin MD, Kao WH, Wahn U, Nickel R. Associations between specific serum IgE response and 6 variants within the genes IL4, IL13, and IL4RA in German children: the German Multicenter Atopy Study. *J Allergy Clin Immunol*. 2004 Mar;113(3):489-95.

Liu XJ, Cao MA, Li WH, Shen CS, Yan SQ, Yuan CS. Alkaloids from Sophora flavescens Aition. *Fitoterapia*. 2010 Sep;81(6):524-7.

Lloyd JU. *American Materia Medica, Therapeutics and Pharmacognosy*. Portland, OR: Eclectic Medical Publications, 1989-1983.

Lloyd-Still JD, Powers CA, Hoffman DR, Boyd-Trull K, Lester LA, Benisek DC, Arterburn LM. Bioavailability and safety of a high dose of docosahexaenoic acid triacylglycerol of algal origin in cystic fibrosis patients: a randomized, controlled study. *Nutrition*. 2006 Jan;22(1):36-46.

Locke GR 3rd, Talley NJ, Fett SL, Zinsmeister AR, Melton LJ 3rd. Prevalence and clinical spectrum of gastroesophageal reflux: a population-based study in Olmsted County, Minnesota. *Gastroenterology*. 1997 May;112(5):1448-56.

Loizzo MR, Saab AM, Tundis R, Statti GA, Menichini F, Lampronti I, Gambari R, Cinatl J, Doerr HW. Phytochemical analysis and in vitro antiviral activities of the essential oils of seven Lebanon species. *Chem Biodivers*. 2008 Mar;5(3):461-70.

Lomax AR, Calder PC. Probiotics, immune function, infection and inflammation: a review of the evidence from studies conducted in humans. *Curr Pharm Des*. 2009;15(13):1428-518.

Longo G, Barbi E, Berti I, Meneghetti R, Pittalis A, Ronfani L, Ventura A. Specific oral tolerance induction in children with very severe cow's milk-induced reactions. *J Allergy Clin Immunol*. 2008 Feb;121(2):343-7.

Lopes EA, Fanelli-Galvani A, Prisco CC, Gonçalves RC, Jacob CM, Cabral AL, Martins MA, Carvalho CR. Assessment of muscle shortening and static posture in children with persistent asthma. *Eur J Pediatr*. 2007 Jul;166(7):715-21.

López N, de Barros-Mazón S, Vilela MM, Silva CM, Ribeiro JD. Genetic and environmental influences on atopic immune response in early life. *J Investig Allergol Clin Immunol*. 1999 Nov-Dec;9(6):392-8.

Lopez-Garcia E, Schulze MB, Meigs JB, Manson JE, Rifai N, Stampfer MJ, Willett WC, Hu FB. Consumption of trans fatty acids is related to plasma biomarkers of inflammation and endothelial dysfunction. *J Nutr*. 2005 Mar;135(3):562-6.

Lu MK, Shih YW, Chang Chien TT, Fang LH, Huang HC, Chen PS. α-Solanine inhibits human melanoma cell migration and invasion by reducing matrix metalloproteinase-2/9 activities. *Biol Pharm Bull*. 2010;33(10):1685-91.

Lucas A, Brooke OG, Cole TJ, Morley R, Bamford MF. Food and drug reactions, wheezing, and eczema in preterm infants. *Arch Dis Child.* 1990 Apr;65(4):411-5. 8; .

Lunardi AC, Marques da Silva CC, Rodrigues Mendes FA, Marques AP, Stelmach R, Fernandes Carvalho CR. Musculoskeletal dysfunction and pain in adults with asthma. *J Asthma.* 2011 Feb;48(1):105-10.

Lykken DT, Tellegen A, DeRubeis R: Volunteer bias in twin research: the rule of two-thirds. *Soc Biol* 1978, 25(1): 1-9. Phillips DI: Twin studies in medical research: can they tell us whether diseases are genetically determined? *Lancet* 1993;341(8851): 1008-1009.

Ma J, Xiao L, Knowles SB. Obesity, insulin resistance and the prevalence of atopy and asthma in US adults. Allergy. 2010 Nov;65(11):1455-63.

Ma XP, Muzhapaer D. Efficacy of sublingual immunotherapy in children with dust mite allergic asthma. *Zhongguo Dang Dai Er Ke Za Zhi.* 2010 May;12(5):344-7.

Mabey R, ed. *The New Age Herbalist.* New York: Simon & Schuster, 1941.

Macdonald TT, Monteleone G. Immunity, inflammation, and allergy in the gut. *Science.* 2005 Mar 25;307(5717):1920-5.

Maciorkowska E, Kaczmarski M, Andrzej K. Endoscopic evaluation of upper gastrointestinal tract mucosa in children with food hypersensitivity. *Med Wieku Rozwoj.* 2000 Jan-Mar;4(1):37-48.

Mackerras D, Cunningham J, Hunt A, Brent P. Re: "effect of supplemental folic acid in pregnancy on childhood asthma: a prospective birth cohort study". *Am J Epidemiol.* 2010 Mar 15;171(6):746-7; author reply 747. 2010 Feb 9.

MacRedmond R, Singhera G, Attridge S, Bahzad M, Fava C, Lai Y, Hallstrand TS, Dorscheid DR. Conjugated linoleic acid improves airway hyper-reactivity in overweight mild asthmatics. *Clin Exp Allergy.* 2010 Jul;40(7):1071-8.

Macsali F, Real FG, Omenaas ER, Bjorge L, Janson C, Franklin K, Svanes C. Oral contraception, body mass index, and asthma: a cross-sectional Nordic-Baltic population survey. *J Allergy Clin Immunol.* 2009 Feb;123(2):391-7.

Madden JA, Plummer SF, Tang J, Garaiova I, Plummer NT, Herbison M, Hunter JO, Shimada T, Cheng L, Shirakawa T. Effect of probiotics on preventing disruption of the intestinal microflora following antibiotic therapy: a double-blind, placebo-controlled pilot study. *Int Immunopharmacol.* 2005 Jun;5(6):1091-7.

Maeda N, Inomata N, Morita A, Kirino M, Ikezawa Z. Correlation of oral allergy syndrome due to plant-derived foods with pollen sensitization in Japan. *Ann Allergy Asthma Immunol.* 2010 Mar;104(3):205-10.

Maes HH, Silberg JL, Neale MC, Eaves LJ. Genetic and cultural transmission of antisocial behavior: an extended twin parent model. *Twin Res Hum Genet.* 2007 Feb;10(1):136-50.

Mai XM, Kull I, Wickman M, Bergström A. Antibiotic use in early life and development of allergic diseases: respiratory infection as the explanation. *Clin Exp Allergy.* 2010 Aug;40(8):1230-7.

Mainardi T, Kapoor S, Bielory L. Complementary and alternative medicine: herbs, phytochemicals and vitamins and their immunologic effects. *J Allergy Clin Immunol.* 2009 Feb;123(2):283-94; quiz 295-6.

Majamaa H, Isolauri E. Probiotics: a novel approach in the management of food allergy. *J Allergy Clin Immunol.* 1997 Feb;99(2):179-85.

Makrides M, Neumann M, Gibson R. Effect of maternal docosahexaenoic acid (DHA) supplementation on breast milk composition. *Europ Jrnl of Clin Nutr.* 1996;50:352-357.

Maliakal PP, Wanwimolruk S. Effect of herbal teas on hepatic drug metabolizing enzymes in rats. *J Pharm Pharmacol.* 2001 Oct;53(10):1323-9.

Mälkönen T, Alanko K, Jolanki R, Luukkonen R, Aalto-Korte K, Lauerma A, Susitaival P. Long-term follow-up study of occupational hand eczema. Br J Dermatol. 2010 Aug 13.

Mallol J, Solé D, Baeza-Bacab M, Aguirre-Camposano V, Soto-Quiros M, Baena-Cagnani C; Latin American ISAAC Group. Regional variation in asthma symptom prevalence in Latin American children. *J Asthma.* 2010 Aug;47(6):644-50.

Maneechotesuwan K, Supawita S, Kasetsinsombat K, Wongkajornsilp A, Barnes PJ. Sputum indoleamine-2, 3-dioxygenase activity is increased in asthmatic airways by using inhaled corticosteroids. *J Allergy Clin Immunol.* 2008 Jan;121(1):43-50.

Månsson HL. Fatty acids in bovine milk fat. *Food Nutr Res.* 2008;52. doi: 10.3402/fnr.v52i0.1821.

Manz F. Hydration and disease. *J Am Coll Nutr.* 2007 Oct;26(5 Suppl):535S-541S.

Marcucci F, Duse M, Frati F, Incorvaia C, Marseglia GL, La Rosa M. The future of sublingual immunotherapy. *Int J Immunopathol Pharmacol.* 2009 Oct-Dec;22(4 Suppl):31-3.

Margioris AN. Fatty acids and postprandial inflammation. *Curr Opin Clin Nutr Metab Care.* 2009 Mar;12(2):129-37.

Maria KW, Behrens T, Brasky TM. Are asthma and allergies in children and adolescents increasing? Results from ISAAC Phase I and Phase II surveys in Munster, Germany. Allergy. 2003;58:572-579.

Martin IR, Wickens K, Patchett K, Kent R, Fitzharris P, Siebers R, Lewis S, Crane J, Holbrook N, Town GI, Smith S. Cat allergen levels in public places in New Zealand. *N Z Med J.* 1998 Sep 25;111(1074):356-8.

Martinez M. Docosahexaenoic acid therapy in docosahexaenoic acid-deficient patients with disorders of peroxisomal biogenesis. *Versicherungsmedizin.* 1996;31 Suppl:145-152

REFERENCES AND BIBLIOGRAPHY

Martínez-Augustin O, Boza JJ, Del Pino JI, Lucena J, Martínez-Valverde A, Gil A. Dietary nucleotides might influence the humoral immune response against cow's milk proteins in preterm neonates. *Biol Neonate.* 1997;71(4):215-23.

Martin-Venegas R, Roig-Perez S, Ferrer R, Moreno JJ. Arachidonic acid cascade and epithelial barrier function during Caco-2 cell differentiation. *J Lipid Res.* 2006 Apr;3.

Maslowski KM, Mackay CR. Diet, gut microbiota and immune responses. *Nat Immunol.* 2011 Jan;12(1):5-9.

Masoli M, Fabian D, Holt S, Beasley R. The global burden of asthma: executive summary of the GINA Dissemination Committee Report. *Allergy.* 2004;59:469-478.

Massey DG, Chien YK, Fournier-Massey G. Mamane: scientific therapy for asthma? *Hawaii Med J.* 1994;53:350-1. 363.

Massicot JG, Cohen SG. Epidemiologic and socioeconomic aspects of allergic diseases. *J Allergy Clin Immunol.* 1986 Nov;78(5 Pt 2):954-8.

Matasar MJ, Neugut AI. Epidemiology of anaphylaxis in the United States. *Curr Allergy Asthma Rep.* 2003;3:30-35.

Matheson MC, Haydn Walters E, Burgess JA, Jenkins MA, Giles GG, Hopper JL, Abramson MJ, Dharmage SC. Childhood immunization and atopic disease into middle-age—a prospective cohort study. *Pediatr Allergy Immunol.* 2010 Mar;21(2 Pt 1):301-6.

Matricardi PM, Bockelbrink A, Beyer K, Keil T, Niggemann B, Grüber C, Wahn U, Lau S. Primary versus secondary immunoglobulin E sensitization to soy and wheat in the Multi-Centre Allergy Study cohort. *Clin Exp Allergy.* 2008 Mar;38(3):493-500.

Matsui EC, Matsui W. Higher serum folate levels are associated with a lower risk of atopy and wheeze. *J Allergy Clin Immunol.* 2009 Jun;123(6):1253-9.e2. 2009 May 5.

Mayes MD. Epidemiologic studies of environmental agents and systemic autoimmune diseases. *Environ Health Perspect.* 1999 Oct;107 Suppl 5:743-8.

McAlindon TE. Nutraceuticals: do they work and when should we use them? *Best Pract Res Clin Rheumatol.* 2006 Feb;20(1):99-115.

McCarney RW, Lasserson TJ, Linde K, Brinkhaus B. An overview of two Cochrane systematic reviews of complementary treatments for chronic asthma: acupuncture and homeopathy. *Respir Med.* 2004 Aug;98(8):687-96.

McCarney RW, Linde K, Lasserson TJ. Homeopathy for chronic asthma. *Cochrane Database Syst Rev.* 2004;(1):CD000353.

McConnaughey E. *Sea Vegetables.* Happy Camp, CA: Naturegraph, 1985.

McDougall J, McDougall M. *The McDougal Plan.* Clinton, NJ: New Win, 1983.

McHugh MK, Symanski E, Pompeii LA, Delclos GL. Prevalence of asthma by industry and occupation in the U.S. working population. *Am J Ind Med.* 2010 May;53(5):463-75.

McHugh MK, Symanski E, Pompeii LA, Delclos GL. Prevalence of asthma among adult females and males in the United States: results from the National Health and Nutrition Examination Survey (NHANES), 2001-2004. *J Asthma.* 2009 Oct;46(8):759-66.

McKeever TM, Lewis SA, Cassano PA, Ocké M, Burney P, Britton J, Smit HA. Patterns of dietary intake and relation to respiratory disease, forced expiratory volume in 1 s, and decline in 5-y forced expiratory volume. *Am J Clin Nutr.* 2010 Aug;92(2):408-15. 2010 Jun 16.

McKenzie H, Main J, Pennington CR, Parratt D. Antibody to selected strains of Saccharomyces cerevisiae (baker's and brewer's yeast) and Candida albicans in Crohn's disease. *Gut.* 1990 May;31(5):536-8.

McLachlan CN. beta-casein A1, ischaemic heart disease mortality, and other illnesses. *Med Hypotheses.* 2001 Feb;56(2):262-72.

McNally ME, Atkinson SA, Cole DE. Contribution of sulfate and sulfoesters to total sulfur intake in infants fed human milk. *J Nutr.* 1991 Aug;121(8):1250-4.

McNaught CE, Woodcock NP, Anderson AD, MacFie J. A prospective randomised trial of probiotics in critically ill patients. *Clin Nutr.* 2005 Apr;24(2):211-9.

Meglio P, Bartone E, Plantamura M, Arabito E, Giampietro PG. A protocol for oral desensitization in children with IgE-mediated cow's milk allergy. *Allergy.* 2004 Sep;59(9):980-7.

Mehra PN, Puri HS. Studies on Gaduchi satwa. *Indian J Pharm.* 1969;31:180-2.

Meier B, Shao Y, Julkunen-Tiitto R, Bettschart A, Sticher O. A chemotaxonomic survey of phenolic compounds in Swiss willow species. *Planta Med.* 1992;58:A698.

Meier B, Sticher O, Julkunen-Tiitto R. Pharmaceutical aspects of the use of willows in herbal remedies. *Planta Med.* 1988;54(6):559-560.

Melcion C, Verroust P, Baud L, Ardaillou N, Morel-Maroger L, Ardaillou R. Protective effect of procyanidolic oligomers on the heterologous phase of glomerulonephritis induced by anti-glomerular basement membrane antibodies. *C R Seances Acad Sci III.* 1982 Dec 6;295(12):721-6.

Mendes FA, Gonçalves RC, Nunes MP, Saraiva-Romanholo BM, Cukier A, Stelmach R, Jacob-Filho W, Martins MA, Carvalho CR. Effects of aerobic training on psychosocial morbidity and symptoms in patients with asthma: a randomized clinical trial. *Chest.* 2010 Aug;138(2):331-7. 2010 Apr 2.

Merchant RE and Andre CA. 2001. A review of recent clinical trials of the nutritional supplement Chlorella pyrenoidosa in the treatment of fibromyalgia, hypertension, and ulcerative colitis. *Altern Ther Health Med.* May-Jun;7(3):79-91.
Messina M. Insights gained from 20 years of soy research. *J Nutr.* 2010 Dec;140(12):2289S-2295S. 2010 Oct 27.
Metsälä J, Lundqvist A, Kaila M, Gissler M, Klaukka T, Virtanen SM. Maternal and perinatal characteristics and the risk of cow's milk allergy in infants up to 2 years of age: a case-control study nested in the Finnish population. *Am J Epidemiol.* 2010 Jun 15;171(12):1310-6.
Meyer A, Kirsch H, Domergue F, Abbadi A, Sperling P, Bauer J, Cirpus P, Zank TK, Moreau H, Roscoe TJ, Zahringer U, Heinz E. Novel fatty acid elongases and their use for the reconstitution of docosahexaenoic acid biosynthesis. *J Lipid Res.* 2004 Oct;45(10):1899-909.
Meyer AL, Elmadfa I, Herbacek I, Micksche M. Probiotic, as well as conventional yogurt, can enhance the stimulated production of proinflammatory cytokines. J Hum Nutr Diet. 2007 Dec;20(6):590-8.
Michaelsen KF. Probiotics, breastfeeding and atopic eczema. *Acta Derm Venereol Suppl (Stockh).* 2005 Nov;(215):21-4.
Michail S. The role of probiotics in allergic diseases. Allergy Asthma Clin Immunol. 2009 Oct 22;5(1):5.
Michalska K, Kisiel W. Sesquiterpene lactones from Taraxacum obovatum. *Planta Med.* 2003 Feb;69(2):181-3.
Michelson PH, Williams LW, Benjamin DK, Barnato AE. Obesity, inflammation, and asthma severity in childhood: data from the National Health and Nutrition Examination Survey 2001-2004. *Ann Allergy Asthma Immunol.* 2009 Nov;103(5):381-5.
Mickleborough TD, Lindley MR, Ray S. Dietary salt, airway inflammation, and diffusion capacity in exercise-induced asthma. *Med Sci Sports Exerc.* 2005 Jun;37(6):904-14.
Mikoluc B, Motkowski R, Karpinska J, Piotrowska-Jastrzebska J. Plasma levels of vitamins A and E, coenzyme Q10, and anti-ox-LDL antibody titer in children treated with an elimination diet due to food hypersensitivity. *Int J Vitam Nutr Res.* 2009 Sep;79(5-6):328-36.
Miller AL. The etiologies, pathophysiology, and alternative/complementary treatment of asthma. *Altern Med Rev.* 2001 Feb;6(1):20-47.
Miller GT. *Living in the Environment.* Belmont, CA: Wadsworth, 1996.
Mindell E, Hopkins V. *Prescription Alternatives.* New Canaan, CT: Keats, 1998.
Miranda H, Outeiro TF. The sour side of neurodegenerative disorders: the effects of protein glycation. *J Pathol.* 2010 May;221(1):13-25.
Mitchell AE, Hong YJ, Koh E, Barrett DM, Bryant DE, Denison RF, Kaffka S. Ten-year comparison of the influence of organic and conventional crop management practices on the content of flavonoids in tomatoes. *J Agric Food Chem.* 2007 Jul 25;55(15):6154-9.
Mittag D, Akkerdaas J, Ballmer-Weber BK, Vogel L, Wensing M, Becker WM, Koppelman SJ, Knulst AC, Helbling A, Hefle SL, Van Ree R, Vieths S. Ara h 8, a Bet v 1-homologous allergen from peanut, is a major allergen in patients with combined birch pollen and peanut allergy. *J Allergy Clin Immunol.* 2004 Dec;114(6):1410-7.
Mittag D, Vieths S, Vogel L, Becker WM, Rihs HP, Helbling A, Wüthrich B, Ballmer-Weber BK. Soybean allergy in patients allergic to birch pollen: clinical investigation and molecular characterization of allergens. *J Allergy Clin Immunol.* 2004 Jan;113(1):148-54.
Miyake Y, Sasaki S, Tanaka K, Hirota Y. Dairy food, calcium and vitamin D intake in pregnancy, and wheeze and eczema in infants. *Eur Respir J.* 2010 Jun;35(6):1228-34. 2009 Oct 19.
Miyazawa T, Itahashi K, Imai T. Management of neonatal cow's milk allergy in high-risk neonates. *Pediatr Int.* 2009 Aug;51(4):544-7.
Moattari A, Aleyasin S, Arabpour M, Sadeghi S. Prevalence of Human Metapneumovirus (hMPV) in Children with Wheezing in Shiraz-Iran. *Iran J Allergy Asthma Immunol.* 2010 Dec;9(4):250-4.
Mokhtar N, Chan SC. Use of complementary medicine amongst asthmatic patients in primary care. *Med J Malaysia.* 2006 Mar;61(1):125-7.
Monarca S, Zerbini I, Simonati C, Gelatti U. Drinking water hardness and chronic degenerative diseases. Part II. Cardiovascular diseases. *Ann. Ig.* 2003;15:41-56.
Moneret-Vautrin DA, Kanny G, Thévenin F. Asthma caused by food allergy. *Rev Med Interne.* 1996;17(7):551-7.
Moneret-Vautrin DA, Morisset M. Adult food allergy. *Curr Allergy Asthma Rep.* 2005 Jan;5(1):80-5.
Monks H, Gowland MH, Mackenzie H, Erlewyn-Lajeunesse M, King R, Lucas JS, Roberts G. How do teenagers manage their food allergies? *Clin Exp Allergy.* 2010 Aug 2.
Moorhead KJ, Morgan HC. *Spirulina: Nature's Superfood.* Kailua-Kona, HI: Nutrex, 1995.
Moreira A, Delgado L, Haahtela T, Fonseca J, Moreira P, Lopes C, Mota J, Santos P, Rytilä P, Castel-Branco MG. Physical training does not increase allergic inflammation in asthmatic children. Eur Respir J. 2008 Dec;32(6):1570-5.
Moreira P, Moreira A, Padrão P, Delgado L. The role of economic and educational factors in asthma: evidence from the Portuguese health survey. *Public Health.* 2008 Apr;122(4):434-9. 2007 Oct 17.

REFERENCES AND BIBLIOGRAPHY

Morel AF, Dias GO, Porto C, Simionatto E, Stuker CZ, Dalcol II. Antimicrobial activity of extractives of Solidago microglossa. *Fitoterapia.* 2006 Sep;77(6):453-5.

Morisset M, Moneret-Vautrin DA, Guenard L, Cuny JM, Frentz P, Hatahet R, Hanss Ch, Beaudouin E, Petit N, Kanny G. Oral desensitization in children with milk and egg allergies obtains recovery in a significant proportion of cases. A randomized study in 60 children with cow's milk allergy and 90 children with egg allergy. *Eur Ann Allergy Clin Immunol.* 2007 Jan;39(1):12-9.

Morisset M, Moneret-Vautrin DA, Kanny G, Guénard L, Beaudouin E, Flabbée J, Hatahet R. Thresholds of clinical reactivity to milk, egg, peanut and sesame in immunoglobulin E-dependent allergies: evaluation by double-blind or single-blind placebo-controlled oral challenges. *Clin Exp Allergy.* 2003 Aug;33(8):1046-51.

Moussaieff A, Shein NA, Tsenter J, Grigoriadis S, Simeonidou C, Alexandrovich AG, Trembovler V, Ben-Neriah Y, Schmitz ML, Fiebich BL, Munoz E, Mechoulam R, Shohami E. Incensole acetate: a novel neuroprotective agent isolated from Boswellia carterii. *J Cereb Blood Flow Metab.* 2008 Jul;28(7):1341-52.

Moyle A. *Nature Cure for Asthma and Hay Fever.* Wellingborough, U.K.: Thorsons, 1978.

Mozaffarian D, Aro A, Willett WC. Health effects of trans-fatty acids: experimental and observational evidence. *Eur J Clin Nutr.* 2009 May;63 Suppl 2:S5-21.

Murray M, Pizzorno J. *Encyclopedia of Natural Medicine.* 2nd Edition. Roseville, CA: Prima Publishing, 1998.

Nadkarni AK, Nadkarni KM. *Indian Materia Medica.* (Vols 1 and 2). Bombay, India: Popular Pradashan, 1908, 1976.

Nagai T, Arai Y, Emori H, Nunome SY, Yabe T, Takeda T, Yamada H. Anti-allergic activity of a Kampo (Japanese herbal) medicine "Sho-seiryu-to (Xiao-Qing-Long-Tang)" on airway inflammation in a mouse model. *Int Immunopharmacol.* 2004 Oct;4(10-11):1353-65.

Nagel G, Linseisen J. Dietary intake of fatty acids, antioxidants and selected food groups and asthma in adults. *Eur J Clin Nutr.* 2005 Jan;59(1):8-15.

Nagel G, Weinmayr G, Kleiner A, Garcia-Marcos L, Strachan DP; ISAAC Phase Two Study Group. Effect of diet on asthma and allergic sensitisation in the International Study on Allergies and Asthma in Childhood (ISAAC) Phase Two. Thorax. 2010 Jun;65(6):516-22.

Naghii MR, Samman S. The role of boron in nutrition and metabolism. *Prog Food Nutr Sci.* 1993 Oct-Dec;17(4):331-49.

Nair PK, Rodriguez S, Ramachandran R, Alamo A, Melnick SJ, Escalon E, Garcia PI Jr, Wnuk SF, Ramachandran C. Immune stimulating properties of a novel polysaccharide from the medicinal plant Tinospora cordifolia. *Int Immunopharmacol.* 2004 Dec 15;4(13):1645-59.

Nakano T, Shimojo N, Morita Y, Arima T, Tomiita M, Kohno Y. Sensitization to casein and beta-lactoglobulin (BLG) in children with cow's milk allergy (CMA). *Arerugi.* 2010 Feb;59(2):117-22.

Napoli, J.E., Brand-Miller, J.C., Conway, P. (2003) Bifidogenic effects of feeding infant formula containing galactooligosaccharides in healthy formula-fed infants. *Asia Pac J Clin Nutr.* 12(Suppl): S60

Nariya M, Shukla V, Jain S, Ravishankar B. Comparison of enteroprotective efficacy of triphala formulations (Indian Herbal Drug) on methotrexate-induced small intestinal damage in rats. *Phytother Res.* 2009 Aug;23(8):1092-8.

Naruszewicz M, Johansson ML, Zapolska-Downar D, Bukowska H. Effect of Lactobacillus plantarum 299v on cardiovascular disease risk factors in smokers. *Am J Clin Nutr.* 2002 Dec;76(6):1249-55.

National Cooperation Group on Childhood Asthma. A nationwide survey in China on prevalence of asthma in urban children. Chin J Pediatr. pp. 123-127.

NDL, BHNRC, ARS, USDA. *Oxygen Radical Absorbance Capacity (ORAC) of Selected Foods - 2007.* Beltsville, MD: USDA-ARS. 2007.

Nentwich I, Michková E, Nevoral J, Urbanek R, Szépfalusi Z. Cow's milk-specific cellular and humoral immune responses and atopy skin symptoms in infants from atopic families fed a partially (pHF) or extensively (eHF) hydrolyzed infant formula. *Allergy.* 2001 Dec;56(12):1144-56.

Newall CA, Anderson LA, Phillipson JD (eds). *Herbal Medicines: A Guide for Health-Care Professionals.* London: Pharmaceut Press; 1996.

Newmark T, Schulick P. *Beyond Aspirin.* Prescott, AZ: Holm, 2000.

Neyestani TR, Shariatzadeh N, Gharavi A, Kalayi A, Khalaji N. Physiological dose of lycopene suppressed oxidative stress and enhanced serum levels of immunoglobulin M in patients with Type 2 diabetes mellitus: a possible role in the prevention of long-term complications. *J Endocrinol Invest.* 2007 Nov;30(10):833-8.

Ngai SP, Jones AY, Hui-Chan CW, Ko FW, Hui DS. Effect of Acu-TENS on post-exercise expiratory lung volume in subjects with asthma-A randomized controlled trial. *Respir Physiol Neurobiol.* 2009 Jul 31;167(3):348-53. 2009 Jun 18.

Nicholls SJ, Lundman P, Harmer JA, Cutri B, Griffiths KA, Rye KA, Barter PJ, Celermajer DS. Consumption of saturated fat impairs the anti-inflammatory properties of high-density lipoproteins and endothelial function. *J Am Coll Cardiol.* 2006 Aug 15;48(4):715-20.

Nicolaou N, Poorafshar M, Murray C, Simpson A, Winell H, Kerry G, Härlin A, Woodcock A, Ahlstedt S, Custovic A. Allergy or tolerance in children sensitized to peanut: prevalence and differentiation using component-resolved diagnostics. *J Allergy Clin Immunol.* 2010 Jan;125(1):191-7.e1-13.

Niederau C, Göpfert E. The effect of chelidonium- and turmeric root extract on upper abdominal pain due to functional disorders of the biliary system. Results from a placebo-controlled double-blind study. *Med Klin.* 1999 Aug 15;94(8):425-30.

Nielsen RG, Bindslev-Jensen C, Kruse-Andersen S, Husby S. Severe gastroesophageal reflux disease and cow milk hypersensitivity in infants and children: disease association and evaluation of a new challenge procedure. J *Pediatr Gastroenterol Nutr.* 2004 Oct;39(4):383-91.

Niggemann B, von Berg A, Bollrath C, Berdel D, Schauer U, Rieger C, Haschke-Becher E, Wahn U. Safety and efficacy of a new extensively hydrolyzed formula for infants with cow's milk protein allergy. *Pediatr Allergy Immunol.* 2008 Jun;19(4):348-54.

Nightingale JA, Rogers DF, Hart LA, Kharitonov SA, Chung KF, Barnes PJ. Effect of inhaled endotoxin on induced sputum in normal, atopic, and atopic asthmatic subjects. *Thorax.* 1998 Jul;53(7):563-71.

Niimi A, Nguyen LT, Usmani O, Mann B, Chung KF. Reduced pH and chloride levels in exhaled breath condensate of patients with chronic cough. *Thorax.* 2004 Jul;59(7):608-12.

Ninan TK, Russell G. Respiratory symptoms and atopy in Aberdeen schoolchildren: evidence from two surveys 25 years apart. BMJ. 1992;304:873-875.

Njoroge GN, Bussmann RW. Traditional management of ear, nose and throat (ENT) diseases in Central Kenya. *J Ethnobiol Ethnomed.* 2006 Dec 27;2:54.

Nobaek S, Johansson ML, Molin G, Ahrné S, Jeppsson B. Alteration of intestinal microflora is associated with reduction in abdominal bloating and pain in patients with irritable bowel syndrome. *Am J Gastroenterol.* 2000 May;95(5):1231-8.

Nodake Y, Fukumoto S, Fukasawa M, Sakakibara R, Yamasaki N. Reduction of the immunogenicity of beta-lactoglobulin from cow's milk by conjugation with a dextran derivative. *Biosci Biotechnol Biochem.* 2010;74(4):721-6.

Noh J, Lee JH, Noh G, Bang SY, Kim HS, Choi WS, Cho S, Lee SS. Characterisation of allergen-specific responses of IL-10-producing regulatory B cells (Br1) in Cow Milk Allergy. *Cell Immunol.* 2010;264(2):143-9.

Noorbakhsh R, Mortazavi SA, Sankian M, Shahidi F, Assarehzadegan MA, Varasteh A. Cloning, expression, characterization, and computational approach for cross-reactivity prediction of manganese superoxide dismutase allergen from pistachio nut. *Allergol Int.* 2010 Sep;59(3):295-304.

Novembre E, Dini L, Bernardini R, Resti M, Vierucci A. Unusual reactions to food additives. *Pediatr Med Chir.* 1992 Jan-Feb;14(1):39-42.

Nowak-Wegrzyn A, Fiocchi A. Is oral immunotherapy the cure for food allergies? *Curr Opin Allergy Clin Immunol.* 2010 Jun;10(3):214-9.

Nsouli TM. Long-term use of nasal saline irrigation: harmful or helpful? *Amer Acad of Allergy, Asthma, and Immunol.* 2009; Abstract O32.

Nurmatov U, Devereux G, Sheikh A. Nutrients and foods for the primary prevention of asthma and allergy: Systematic review and meta-analysis. *J Allergy Clin Immunol.* 2010 Dec 23.

Nusem D, Panasoff J. Beer anaphylaxis. *Isr Med Assoc J.* 2009 Jun;11(6):380-1.

Nwaru BI, Erkkola M, Ahonen S, Kaila M, Haapala AM, Kronberg-Kippilä C, Salmelin R, Veijola R, Ilonen J, Simell O, Knip M, Virtanen SM. Age at the introduction of solid foods during the first year and allergic sensitization at age 5 years. *Pediatrics.* 2010 Jan;125(1):50-9. 2009 Dec 7.

O'Connor J., Bensky D. (ed). *Shanghai College of Traditional Chinese Medicine: Acupuncture: A Comprehensive Text.* Seattle: Eastland Press, 1981.

Odamaki T, Xiao JZ, Iwabuchi N, Sakamoto M, Takahashi N, Kondo S, Miyaji K, Iwatsuki K, Togashi H, Enomoto T, Benno Y. Influence of Bifidobacterium longum BB536 intake on faecal microbiota in individuals with Japanese cedar pollinosis during the pollen season. *J Med Microbiol.* 2007 Oct;56(Pt 10):1301-8.

Oehme FW (ed.). *Toxicity of heavy metals in the environment. Part 1.* New York: M.Dekker, 1979.

Ogawa T, Hashikawa S, Asai Y, Sakamoto H, Yasuda K, Makimura Y. A new synbiotic, Lactobacillus casei subsp. casei together with dextran, reduces murine and human allergic reaction. *FEMS Immunol Med Microbiol.* 2006 Apr;46(3):400-9.

Oh CK, Lücker PW, Wetzelsberger N, Kuhlmann F. The determination of magnesium, calcium, sodium and potassium in assorted foods with special attention to the loss of electrolytes after various forms of food preparations. *Mag.-Bull.* 1986;8:297-302.

Oh SY, Chung J, Kim MK, Kwon SO, Cho BH. Antioxidant nutrient intakes and corresponding biomarkers associated with the risk of atopic dermatitis in young children. *Eur J Clin Nutr.* 2010 Mar;64(3):245-52. 2010 Jan 27.

REFERENCES AND BIBLIOGRAPHY

Ok IS, Kim SH, Kim BK, Lee JC, Lee YC. Pinellia ternata, Citrus reticulata, and their combinational prescription inhibit eosinophil infiltration and airway hyperresponsiveness by suppressing CCR3+ and Th2 cytokines production in the ovalbumin-induced asthma model. *Mediators Inflamm.* 2009;2009:413270.

Ołdak E, Kurzatkowska B, Stasiak-Barmuta A. Natural course of sensitization in children: follow-up study from birth to 6 years of age, I. Evaluation of total serum IgE and specific IgE antibodies with regard to atopic family history. *Rocz Akad Med Bialymst.* 2000;45:87-95.

O'Neil C, Helbling AA, Lehrer SB. Allergic reactions to fish. *Clin Rev Allergy.* 1993 Summer;11(2):183-200.

O'Neil C, Helbling AA, Lehrer SB. Allergic reactions to fish. *Clin Rev Allergy.* 1993;11(2):183-200.

Oreskovic NM, Sawicki GS, Kinane TB, Winickoff JP, Perrin JM. Travel patterns to school among children with asthma. *Clin Pediatr.* 2009 Jul;48(6):632-40. 2009 May 6.

Ortiz-Andrellucchi A, Sánchez-Villegas A, Rodríguez-Gallego C, Lemes A, Molero T, Soria A, Peña-Quintana L, Santana M, Ramírez O, García J, Cabrera F, Cobo J, Serra-Majem L. Immunomodulatory effects of the intake of fermented milk with Lactobacillus casei DN114001 in lactating mothers and their children. *Br J Nutr.* 2008 Oct;100(4):834-45.

Osguthorpe JD. Immunotherapy. *Curr Opin Otolaryngol Head Neck Surg.* 2010 Jun;18(3):206-12.

Otto SJ, van Houwelingen AC, Hornstra G. The effect of supplementation with docosahexaenoic and arachidonic acid derived from single cell oils on plasma and erythrocyte fatty acids of pregnant women in the second trimester. *Prostaglandins Leukot Essent Fatty Acids.* 2000 Nov;63(5):323-8.

Ou CC, Tsao SM, Lin MC, Yin MC. Protective action on human LDL against oxidation and glycation by four organosulfur compounds derived from garlic. *Lipids.* 2003 Mar;38(3):219-24.

Ouwehand AC, Bergsma N, Parhiala R, Lahtinen S, Gueimonde M, Finne-Soveri H, Strandberg T, Pitkälä K, Salminen S. Bifidobacterium microbiota and parameters of immune function in elderly subjects. *FEMS Immunol Med Microbiol.* 2008 Jun;53(1):18-25.

Ouwehand AC, Nermes M, Collado MC, Rautonen N, Salminen S, Isolauri E. Specific probiotics alleviate allergic rhinitis during the birch pollen season. *World J Gastroenterol.* 2009 Jul 14;15(26):3261-8.

Ouwehand AC, Tiihonen K, Saarinen M, Putaala H, Rautonen N. Influence of a combination of Lactobacillus acidophilus NCFM and lactitol on healthy elderly: intestinal and immune parameters. *Br J Nutr.* 2009 Feb;101(3):367-75.

Ozdemir O. Any benefits of probiotics in allergic disorders? *Allergy Asthma Proc.* 2010 Mar;31(2):103-11.

Paganelli R, Pallone F, Montano S, Le Moli S, Matricardi PM, Fais S, Paoluzi P, D'Amelio R, Aiuti F. Isotypic analysis of antibody response to a food antigen in inflammatory bowel disease. *Int Arch Allergy Appl Immunol.* 1985;78(1):81-5.

Pahud JJ, Schwarz K. Research and development of infant formulae with reduced allergenic properties. *Ann Allergy.* 1984 Dec;53(6 Pt 2):609-14.

Pakhale S, Doucette S, Vandemheen K, Boulet LP, McIvor RA, Fitzgerald JM, Hernandez P, Lemiere C, Sharma S, Field SK, Alvarez GG, Dales RE, Aaron SD. A comparison of obese and nonobese people with asthma: exploring an asthma-obesity interaction. *Chest.* 2010 Jun;137(6):1316-23. 2010 Feb 12.

Palacin A, Bartra J, Muñoz R, Diaz-Perales A, Valero A, Salcedo G. Anaphylaxis to wheat flour-derived foodstuffs and the lipid transfer protein syndrome: a potential role of wheat lipid transfer protein Tri a 14. *Int Arch Allergy Immunol.* 2010;152(2):178-83.

Palacios R, Sugawara I. Hydrocortisone abrogates proliferation of T cells in autologous mixed lymphocyte reaction by rendering the interleukin-2 Producer T cells unresponsive to interleukin-1 and unable to synthesize the T-cell growth factor. *Scand J Immunol.* 1982 Jan;15(1):25-31. 7.

Palacios R. HLA-DR antigens render interleukin-2-producer T lymphocytes sensitive to interleukin-1. *Scand J Immunol.* 1981 Sep;14(3):321-6.

Palmer DJ, Gold MS, Makrides M. Effect of cooked and raw egg consumption on ovalbumin content of human milk: a randomized, double-blind, cross-over trial. *Clin Exp Allergy.* 2005 Feb;35(2):173-8.

Panghal S, Mallapur SS, Kumar M, Ram V, Singh BK. Antiinflammatory Activity of Piper longum Fruit Oil. *Indian J Pharm Sci.* 2009 Jul;71(4):454-6.

Panzani R, Ariano R, Mistrello G. Cypress pollen does not cross-react to plant-derived foods. *Eur Ann Allergy Clin Immunol.* 2010 Jun;42(3):125-6.

Parcell S. Sulfur in human nutrition and applications in medicine. *Altern Med Rev.* 2002 Feb;7(1):22-44.

Park BJ, Tsunetsugu Y, Kasetani T, Kagawa T, Miyazaki Y. The physiological effects of Shinrin-yoku (taking in the forest atmosphere or forest bathing): evidence from field experiments in 24 forests across Japan. *Environ Health Prev Med.* 2010 Jan;15(1):18-26.

Parra D, De Morentin BM, Cobo JM, Mateos A, Martinez JA. Monocyte function in healthy middle-aged people receiving fermented milk containing Lactobacillus casei. *J Nutr Health Aging.* 2004;8(4):208-11.

Parra MD, Martínez de Morentin BE, Cobo JM, Mateos A, Martínez JA. Daily ingestion of fermented milk containing Lactobacillus casei DN114001 improves innate-defense capacity in healthy middle-aged people. *J Physiol Biochem.* 2004 Jun;60(2):85-91.
Partridge MR, Dockrell M, Smith NM: The use of complementary medicines by those with asthma. Respir Med 2003, 97:436-438.
Pastorello EA, Farioli L, Conti A, Pravettoni V, Bonomi S, Iametti S, Fortunato D, Scibilia J, Bindslev-Jensen C, Ballmer-Weber B, Robino AM, Ortolani C. Wheat IgE-mediated food allergy in European patients: alpha-amylase inhibitors, lipid transfer proteins and low-molecular-weight glutenins. Allergenic molecules recognized by double-blind, placebo-controlled food challenge. *Int Arch Allergy Immunol.* 2007;144(1):10-22.
Pastorello EA, Pompei C, Pravettoni V, Farioli L, Calamari AM, Scibilia J, Robino AM, Conti A, Iametti S, Fortunato D, Bonomi S, Ortolani C. Lipid-transfer protein is the major maize allergen maintaining IgE-binding activity after cooking at 100 degrees C, as demonstrated in anaphylactic patients and patients with positive double-blind, placebo-controlled food challenge results. *J Allergy Clin Immunol.* 2003 Oct;112(4):775-83.
Patchett K, Lewis S, Crane J, Fitzharris P. Cat allergen (Fel d 1) levels on school children's clothing and in primary school classrooms in Wellington, New Zealand. *J Allergy Clin Immunol.* 1997 Dec;100(6 Pt 1):755-9.
Patel DS, Rafferty GF, Lee S, Hannam S, Greenough A. Work of breathing and volume targeted ventilation in respiratory distress. *Arch Dis Child Fetal Neonatal Ed.* 2010 Nov;95(6):F443-6.
Patriarca G, Nucera E, Pollastrini E, Roncallo C, De Pasquale T, Lombardo C, Pedone C, Gasbarrini G, Buonomo A, Schiavino D. Oral specific desensitization in food-allergic children. *Dig Dis Sci.* 2007 Jul;52(7):1662-72.
Patriarca G, Nucera E, Roncallo C, Pollastrini E, Bartolozzi F, De Pasquale T, Buonomo A, Gasbarrini G, Di Campli C, Schiavino D. Oral desensitizing treatment in food allergy: clinical and immunological results. *Aliment Pharmacol Ther.* 2003 Feb;17(3):459-65.
Patwardhan B, Gautam M. Botanical immunodrugs: scope and opportunities. *Drug Discov Today.* 2005 Apr 1;10(7):495-502.
Payment P, Franco E, Richardson L, Siemiatyck, J. Gastrointestinal health effects associated with the consumption of drinking water produced by point-of-use domestic reverse-osmosis filtration units. *Appl. Environ. Microbiol.* 1991;57:945-948.
Peat JK, van den Berg RH, Green WF, Mellis CM, Leeder SR, Woolcock AJ. Changing prevalence of asthma in Australian children. *BMJ.* 1994;308:1591-1596.
Pehowich DJ, Gomes AV, Barnes JA. Fatty acid composition and possible health effects of coconut constituents. *West Indian Med J.* 2000 Jun;49(2):128-33.
Perez-Galvez A, Martin HD, Sies H, Stahl W. Incorporation of carotenoids from paprika oleoresin into human chylomicrons. *Br J Nutr.* 2003 Jun;89(6):787-93.
Perez-Pena R. Secrets of the Mummy's Medicine Chest. *NY Times.* 2005 Sept 10.
Pessi T, Sütas Y, Hurme M, Isolauri E. Interleukin-10 generation in atopic children following oral Lactobacillus rhamnosus GG. *Clin Exp Allergy.* 2000 Dec;30(12):1804-8.
Peters JI, McKinney JM, Smith B, Wood P, Forkner E, Galbreath AD. Impact of obesity in asthma: evidence from a large prospective disease management study. *Ann Allergy Asthma Immunol.* 2011 Jan;106(1):30-5.
Peterson CG, Hansson T, Skott A, Bengtsson U, Ahlstedt S, Magnussons J. Detection of local mast-cell activity in patients with food hypersensitivity. *J Investig Allergol Clin Immunol.* 2007;17(5):314-20.
Peterson KA, Samuelson WM, Ryujin DT, Young DC, Thomas KL, Hilden K, Fang JC. The role of gastroesophageal reflux in exercise-triggered asthma: a randomized controlled trial. *Dig Dis Sci.* 2009 Mar;54(3):564-71. 2008 Aug 8.
Petlevski R, Hadzija M, Slijepcević M, Juretić D, Petrik J. Glutathione S-transferases and malondialdehyde in the liver of NOD mice on short-term treatment with plant mixture extract P-9801091. *Phytother Res.* 2003 Apr;17(4):311-4.
Pfefferle PI, Sel S, Ege MJ, Büchele G, Blümer N, Krauss-Etschmann S, Herzum I, Albers CE, Lauener RP, Roponen M, Hirvonen MR, Vuitton DA, Riedler J, Brunekreef B, Dalphin JC, Braun-Fahrländer C, Pekkanen J, von Mutius E, Renz H; PASTURE Study Group. Cord blood allergen-specific IgE is associated with reduced IFN-gamma production by cord blood cells: the Protection against Allergy-Study in Rural Environments (PASTURE) Study. *J Allergy Clin Immunol.* 2008 Oct;122(4):711-6.
Pfundstein B, El Desouky SK, Hull WE, Haubner R, Erben G, Owen RW. Polyphenolic compounds in the fruits of Egyptian medicinal plants (Terminalia bellerica, Terminalia chebula and Terminalia horrida): characterization, quantitation and determination of antioxidant capacities. *Phytochemistry.* 2010 Jul;71(10):1132-48.
Physicians' Desk Reference. Montvale, NJ: Thomson, 2003-2008.
Pierce SK, Klinman NR. Antibody-specific immunoregulation. *J Exp Med.* 1977 Aug 1;146(2):509-19.
Piirainen L, Haahtela S, Helin T, Korpela R, Haahtela T, Vaarala O. Effect of Lactobacillus rhamnosus GG on rBet v1 and rMal d1 specific IgA in the saliva of patients with birch pollen allergy. *Ann Allergy Asthma Immunol.* 2008 Apr;100(4):338-42.
Pike MG, Heddle RJ, Boulton P, Turner MW, Atherton DJ. Increased intestinal permeability in atopic eczema. *J Invest Dermatol.* 1986 Feb;86(2):101-4.

REFERENCES AND BIBLIOGRAPHY

Pines JM, Prabhu A, Hilton JA, Hollander JE, Datner EM. The effect of emergency department crowding on length of stay and medication treatment times in discharged patients with acute asthma. *Acad Emerg Med.* 2010 Aug;17(8):834-9.

Pitten FA, Scholler M, Krüger U, Effendy I, Kramer A. Filamentous fungi and yeasts on mattresses covered with different encasings. Eur J Dermatol. 2001 Nov-Dec;11(6):534-7.

Pitt-Rivers R, Trotter WR. *The Thyroid Gland.* London: Butterworth Publ, 1954.

Plaschke P, Janson C, Norrman E, Björnsson E, Ellbjär S, Järvholm B. Association between atopic sensitization and asthma and bronchial hyperresponsiveness in swedish adults: pets, and not mites, are the most important allergens. *J Allergy Clin Immunol.* 1999 Jul;104(1):58-65.

Plaut TE, Jones TB. *Dr. Tom Plaut's Asthma guide for people of all ages.* Amherst, MA: Pedipress, 1999.

Plaza V, Miguel E, Bellido-Casado J, Lozano MP, Ríos L, Bolíbar I. [Usefulness of the Guidelines of the Spanish Society of Pulmonology and Thoracic Surgery (SEPAR) in identifying the causes of chronic cough]. Arch Bronconeumol. 2006 Feb;42(2):68-73.

Plohmann B, Bader G, Hiller K, Franz G. Immunomodulatory and antitumoral effects of triterpenoid saponins. *Pharmazie.* 1997 Dec;52(12):953-7.

Pobłocka-Olech L, Krauze-Baranowska M. SPE-HPTLC of procyanidins from the barks of different species and clones of Salix. *J Pharm Biomed Anal.* 2008 Nov 4;48(3):965-8.

Pohjavuori E, Viljanen M, Korpela R, Kuitunen M, Tiittanen M, Vaarala O, Savilahti E. Lactobacillus GG effect in increasing IFN-gamma production in infants with cow's milk allergy. *J Allergy Clin Immunol.* 2004 Jul;114(1):131-6.

Polito A, Aboab J, Annane D. The hypothalamic pituitary adrenal axis in sepsis. *Novartis Found Symp.* 2007;280:182-203.

Polk S, Sunyer J, Muñoz-Ortiz L, Barnes M, Torrent M, Figueroa C, Harris J, Vall O, Antó JM, Cullinan P. A prospective study of Fel d1 and Der p1 exposure in infancy and childhood wheezing. *Am J Respir Crit Care Med.* 2004 Aug 1;170(3):273-8.

Pollini F, Capristo C, Boner AL. Upper respiratory tract infections and atopy. *Int J Immunopathol Pharmacol.* 2010 Jan-Mar;23(1 Suppl):32-7.

Ponsonby AL, McMichael A, van der Mei I. Ultraviolet radiation and autoimmune disease: insights from epidemiological research. *Toxicology.* 2002 Dec 27;181-182:71-8.

Postlethwait EM. Scavenger receptors clear the air. *J Clin Invest.* 2007 Mar;117(3):601-4.

Postma DS. Gender Differences in Asthma Development and Progression. *Gender Medicine.* 2007;4:S133-146.

Potterton D. (Ed.) *Culpeper's Color Herbal.* New York: Sterling, 1983.

Poulos LM, Waters AM, Correll PK, Loblay RH, Marks GB. Trends in hospitalizations for anaphylaxis, angioedema, and urticaria in Australia, 1993-1994 to 2004-2005. *J Allergy Clin Immunol.* 2007 Oct;120(4):878-84.

Prescott SL, Wickens K, Westcott L, Jung W, Currie H, Black PN, Stanley TV, Mitchell EA, Fitzharris P, Siebers R, Wu L, Crane J; Probiotic Study Group. Supplementation with Lactobacillus rhamnosus or Bifidobacterium lactis probiotics in pregnancy increases cord blood interferon-gamma and breast milk transforming growth factor-beta and immunoglobin A detection. *Clin Exp Allergy.* 2008 Oct;38(10):1606-14.

Priftis KN, Panagiotakos DB, Anthracopoulos MB, Papadimitriou A, Nicolaidou P. Aims, methods and preliminary findings of the Physical Activity, Nutrition and Allergies in Children Examined in Athens (PANACEA) epidemiological study. *BMC Public Health.* 2007 Jul 4;7:140.

Prioult G, Fliss I, Pecquet S. Effect of probiotic bacteria on induction and maintenance of oral tolerance to beta-lactoglobulin in gnotobiotic mice. *Clin Diagn Lab Immunol.* 2003 Sep;10(5):787-92.

Prucksunand C, Indrasukhsri B, Leethochawalit M, Hungspreugs K. Phase II clinical trial on effect of the long turmeric (Curcuma longa Linn) on healing of peptic ulcer. *Southeast Asian J Trop Med Public Health.* 2001 Mar;32(1):208-15.

Pruthi S, Thapa MM. Infectious and inflammatory disorders. *Magn Reson Imaging Clin N Am.* 2009 Aug;17(3):423-38, v.

Qin HL, Zheng JJ, Tong DN, Chen WX, Fan XB, Hang XM, Jiang YQ. Effect of Lactobacillus plantarum enteral feeding on the gut permeability and septic complications in the patients with acute pancreatitis. *Eur J Clin Nutr.* 2008 Jul;62(7):923-30.

Qu C, Srivastava K, Ko J, Zhang TF, Sampson HA, Li XM. Induction of tolerance after establishment of peanut allergy by the food allergy herbal formula-2 is associated with up-regulation of interferon-gamma. *Clin Exp Allergy.* 2007 Jun;37(6):846-55.

Radon K, Danuser B, Iversen M, Jörres R, Monso E, Opravil U, Weber C, Donham KJ, Nowak D. Respiratory symptoms in European animal farmers. *Eur Respir J.* 2001 Apr;17(4):747-54.

Raherison C, Pénard-Morand C, Moreau D, Caillaud D, Charpin D, Kopferschmitt C, Lavaud F, Taytard A, Maesano IA. Smoking exposure and allergic sensitization in children according to maternal allergies. *Ann Allergy Asthma Immunol.* 2008 Apr;100(4):351-7.

Rahman MM, Bhattacharya A, Fernandes G. Docosahexaenoic acid is more potent inhibitor of osteoclast differentiation in RAW 264.7 cells than eicosapentaenoic acid. *J Cell Physiol.* 2008 Jan;214(1):201-9.

Raithel M, Weidenhiller M, Abel R, Baenkler HW, Hahn EG. Colorectal mucosal histamine release by mucosa oxygenation in comparison with other established clinical tests in patients with gastrointestinally mediated allergy. *World J Gastroenterol.* 2006 Aug 7;12(29):4699-705.

Raloff J. III Winds. *Science News:* 2001;160(14):218.

Rampton DS, Murdoch RD, Sladen GE. Rectal mucosal histamine release in ulcerative colitis. *Clin Sci (Lond).* 1980 Nov;59(5):389-91.

Rancé F, Kanny G, Dutau G, Moneret-Vautrin DA. Food allergens in children. *Arch Pediatr.* 1999;6(Suppl 1):61S-66S.

Randal Bollinger R, Barbas AS, Bush EL, Lin SS, Parker W. Biofilms in the large bowel suggest an apparent function of the human vermiform appendix. *J Theor Biol.* 2007 Dec 21;249(4):826-31.

Ranjbaran Z, Keefer L, Stepanski E, Farhadi A, Keshavarzian A. The relevance of sleep abnormalities to chronic inflammatory conditions. *Inflamm Res.* 2007 Feb;56(2):51-7.

Rao SK, Rao PS, Rao BN. Preliminary investigation of the radiosensitizing activity of guduchi (Tinospora cordifolia) in tumor-bearing mice. *Phytother Res.* 2008 Nov;22(11):1482-9.

Rapin JR, Wiernsperger N. Possible links between intestinal permeablity and food processing: A potential therapeutic niche for glutamine. *Clinics (Sao Paulo).* 2010 Jun;65(6):635-43.

Rappoport J. Both sides of the pharmaceutical death coin. *Townsend Letter for Doctors and Patients.* 2006 Oct.

Rauha JP, Remes S, Heinonen M, Hopia A, Kähkönen M, Kujala T, Pihlaja K, Vuorela H, Vuorela P. Antimicrobial effects of Finnish plant extracts containing flavonoids and other phenolic compounds. *Int J Food Microbiol.* 2000 May 25;56(1):3-12.

Rauma A. Antioxidant status in vegetarians versus omnivores. *Nutrition.* 2003;16(2): 111-119.

Rautava S, Isolauri E. Cow's milk allergy in infants with atopic eczema is associated with aberrant production of interleukin-4 during oral cow's milk challenge. *J Pediatr Gastroenterol Nutr.* 2004 Nov;39(5):529-35.

Reger D, Goode S, Mercer E. *Chemistry: Principles & Practice.* Fort Worth, TX: Harcourt Brace, 1993.

Reha CM, Ebru A. Specific immunotherapy is effective in the prevention of new sensitivities. *Allergol Immunopathol (Madr).* 2007 Mar-Apr;35(2):44-51.

Reuter A, Lidholm J, Andersson K, Ostling J, Lundberg M, Scheurer S, Enrique E, Cistero-Bahima A, San Miguel-Moncin M, Ballmer-Weber BK, Vieths S. A critical assessment of allergen component-based in vitro diagnosis in cherry allergy across Europe. *Clin Exp Allergy.* 2006 Jun;36(6):815-23.

Reznik M, Sharif I, Ozuah PO. Rubbing ointments and asthma morbidity in adolescents. *J Altern Complement Med.* 2004 Dec;10(6):1097-9. Uu

Riccia DN, Bizzini F, Perilli MG, Polimeni A, Trinchieri V, Amicosante G, Cifone MG. Anti-inflammatory effects of *Lactobacillus brevis* (CD2) on periodontal disease. *Oral Dis.* 2007 Jul;13(4):376-85.

Riccioni G, Barbara M, Bucciarelli T, di Ilio C, D'Orazio N. Antioxidant vitamin supplementation in asthma. *Ann Clin Lab Sci.* 2007 Winter;37(1):96-101.

Riccioni G, Bucciarelli T, Mancini B, Di Ilio C, Della Vecchia R, D'Orazio N. Plasma lycopene and antioxidant vitamins in asthma: the PLAVA study. *J Asthma.* 2007 Jul-Aug;44(6):429-32.

Riccioni G, Di Stefano F, De Benedictis M, Verna N, Cavallucci E, Paolini F, Di Sciascio MB, Della Vecchia R, Schiavone C, Boscolo P, Conti P, Di Gioacchino M. Seasonal variability of non-specific bronchial responsiveness in asthmatic patients with allergy to house dust mites. *Allergy Asthma Proc.* 2001 Jan-Feb;22(1):5-9.

Riccioni G, D'Orazio N. The role of selenium, zinc and antioxidant vitamin supplementation in the treatment of bronchial asthma: adjuvant therapy or not? *Expert Opin Investig Drugs.* 2005 Sep;14(9):1145-55.

Rimkiene S, Ragazinskiene O, Savickiene N. The cumulation of Wild pansy (Viola tricolor L.) accessions: the possibility of species preservation and usage in medicine. *Medicina (Kaunas).* 2003;39(4):411-6.

Rinne M, Kalliomaki M, Arvilommi H, Salminen S, Isolauri E. Effect of probiotics and breastfeeding on the bifidobacterium and lactobacillus/enterococcus microbiota and humoral immune responses. *J Pediatr.* 2005 Aug;147(2):186-91.

Río ME, Zago Beatriz L, Garcia H, Winter L. The nutritional status change the effectiveness of a dietary supplement of lactic bacteria on the emerging of respiratory tract diseases in children. *Arch Latinoam Nutr.* 2002 Mar;52(1):29-34.

Robert AM, Groult N, Six C, Robert L. The effect of procyanidolic oligomers on mesenchymal cells in culture II—Attachment of elastic fibers to the cells. *Pathol Biol.* 1990 Jun;38(6):601-7.

Roberts G, Lack G. Diagnosing peanut allergy with skin prick and specific IgE testing. *J Allergy Clin Immunol.* 2005 Jun;115(6):1291-6.

Robinson L, Cherewatenko VS, Reeves S. *Epicor: The Key to a Balanced Immune System.* Sherman Oaks, CA: Health Point, 2009.

Rodriguez J, Crespo JF, Burks W, Rivas-Plata C, Fernandez-Anaya S, Vives R, Daroca P. Randomized, double-blind, crossover challenge study in 53 subjects reporting adverse reactions to melon (Cucumis melo). *J Allergy Clin Immunol.* 2000 Nov;106(5):968-72.

Rodriguez-Fragoso L, Reyes-Esparza J, Burchiel SW, Herrera-Ruiz D, Torres E. Risks and benefits of commonly used herbal medicines in Mexico. *Toxicol Appl Pharmacol.* 2008 Feb 15;227(1):125-35.

REFERENCES AND BIBLIOGRAPHY

Rodríguez-Ortiz PG, Muñoz-Mendoza D, Arias-Cruz A, González-Díaz SN, Herrera-Castro D, Vidaurri-Ojeda AC. Epidemiological characteristics of patients with food allergy assisted at Regional Center of Allergies and Clinical Immunology of Monterrey. *Rev Alerg Mex.* 2009 Nov-Dec;56(6):185-91.

Roduit C, Scholtens S, de Jongste JC, Wijga AH, Gerritsen J, Postma DS, Brunekreef B, Hoekstra MO, Aalberse R, Smit HA. Asthma at 8 years of age in children born by caesarean section. *Thorax.* 2009 Feb;64(2):107-13.

Roessler A, Friedrich U, Vogelsang H, Bauer A, Kaatz M, Hipler UC, Schmidt I, Jahreis G. The immune system in healthy adults and patients with atopic dermatitis seems to be affected differently by a probiotic intervention. *Clin Exp Allergy.* 2008 Jan;38(1):93-102.

Roger A, Justicia JL, Navarro LÁ, Eseverri JL, Ferrès J, Malet A, Alvà V. Observational study of the safety of an ultra-rush sublingual immunotherapy regimen to treat rhinitis due to house dust mites. *Int Arch Allergy Immunol.* 2011;154(1):69-75. 2010 Jul 27.

Romeo J, Wärnberg J, Nova E, Díaz LE, González-Gross M, Marcos A. Changes in the immune system after moderate beer consumption. *Ann Nutr Metab.* 2007;51(4):359-66.

Romieu I, Barraza-Villarreal A, Escamilla-Núñez C, Texcalac-Sangrador JL, Hernandez-Cadena L, Díaz-Sánchez D, De Batlle J, Del Rio-Navarro BE. Dietary intake, lung function and airway inflammation in Mexico City school children exposed to air pollutants. *Respir Res.* 2009 Dec 10;10:122.

Ronteltap A, van Schaik J, Wensing M, Rynja FJ, Knulst AC, de Vries JH. Sensory testing of recipes masking peanut or hazelnut for double-blind placebo-controlled food challenges. *Allergy.* 2004 Apr;59(4):457-60. Clark S, Bock SA, Gaeta TJ, Brenner BE, Cydulka RK, Camargo CA; Multicenter Airway Research Collaboration-8 Investigators. Multicenter study of emergency department visits for food allergies. *J Allergy Clin Immunol.* 2004 Feb;113(2):347-52.

Rook GA, Hernandez-Pando R. Pathogenetic role, in human and murine tuberculosis, of changes in the peripheral metabolism of glucocorticoids and antiglucocorticoids. *Psychoneuroendocrinology.* 1997;22 Suppl 1:S109-13.

Ros E, Mataix J. Fatty acid composition of nuts—implications for cardiovascular health. *Br J Nutr.* 2006 Nov;96 Suppl 2:S29-35.

Rosenfeldt V, Benfeldt E, Valerius NH, Paerregaard A, Michaelsen KF. Effect of probiotics on gastrointestinal symptoms and small intestinal permeability in children with atopic dermatitis. *J Pediatr.* 2004 Nov;145(5):612-6.

Rosenkranz SK, Swain KE, Rosenkranz RR, Beckman B, Harms CA. Modifiable lifestyle factors impact airway health in non-asthmatic prepubescent boys but not girls. *Pediatr Pulmonol.* 2010 Dec 30.

Rozycki VR, Baigorria CM, Freyre MR, Bernard CM, Zannier MS, Charpentier M. Nutrient content in vegetable species from the Argentine Chaco. *Arch Latinoam Nutr.* 1997 Sep;47(3):265-70.

Rubin E., Farber JL. *Pathology.* 3rd Ed. Philadelphia: Lippincott-Raven, 1999.

Rudders SA, Espinola JA, Camargo CA Jr. North-south differences in US emergency department visits for acute allergic reactions. *Ann Allergy Asthma Immunol.* 2010 May;104(5):413-6.

Rynard PB, Palij B, Galloway CA, Roughley FR. Resperin inhalation treatment for chronic respiratory diseases. *Can Fam Physician.* 1968 Oct;14(10):70-1.

Saarinen KM, Juntunen-Backman K, Järvenpää AL, Klemetti P, Kuitunen P, Lope L, Renlund M, Siivola M, Vaarala O, Savilahti E. Breast-feeding and the development of cows' milk protein allergy. *Adv Exp Med Biol.* 2000;478:121-30.

Sahagún-Flores JE, López-Peña LS, de la Cruz-Ramírez Jaimes J, García-Bravo MS, Peregrina-Gómez R, de Alba-García JE. Eradication of Helicobacter pylori: triple treatment scheme plus Lactobacillus vs. triple treatment alone. *Cir Cir.* 2007 Sep-Oct;75(5):333-6.

Sahakian NM, White SK, Park JH, Cox-Ganser JM, Kreiss K. Identification of mold and dampness-associated respiratory morbidity in 2 schools: comparison of questionnaire survey responses to national data. *J Sch Health.* 2008 Jan;78(1):32-7.

Sahin-Yilmaz A, Nocon CC, Corey JP. Immunoglobulin E-mediated food allergies among adults with allergic rhinitis. *Otolaryngol Head Neck Surg.* 2010 Sep;143(3):379-85.

Salem N, Wegher B, Mena P, Uauy R. Arachidonic and docosahexaenoic acids are biosynthesized from their 18-carbon precursors in human infants. *Proc Natl Acad Sci.* 1996;93:49-54.

Salim AS. Sulfhydryl-containing agents in the treatment of gastric bleeding induced by nonsteroidal anti-inflammatory drugs. *Can J Surg.* 1993 Feb;36(1):53-8.

Salmi H, Kuitunen M, Viljanen M, Lapatto R. Cow's milk allergy is associated with changes in urinary organic acid concentrations. *Pediatr Allergy Immunol.* 2010 Mar;21(2 Pt 2):e401-6.

Salminen S, Isolauri E, Salminen E. Clinical uses of probiotics for stabilizing the gut mucosal barrier: successful strains and future challenges. *Antonie Van Leeuwenhoek.* 1996 Oct;70(2-4):347-58.

Salom IL, Silvis SE, Doscherholmen A. Effect of cimetidine on the absorption of vitamin B12. *Scand J Gastroenterol.* 1982;17:129-31.

Salome CM, Marks GB. Sex, asthma and obesity: an intimate relationship? *Clin Exp Allergy.* 2011 Jan;41(1):6-8.

Salpietro CD, Gangemi S, Briuglia S, Meo A, Merlino MV, Muscolino G, Bisignano G, Trombetta D, Saija A. The almond milk: a new approach to the management of cow-milk allergy/intolerance in infants. *Minerva Pediatr.* 2005 Aug;57(4):173-80.

Salvi SS, Barnes PJ. Chronic obstructive pulmonary disease in non-smokers. *Lancet.* 2009 Aug 29;374(9691):733-43.

Sancho AI, Hoffmann-Sommergruber K, Alessandri S, Conti A, Giuffrida MG, Shewry P, Jensen BM, Skov P, Vieths S. Authentication of food allergen quality by physicochemical and immunological methods. *Clin Exp Allergy.* 2010 Jul;40(7):973-86.

Santos A, Dias A, Pinheiro JA. Predictive factors for the persistence of cow's milk allergy. *Pediatr Allergy Immunol.* 2010 Apr 27.

Sanz Ortega J, Martorell Aragonés A, Michavila Gómez A, Nieto García A; Grupo de Trabajo para el Estudio de la Alergia Alimentaria. Incidence of IgE-mediated allergy to cow's milk proteins in the first year of life. *An Esp Pediatr.* 2001 Jun;54(6):536-9.

Sato Y, Akiyama H, Matsuoka H, Sakata K, Nakamura R, Ishikawa S, Inakuma T, Totsuka M, Sugita-Konishi Y, Ebisawa M, Teshima R. Dietary carotenoids inhibit oral sensitization and the development of food allergy. *J Agric Food Chem.* 2010 Jun 23;58(12):7180-6.

Satyanarayana S, Sushruta K, Sarma GS, Srinivas N, Subba Raju GV. Antioxidant activity of the aqueous extracts of spicy food additives—evaluation and comparison with ascorbic acid in in-vitro systems. *J Herb Pharmacother.* 2004;4(2):1-10.

Savage JH, Kaeding AJ, Matsui EC, Wood RA. The natural history of soy allergy. *J Allergy Clin Immunol.* 2010 Mar;125(3):683-6.

Savilahti EM, Karinen S, Salo HM, Klemetti P, Saarinen KM, Klemola T, Kuitunen M, Hautaniemi S, Savilahti E, Vaarala O. Combined T regulatory cell and Th2 expression profile identifies children with cow's milk allergy. *Clin Immunol.* 2010 Jul;136(1):16-20.

Savilahti EM, Rantanen V, Lin JS, Karinen S, Saarinen KM, Goldis M, Mäkelä MJ, Hautaniemi S, Savilahti E, Sampson HA. Early recovery from cow's milk allergy is associated with decreasing IgE and increasing IgG4 binding to cow's milk epitopes. *J Allergy Clin Immunol.* 2010 Jun;125(6):1315-1321.e9.

Sazanova NE, Varnacheva LN, Novikova AV, Pletneva NB. Immunological aspects of food intolerance in children during first years of life. *Pediatriia.* 1992;(3):14-8.

Scadding G, Bjarnason I, Brostoff J, Levi AJ, Peters TJ. Intestinal permeability to 51Cr-labelled ethylenediaminetetraacetate in food-intolerant subjects. *Digestion.* 1989;42(2):104-9.

Scalabrin DM, Johnston WH, Hoffman DR, P'Pool VL, Harris CL, Mitmesser SH. Growth and tolerance of healthy term infants receiving hydrolyzed infant formulas supplemented with Lactobacillus rhamnosus GG: randomized, double-blind, controlled trial. *Clin Pediatr (Phila).* 2009 Sep;48(7):734-44.

Schauenberg P, Paris F. *Guide to Medicinal Plants.* New Canaan, CT: Keats Publ, 1977.

Schauss AG, Wu X, Prior RL, Ou B, Huang D, Owens J, Agarwal A, Jensen GS, Hart AN, Shanbrom E. Antioxidant capacity and other bioactivities of the freeze-dried Amazonian palm berry, Euterpe oleraceae mart. (acai). *J Agric Food Chem.* 2006 Nov 1;54(22):8604-10.

Schempp H, Weiser D, Elstner EF. Biochemical model reactions indicative of inflammatory processes. Activities of extracts from Fraxinus excelsior and Populus tremula. *Arzneimittelforschung.* 2000 Apr;50(4):362-72.

Schillaci D, Arizza V, Dayton T, Camarda L, Di Stefano V. In vitro anti-biofilm activity of Boswellia spp. oleogum resin essential oils. *Lett Appl Microbiol.* 2008 Nov;47(5):433-8.

Schmid B, Kötter I, Heide L. Pharmacokinetics of salicin after oral administration of a standardised willow bark extract. *Eur J Clin Pharmacol.* 2001 Aug;57(5):387-91.

Schmitt DA, Maleki SJ (2004) Comparing the effects of boiling, frying and roasting on the allergenicity of peanuts. *J Allergy Clin Immunol.* 113: S155.

Schnappinger M, Sausenthaler S, Linseisen J, Hauner H, Heinrich J. Fish consumption, allergic sensitisation and allergic diseases in adults. *Ann Nutr Metab.* 2009;54(1):67-74.

Schönfeld P. Phytanic Acid toxicity: implications for the permeability of the inner mitochondrial membrane to ions. *Toxicol Mech Methods.* 2004;14(1-2):47-52.

Schottner M, Gansser D, Spiteller G. Lignans from the roots of Urtica dioica and their metabolites bind to human sex hormone binding globulin (SHBG). *Planta Med.* 1997;65:529-532.

Schouten B, van Esch BC, Hofman GA, Boon L, Knippels LM, Willemsen LE, Garssen J. Oligosaccharide-induced whey-specific CD25(+) regulatory T-cells are involved in the suppression of cow milk allergy in mice. *J Nutr.* 2010 Apr;140(4):835-41.

Schroecksnadel S, Jenny M, Fuchs D. Sensitivity to sulphite additives. *Clin Exp Allergy.* 2010 Apr;40(4):688-9.

Schulick P. *Ginger: Common Spice & Wonder Drug.* Brattleboro, VT: Herbal Free Perss, 1996.

Schulz V, Hansel R, Tyler VE. *Rational Phytotherapy.* Berlin: Springer-Verlag; 1998.

Schumacher P. *Biophysical Therapy Of Allergies.* Stuttgart: Thieme, 2005.

Schütz K, Carle R, Schieber A. Taraxacum—a review on its phytochemical and pharmacological profile. *J Ethnopharmacol.* 2006 Oct 11;107(3):313-23.

REFERENCES AND BIBLIOGRAPHY

Schwab D, Hahn EG, Raithel M. Enhanced histamine metabolism: a comparative analysis of collagenous colitis and food allergy with respect to the role of diet and NSAID use. *Inflamm Res.* 2003 Apr;52(4):142-7.

Schwab D, Müller S, Aigner T, Neureiter D, Kirchner T, Hahn EG, Raithel M. Functional and morphologic characterization of eosinophils in the lower intestinal mucosa of patients with food allergy. *Am J Gastroenterol.* 2003 Jul;98(7):1525-34.

Schwelberger HG. Histamine intolerance: a metabolic disease? *Inflamm Res.* 2010 Mar;59 Suppl 2:S219-21.

Scott-Taylor TH, O'B Hourihane J, Strobel S. Correlation of allergen-specific IgG subclass antibodies and T lymphocyte cytokine responses in children with multiple food allergies. *Pediatr Allergy Immunol.* 2010 Sep;21(6):935-44.

Scurlock AM, Jones SM. An update on immunotherapy for food allergy. *Curr Opin Allergy Clin Immunol.* 2010 Dec;10(6):587-93.

Sealey-Voyksner JA, Khosla C, Voyksner RD, Jorgenson JW. Novel aspects of quantitation of immunogenic wheat gluten peptides by liquid chromatography-mass spectrometry. *J Chromatogr A.* 2010 Jun 18;1217(25):4167-83.

Senior F. Fallout. *New York Magazine.* Fall: 2003.

Senna G, Gani F, Leo G, Schiappoli M. Alternative tests in the diagnosis of food allergies. *Recenti Prog Med.* 2002 May;93(5):327-34.

Seo K, Jung S, Park M, Song Y, Choung S. Effects of leucocyanidines on activities of metabolizing enzymes and antioxidant enzymes. *Biol Pharm Bull.* 2001 May;24(5):592-3.

Seo SW, Koo HN, An HJ, Kwon KB, Lim BC, Seo EA, Ryu DG, Moon G, Kim HY, Kim HM, Hong SH. Taraxacum officinale protects against cholecystokinin-induced acute pancreatitis in rats. *World J Gastroenterol.* 2005 Jan 28;11(4):597-9.

Seppo L, Korpela R, Lönnerdal B, Metsäniitty L, Juntunen-Backman K, Klemola T, Paganus A, Vanto T. A follow-up study of nutrient intake, nutritional status, and growth in infants with cow milk allergy fed either a soy formula or an extensively hydrolyzed whey formula. *Am J Clin Nutr.* 2005 Jul;82(1):140-5.

Serra A, Cocuzza S, Poli G, La Mantia I, Messina A, Pavone P. Otologic findings in children with gastroesophageal reflux. *Int J Pediatr Otorhinolaryngol.* 2007 Nov;71(11):1693-7. 2007 Aug 22.

Sevar R. Audit of outcome in 455 consecutive patients treated with homeopathic medicines. *Homeopathy.* 2005 Oct;94(4):215-21.

Shahani KM, Meshbesher BF, Mangalampalli V. *Cultivate Health From Within.* Danbury, CT: Vital Health Publ, 2005.

Shaheen S, Potts J, Gnatiuc L, Makowska J, Kowalski ML, Joos G, van Zele T, van Durme Y, De Rudder I, Wöhrl S, Godnic-Cvar J, Skadhauge L, Thomsen G, Zuberbier T, Bergmann KC, Heinzerling L, Gjomarkaj M, Bruno A, Pace E, Bonini S, Fokkens W, Weersink EJ, Loureiro C, Todo-Bom A, Villanueva CM, Sanjuas C, Zock JP, Janson C, Burney P; Selenium and Asthma Research Integration project; GA2LEN. The relation between paracetamol use and asthma: a GA2LEN European case-control study. *Eur Respir J.* 2008 Nov;32(5):1231-6.

Shaheen SO, Newson RB, Rayman MP, Wong AP, Tumilty MK, Phillips JM, Potts JF, Kelly FJ, White PT, Burney PG. Randomised, double blind, placebo-controlled trial of selenium supplementation in adult asthma. *Thorax.* 2007 Jun;62(6):483-90.

Shakib F, Brown HM, Phelps A, Redhead R. Study of IgG sub-class antibodies in patients with milk intolerance. *Clin Allergy.* 1986 Sep;16(5):451-8.

Sharma P, Sharma BC, Puri V, Sarin SK. An open-label randomized controlled trial of lactulose and probiotics in the treatment of minimal hepatic encephalopathy. *Eur J Gastroent Hepatol.* 2008 Jun;20(6):506-11.

Sharma SC, Sharma S, Gulati OP. Pycnogenol inhibits the release of histamine from mast cells. *Phytother Res.* 2003 Jan;17(1):66-9.

Sharnan J, Kumar L, Singh S. Comparison of results of skin prick tests, enzyme-linked immunosorbent assays and food challenges in children with respiratory allergy. *J Trop Pediatr.* 2001 Dec;47(6):367-8.

Shawcross DL, Wright G, Olde Damink SW, Jalan R. Role of ammonia and inflammation in minimal hepatic encephalopathy. *Metab Brain Dis.* 2007 Mar;22(1):125-38.

Shea KM, Trucker RT, Weber RW, Peden DB. Climate change and allergic disease. *Clin Rev Allergy Immunol.* 2008;6:443-453.

Shea-Donohue T, Stiltz J, Zhao A, Notari L. Mast Cells. *Curr Gastroenterol Rep.* 2010 Aug 14.

Shen FY, Lee MS, Jung SK. Effectiveness of pharmacopuncture for asthma: a systematic review and meta-analysis. *Evid Based Complement Alternat Med.* 2011;2011. pii: 678176.

Sheth SS, Waserman S, Kagan R, Alizadehfar R, Primeau MN, Elliot S, St Pierre Y, Wickett R, Joseph L, Harada L, Dufresne C, Allen M, Allen M, Godefroy SB, Clarke AE. Role of food labels in accidental exposures in food-allergic individuals in Canada. *Ann Allergy Asthma Immunol.* 2010 Jan;104(1):60-5.

Shi S, Zhao Y, Zhou H, Zhang Y, Jiang X, Huang K. Identification of antioxidants from Taraxacum mongolicum by high-performance liquid chromatography-diode array detection-radical-scavenging detection-electrospray ionization mass spectrometry and nuclear magnetic resonance experiments. *J Chromatogr A.* 2008 Oct 31;1209(1-2):145-52.

Shi S, Zhou H, Zhang Y, Huang K, Liu S. Chemical constituents from Neo-Taraxacum siphonathum. *Zhongguo Zhong Yao Za Zhi.* 2009 Apr;34(8):1002-4.

Shi SY, Zhou CX, Xu Y, Tao QF, Bai H, Lu FS, Lin WY, Chen HY, Zheng W, Wang LW, Wu YH, Zeng S, Huang KX, Zhao Y, Li XK, Qu J. Studies on chemical constituents from herbs of Taraxacum mongolicum. *Zhongguo Zhong Yao Za Zhi.* 2008 May;33(10):1147-57.

Shibata H, Nabe T, Yamamura H, Kohno S. l-Ephedrine is a major constituent of Mao-Bushi-Saishin-To, one of the formulas of Chinese medicine, which shows immediate inhibition after oral administration of passive cutaneous anaphylaxis in rats. *Inflamm Res.* 2000 Aug;49(8):398-403.

Shichinohe K, Shimizu M, Kurokawa K. Effect of M-711 on experimental asthma in rats. *J Vet Med Sci.* 1996 Jan;58(1):55-9.

Shimauchi H, Mayanagi G, Nakaya S, Minamibuchi M, Ito Y, Yamaki K, Hirata H. Improvement of periodontal condition by probiotics with *Lactobacillus salivarius* WB21: a randomized, double-blind, placebo-controlled study. *J Clin Periodontol.* 2008 Oct;35(10):897-905.

Shimoi T, Ushiyama H, Kan K, Saito K, Kamata K, Hirokado M. Survey of glycoalkaloids content in the various potatoes. *Shokuhin Eiseigaku Zasshi.* 2007 Jun;48(3):77-82.

Shishehbor F, Behroo L, Ghafouriyan Broujerdnia M, Namjoyan F, Latifi SM. Quercetin effectively quells peanut-induced anaphylactic reactions in the peanut sensitized rats. *Iran J Allergy Asthma Immunol.* 2010 Mar;9(1):27-34.

Shishodia S, Harikumar KB, Dass S, Ramawat KG, Aggarwal BB. The guggul for chronic diseases: ancient medicine, modern targets. *Anticancer Res.* 2008 Nov-Dec;28(6A):3647-64.

Shivpuri DN, Menon MP, Parkash D. Preliminary studies in Tylophora indica in the treatment of asthma and allergic rhinitis. *J Assoc Physicians India.* 1968 Jan;16(1):9-15.

Shivpuri DN, Menon MP, Prakash D. A crossover double-blind study on Tylophora indica in the treatment of asthma and allergic rhinitis. *J Allergy.* 1969 Mar;43(3):145-50.

Shivpuri DN, Singhal SC, Parkash D. Treatment of asthma with an alcoholic extract of Tylophora indica: a cross-over, double-blind study. *Ann Allergy.* 1972; 30:407-12.

Shoaf, K., Muvey, G.L., Armstrong, G.D., Hutkins, R.W. (2006) Prebiotic galactooligosaccharides reduce adherence of enteropathogenic Escherichia coli to tissue culture cells. *Infect Immun.* Dec;74(12):6920-8.

Sicherer SH, Muñoz-Furlong A, Godbold JH, Sampson HA. US prevalence of self-reported peanut, tree nut, and sesame allergy: 11-year follow-up. *J Allergy Clin Immunol.* 2010 Jun;125(6):1322-6.

Sicherer SH, Noone SA, Koerner CB, Christie L, Burks AW, Sampson HA. Hypoallergenicity and efficacy of an amino acid-based formula in children with cow's milk and multiple food hypersensitivities. *J Pediatr.* 2001 May;138(5):688-93.

Sicherer SH, Sampson HA. Food allergy. *J Allergy Clin Immunol.* 2010 Feb;125(2 Suppl 2):S116-25.

Sidoroff V, Hyvärinen M, Piippo-Savolainen E, Korppi M. Lung function and overweight in school aged children after early childhood wheezing. *Pediatr Pulmonol.* 2010 Dec 30.

Sigstedt SC, Hooten CJ, Callewaert MC, Jenkins AR, Romero AE, Pullin MJ, Kornienko A, Lowrey TK, Slambrouck SV, Steelant WF. Evaluation of aqueous extracts of Taraxacum officinale on growth and invasion of breast and prostate cancer cells. *Int J Oncol.* 2008 May;32(5):1085-90.

Silman AJ, MacGregor AJ, Thomson W, Holligan S, Carthy D, Farhan A, Ollier WE. Twin concordance rates for rheumatoid arthritis: results from a nationwide study. *Br J Rheumatol.* 1993 Oct;32(10):903-7.

Silva MF, Kamphorst AO, Hayashi EA, Belllo M, Carvalho CR, Faria AM, Sabino KC, Coelho MG, Nobrega A, Tavares D, Silva AC. Innate profiles of cytokines implicated on oral tolerance correlate with low- or high-suppression of humoral response. *Immunology.* 2010 Jul;130(3):447-57.

Simeone D, Miele E, Boccia G, Marino A, Troncone R, Staiano A. Prevalence of atopy in children with chronic constipation. *Arch Dis Child.* 2008 Dec;93(12):1044-7.

Simões EA, Carbonell-Estrany X, Rieger CH, Mitchell I, Fredrick L, Groothuis JR; Palivizumab Long-Term Respiratory Outcomes Study Group. The effect of respiratory syncytial virus on subsequent recurrent wheezing in atopic and nonatopic children. *J Allergy Clin Immunol.* 2010 Aug;126(2):256-62. 2010 Jul 10.

Simons FER. What's in a name? The allergic rhinitis-asthma connection. *Clin Exp All Rev.* 2003;3:9-17.

Simonte SJ, Ma S, Mofidi S, Sicherer SH. Relevance of casual contact with peanut butter in children with peanut allergy. *J Allergy Clin Immunol.* 2003 Jul;112(1):180-2.

Simopoulos AP. Essential fatty acids in health and chronic disease. *Am J Clin Nutr.* 1999 Sep;70(3 Suppl):560S-569S.

Simpson AB, Yousef E, Hossain J. Association between peanut allergy and asthma morbidity. *J Pediatr.* 2010 May;156(5):777-81.

Simpson A, Tan VY, Winn J, Svensén M, Bishop CM, Heckerman DE, Buchan I, Custovic A. Beyond atopy: multiple patterns of sensitization in relation to asthma in a birth cohort study. *Am J Respir Crit Care Med.* 2010 Jun 1;181(11):1200-6.

Singer P, Shapiro H, Theilla M, Anbar R, Singer J, Cohen J. Anti-inflammatory properties of omega-3 fatty acids in critical illness: novel mechanisms and an integrative perspective. *Intensive Care Med.* 2008 Sep;34(9):1580-92.

Singh BB, Khorsan R, Vinjamury SP, Der-Martirosian C, Kizhakkeveettil A, Anderson TM. Herbal treatments of asthma: a systematic review. *J Asthma.* 2007 Nov;44(9):685-98.

REFERENCES AND BIBLIOGRAPHY

Singh S, Khajuria A, Taneja SC, Johri RK, Singh J, Qazi GN. Boswellic acids: A leukotriene inhibitor also effective through topical application in inflammatory disorders. *Phytomedicine*. 2008 Jun;15(6-7):400-7.

Singh V, Jain NK. Asthma as a cause for, rather than a result of, gastroesophageal reflux. *J Asthma*. 1983;20(4):241-3. 3.

Sirvent S, Palomares O, Vereda A, Villalba M, Cuesta-Herranz J, Rodríguez R. nsLTP and profilin are allergens in mustard seeds: cloning, sequencing and recombinant production of Sin a 3 and Sin a 4. *Clin Exp Allergy*. 2009 Dec;39(12):1929-36.

Skamstrup Hansen K, Vieths S, Vestergaard H, Skov PS, Bindslev-Jensen C, Poulsen LK. Seasonal variation in food allergy to apple. *J Chromatogr B Biomed Sci Appl*. 2001 May 25;756(1-2):19-32.

Skripak JM, Nash SD, Rowley H, Brereton NH, Oh S, Hamilton RG, Matsui EC, Burks AW, Wood RA. A randomized, double-blind, placebo-controlled study of milk oral immunotherapy for cow's milk allergy. *J Allergy Clin Immunol*. 2008 Dec;122(6):1154-60.

Sletten GB, Halvorsen R, Egaas E, Halstensen TS. Changes in humoral responses to beta-lactoglobulin in tolerant patients suggest a particular role for IgG4 in delayed, non-IgE-mediated cow's milk allergy. *Pediatr Allergy Immunol*. 2006 Sep;17(6):435-43.

Smith J. *Genetic Roulette: The Documented Health Risks of Genetically Engineered Foods*. White River Jct, Vermont: Chelsea Green, 2007.

Smith K, Warholak T, Armstrong E, Leib M, Rehfeld R, Malone D. Evaluation of risk factors and health outcomes among persons with asthma. *J Asthma*. 2009 Apr;46(3):234-7.

Smith LJ, Holbrook JT, Wise R, Blumenthal M, Dozor AJ, Mastronarde J, Williams L; American Lung Association Asthma Clinical Research Centers. Dietary intake of soy genistein is associated with lung function in patients with asthma. *J Asthma*. 2004;41(8):833-43.

Smith S, Sullivan K. Examining the influence of biological and psychological factors on cognitive performance in chronic fatigue syndrome: a randomized, double-blind, placebo-controlled, crossover study. *Int J Behav Med*. 2003;10(2):162-73.

Sofic E, Denisova N, Youdim K, Vatrenjak-Velagic V, De Filippo C, Mehmedagic A, Causevic A, Cao G, Joseph JA, Prior RL. Antioxidant and pro-oxidant capacity of catecholamines and related compounds. Effects of hydrogen peroxide on glutathione and sphingomyelinase activity in pheochromocytoma PC12 cells: potential relevance to age-related diseases. *J Neural Transm*. 2001;108(5):541-57.

Soleo L, Colosio C, Alinovi R, Guarneri D, Russo A, Lovreglio P, Vimercati L, Birindelli S, Cortesi I, Flore C, Carta P, Colombi A, Parrinello G, Ambrosi L. Immunologic effects of exposure to low levels of inorganic mercury. *Med Lav*. 2002 May-Jun;93(3):225-32.

Sompamit K, Kukongviriyapan U, Nakmareong S, Pannangpetch P, Kukongviriyapan V. Curcumin improves vascular function and alleviates oxidative stress in non-lethal lipopolysaccharide-induced endotoxaemia in mice. *Eur J Pharmacol*. 2009 Aug 15;616(1-3):192-9.

Sonibare MA, Gbile ZO. Ethnobotanical survey of anti-asthmatic plants in South Western Nigeria. *Afr J Tradit Complement Altern Med*. 2008 Jun 18;5(4):340-5.

Sontag SJ, O'Connell S, Khandelwal S, Greenlee H, Schnell T, Nemchausky B, Chejfec G, Miller T, Seidel J, Sonnenberg A. Asthmatics with gastroesophageal reflux: long term results of a randomized trial of medical and surgical antireflux therapies. *Am J Gastroenterol*. 2003 May;98(5):987-99.

Sosa M, Saavedra P, Valero C, Guañabens N, Nogués X, del Pino-Montes J, Mosquera J, Alegre J, Gómez-Alonso C, Muñoz-Torres M, Quesada M, Pérez-Cano R, Jódar E, Torrijos A, Lozano-Tonkin C, Díaz-Curiel M; GIUMO Study Group. Inhaled steroids do not decrease bone mineral density but increase risk of fractures: data from the GIUMO Study Group. J Clin Densitom. 2006 Apr-Jun;9(2):154-8.

Soyka F, Edmonds A. *The Ion Effect: How Air Electricity Rules your Life and Health*. Bantam, New York: Bantam, 1978.

Spence A. *Basic Human Anatomy*. Menlo Park, CA: Benjamin/Commings, 1986.

Spiller G. *The Super Pyramid*. New York: HRS Press, 1993.

Sporik R, Squillace SP, Ingram JM, Rakes G, Honsinger RW, Platts-Mills TA. Mite, cat, and cockroach exposure, allergen sensitisation, and asthma in children: a case-control study of three schools. *Thorax*. 1999 Aug;54(8):675-80.

Srivastava K, Zou ZM, Sampson HA, Dansky H, Li XM. Direct Modulation of Airway Reactivity by the Chinese Anti-Asthma Herbal Formula ASHMI. *J Allergy Clin Immunol*. 2005;115:S7.

Srivastava KD, Qu C, Zhang T, Goldfarb J, Sampson HA, Li XM. Food Allergy Herbal Formula-2 silences peanut-induced anaphylaxis for a prolonged posttreatment period via IFN-gamma-producing CD8+ T cells. *J Allergy Clin Immunol*. 2009 Feb;123(2):443-51.

Srivastava KD, Zhang TF, Qu C, Sampson HA, Li XM. Silencing Peanut Allergy: A Chinese Herbal Formula, FAHF-2, Completely Blocks Peanut-induced Anaphylaxis for up to 6 Months Following Therapy in a Murine Model Of Peanut Allergy. *J Allergy Clin Immunol*. 2006;117:S328.

Staden U, Rolinck-Werninghaus C, Brewe F, Wahn U, Niggemann B, Beyer K. Specific oral tolerance induction in food allergy in children: efficacy and clinical patterns of reaction. *Allergy*. 2007 Nov;62(11):1261-9.

Stahl SM. Selective histamine H1 antagonism: novel hypnotic and pharmacologic actions challenge classical notions of antihistamines. CNS Spectr. 2008 Dec;13(12):1027-38.

State Pharmacopoeia Commission of The People's Republic of China. *Pharmacopoeia of the People's Republic of China*. Beijing: Chemical Industry Press; 2005.

Steinman HA, Le Roux M, Potter PC. Sulphur dioxide sensitivity in South African asthmatic children. *S Afr Med J.* 1993 Jun;83(6):387-90.

Stenberg JA, Hambäck PA, Ericson L. Herbivore-induced "rent rise" in the host plant may drive a diet breadth enlargement in the tenant. *Ecology*. 2008 Jan;89(1):126-33.

Stengler M. *The Natural Physician's Healing Therapies*. Stamford, CT: Bottom Line Books, 2008.

Stensrud T, Carlsen KH. Can one single test protocol for provoking exercise-induced bronchoconstriction also be used for assessing aerobic capacity? *Clin Respir J.* 2008 Jan;2(1):47-53.

Steurer-Stey C, Russi EW, Steurer J: Complementary and alternative medicine in asthma: do they work? *Swiss Med Wkly*. 2002, 132:338-344.

Stillerman A, Nachtsheim C, Li W, Albrecht M, Waldman J. Efficacy of a novel air filtration pillow for avoidance of perennial allergens in symptomatic adults. *Ann Allergy Asthma Immunol*. 2010 May;104(5):440-9.

Stirapongsasuti P, Tanglertsampan C, Aunhachoke K, Sangasapaviliya A. Anaphylactic reaction to phuk-waan-ban in a patient with latex allergy. *J Med Assoc Thai*. 2010 May;93(5):616-9.

Størdal K, Johannesdottir GB, Bentsen BS, Knudsen PK, Carlsen KC, Closs O, Handeland M, Holm HK, Sandvik L. Acid suppression does not change respiratory symptoms in children with asthma and gastro-oesophageal reflux disease. *Arch Dis Child*. 2005 Sep;90(9):956-60.

Stratiki Z, Costalos C, Sevastiadou S, Kastanidou O, Skouroliakou M, Giakoumatou A, Petrohilou V. The effect of a bifidobacter supplemented bovine milk on intestinal permeability of preterm infants. *Early Hum Dev*. 2007 Sep;83(9):575-9.

Strinnholm A, Brulin C, Lindh V. Experiences of double-blind, placebo-controlled food challenges (DBPCFC): a qualitative analysis of mothers' experiences. *J Child Health Care*. 2010 Jun;14(2):179-88.

Stutius LM, Sheehan WJ, Rangsithienchai P, Bharmanee A, Scott JE, Young MC, Dioun AF, Schneider LC, Phipatanakul W. Characterizing the relationship between sesame, coconut, and nut allergy in children. *Pediatr Allergy Immunol*. 2010 Dec;21(8):1114-8.

Sugawara G, Nagino M, Nishio H, Ebata T, Takagi K, Asahara T, Nomoto K, Nimura Y. Perioperative synbiotic treatment to prevent postoperative infectious complications in biliary cancer surgery: a randomized controlled trial. *Ann Surg*. 2006 Nov;244(5):706-14.

Sulman FG, Levy D, Lunkan L, Pfeifer Y, Tal E. New methods in the treatment of weather sensitivity. *Fortschr Med*. 1977 Mar 17;95(11):746-52.

Sulman FG. Migraine and headache due to weather and allied causes and its specific treatment. *Ups J Med Sci Suppl*. 1980;31:41-4.

Sumantran VN, Kulkarni AA, Harsulkar A, Wele A, Koppikar SJ, Chandwaskar R, Gaire V, Dalvi M, Wagh UV. Hyaluronidase and collagenase inhibitory activities of the herbal formulation Triphala guggulu. *J Biosci*. 2007 Jun;32(4):755-61.

Sumiyoshi M, Sakanaka M, Kimura Y. Effects of Red Ginseng extract on allergic reactions to food in Balb/c mice. *J Ethnopharmacol*. 2010 Aug 14.

Sung JH, Lee JO, Son JK, Park NS, Kim MR, Kim JG, Moon DC. Cytotoxic constituents from Solidago virga-aurea var. gigantea MIQ. *Arch Pharm Res*. 1999 Dec;22(6):633-7.

Suomalainen H, Isolauri E. New concepts of allergy to cow's milk. *Ann Med*. 1994 Aug;26(4):289-96.

Sur S, Camara M, Buchmeier A, Morgan S, Nelson HS. Double-blind trial of pyridoxine (vitamin B6) in the treatment of steroid-dependent asthma. Ann Allergy. 1993 Feb;70(2):147-52.

Sütas Y, Kekki OM, Isolauri E. Late onset reactions to oral food challenge are linked to low serum interleukin-10 concentrations in patients with atopic dermatitis and food allergy. *Clin Exp Allergy*. 2000 Aug;30(8):1121-8.

Svanes C, Heinrich J, Jarvis D, Chinn S, Omenaas E, Gulsvik A, Künzli N, Burney P. Pet-keeping in childhood and adult asthma and hay fever: European community respiratory health survey. *J Allergy Clin Immunol*. 2003 Aug;112(2):289-300.

Svendsen AJ, Holm NV, Kyvik K, *et al*. Relative importance of genetic effects in rheumatoid arthritis: historical cohort study of Danish nationwide twin population. *BMJ* 2002;324(7332): 264-266.

Sweeney B, Vora M, Ulbricht C, Basch E. Evidence-based systematic review of dandelion (Taraxacum officinale) by natural standard research collaboration. *J Herb Pharmacother*. 2005;5(1):79-93.

Swiderska-Kiełbik S, Krakowiak A, Wiszniewska M, Dudek W, Walusiak-Skorupa J, Krawczyk-Szulc P, Michowicz A, Pałczyński C. Health hazards associated with occupational exposure to birds. *Med Pr*. 2010;61(2):213-22.

REFERENCES AND BIBLIOGRAPHY

Szyf M, McGowan P, Meaney MJ. The social environment and the epigenome. *Environ Mol Mutagen.* 2008 Jan;49(1):46-60.

Takada Y, Ichikawa H, Badmaev V, Aggarwal BB. Acetyl-11-keto-beta-boswellic acid potentiates apoptosis, inhibits invasion, and abolishes osteoclastogenesis by suppressing NF-kappa B and NF-kappa B-regulated gene expression. *J Immunol.* 2006 Mar 1;176(5):3127-40.

Takahashi N, Eisenhuth G, Lee I, Schachtele C, Laible N, Binion S. Nonspecific antibacterial factors in milk from cows immunized with human oral bacterial pathogens. *J Dairy Sci.* 1992 Jul;75(7):1810-20.

Takasaki M, Konoshima T, Tokuda H, Masuda K, Arai Y, Shiojima K, Ageta H. Anti-carcinogenic activity of Taraxacum plant. I. *Biol Pharm Bull.* 1999 Jun;22(6):602-5.

Takeda K, Suzuki T, Shimada SI, Shida K, Nanno M, Okumura K. Interleukin-12 is involved in the en-hancement of human natural killer cell activity by Lactobacillus casei Shirota. *Clin Exp Immunol.* 2006 Oct;146(1):109-15.

Tamaoki J, Chiyotani A, Sakai A, Takemura H, Konno K. Effect of menthol vapour on airway hyperresponsiveness in patients with mild asthma. *Respir Med.* 1995 Aug;89(7):503-4.

Tamura M, Shikina T, Morihana T, Hayama M, Kajimoto O, Sakamoto A, Kajimoto Y, Watanabe O, Nonaka C, Shida K, Nanno M. Effects of probiotics on allergic rhinitis induced by Japanese cedar pol-len: randomized double-blind, placebo-controlled clinical trial. *Int Arch Allergy Imml.* 2007;143(1):75-82.

Taniguchi C, Homma M, Takano O, Hirano T, Oka K, Aoyagi Y, Niitsuma T, Hayashi T. Pharmacological effects of urinary products obtained after treatment with saiboku-to, a herbal medicine for bronchial asthma, on type IV allergic reaction. *Planta Med.* 2000 Oct;66(7):607-11.

Tapiero H, Ba GN, Couvreur P, Tew KD. Polyunsaturated fatty acids (PUFA) and eicosanoids in human health and pathologies. *Biomed Pharmacother.* 2002 Jul;56(5):215-22.

Tapsell LC, Hemphill I, Cobiac L, Patch CS, Sullivan DR, Fenech M, Roodenrys S, Keogh JB, Clifton PM, Williams PG, Fazio VA, Inge KE. Health benefits of herbs and spices: the past, the present, the future. *Med J Aust.* 2006 Aug 21;185(4 Suppl):S4-24.

Tasli L, Mat C, De Simone C, Yazici H. Lactobacilli lozenges in the management of oral ulcers of Behçet's syndrome. *Clin Exp Rheumatol.* 2006 Sep-Oct;24(5 Suppl 42):S83-6.

Taussig SJ, Batkin S. Bromelain, the enzyme complex of pineapple (Ananas comosus) and its clinical application. An update. *J Ethnopharmacol.* 1988 Feb-Mar;22(2):191-203.

Taylor AL, Dunstan JA, Prescott SL. Probiotic supplementation for the first 6 months of life fails to reduce the risk of atopic dermatitis and increases the risk of allergen sensitization in high-risk children: a randomized controlled trial. *J Allergy Clin Immunol.* 2007 Jan;119(1):184-91.

Taylor AL, Hale J, Wiltschut J, Lehmann H, Dunstan JA, Prescott SL. Effects of probiotic supplementation for the first 6 months of life on allergen- and vaccine-specific immune responses. *Clin Exp Allergy.* 2006 Oct;36(10):1227-35.

Taylor RB, Lindquist N, Kubanek J, Hay ME. Intraspecific variation in palatability and defensive chemistry of brown seaweeds: effects on herbivore fitness. *Oecologia.* 2003 Aug;136(3):412-23.

Teitelbaum J. *From Fatigue to Fantastic.* New York: Avery, 2001.

Terheggen-Lagro SW, Khouw IM, Schaafsma A, Wauters EA. Safety of a new extensively hydrolysed formula in children with cow's milk protein allergy: a double blind crossover study. *BMC Pediatr.* 2002 Oct 14;2:10.

Terracciano L, Bouygue GR, Sarratud T, Veglia F, Martelli A, Fiocchi A. Impact of dietary regimen on the duration of cow's milk allergy: a random allocation study. *Clin Exp Allergy.* 2010 Apr;40(4):637-42.

Tesse R, Schieck M, Kabesch M. Asthma and endocrine disorders: Shared mechanisms and genetic pleiotropy. *Mol Cell Endocrinol.* 2010 Dec 4. [ahead of print] .

Thakkar K, Boatright RO, Gilger MA, El-Serag HB. Gastroesophageal reflux and asthma in children: a systematic review. *Pediatrics.* 2010 Apr;125(4):e925-30. 2010 Mar 29.

Tham KW, Zuraimi MS, Koh D, Chew FT, Ooi PL. Associations between home dampness and presence of molds with asthma and allergic symptoms among young children in the tropics. *Pediatr Allergy Immunol.* 2007 Aug;18(5):418-24.

Thampithak A, Jaisin Y, Meesarapee B, Chongthammakun S, Piyachaturawat P, Govitrapong P, Supavilai P, Sanvarinda Y. Transcriptional regulation of iNOS and COX-2 by a novel compound from Curcuma comosa in lipopolysaccharide-induced microglial activation. *Neurosci Lett.* 2009 Sep 22;462(2):171-5.

Theler B, Brockow K, Ballmer-Weber BK. Clinical presentation and diagnosis of meat allergy in Switzerland and Southern Germany. *Swiss Med Wkly.* 2009 May 2;139(17-18):264-70.

Theofilopoulos AN, Kono DH: The genes of systemic autoimmunity. *Proc Assoc Am Physicians.* 1999;111(3): 228-240.

Thiruvengadam KV, Haranath K, Sudarsan S, Sekar TS, Rajagopal KR, Zacharian MG, Devarajan TV. Tylophora indica in bronchial asthma (a controlled comparison with a standard anti-asthmatic drug). *J Indian Med Assoc.* 1978 Oct 1;71(7):172-6.

Thomas M. Are breathing exercises an effective strategy for people with asthma? *Nurs Times.* 2009 Mar 17-23;105(10):22-7.

Thomas, R.G., Gebhardt, S.E. 2008. Nutritive value of pomegranate fruit and juice. *Maryland Dietetic Association Annual Meeting, USDA-ARS.* 2008 April 11.

Thompson T, Lee AR, Grace T. Gluten contamination of grains, seeds, and flours in the United States: a pilot study. *J Am Diet Assoc.* 2010 Jun;110(6):937-40.
Tierra L. *The Herbs of Life.* Freedom, CA: Crossing Press, 1992.
Tierra M. *The Way of Herbs.* New York: Pocket Books, 1990.
Tisserand R. *The Art of Aromatherapy.* New York: Inner Traditions, 1979.
Tiwari M. *Ayurveda: A Life of Balance.* Rochester, VT: Healing Arts, 1995.
Tlaskalová-Hogenová H, Stepánková R, Hudcovic T, Tucková L, Cukrowska B, Lodinová-Zádníková R, Kozáková H, Rossmann P, Bártová J, Sokol D, Funda DP, Borovská D, Reháková Z, Sinkora J, Hofman J, Drastich P, Kokesová A. Commensal bacteria (normal microflora), mucosal immunity and chronic inflammatory and autoimmune diseases. *Immunol Lett.* 2004 May 15;93(2-3):97-108.
Todd GR, Acerini CL, Ross-Russell R, Zahra S, Warner JT, McCance D. Survey of adrenal crisis associated with inhaled corticosteroids in the United Kingdom. *Arch Dis Child.* 2002 Dec;87(6):457-61.
Tonkal AM, Morsy TA. An update review on Commiphora molmol and related species. *J Egypt Soc Parasitol.* 2008 Dec;38(3):763-96.
Topçu G, Erenler R, Cakmak O, Johansson CB, Celik C, Chai HB, Pezzuto JM. Diterpenes from the berries of Juniperus excelsa. *Phytochemistry.* 1999 Apr;50(7):1195-9.
Tordesillas L, Pacios LF, Palacín A, Cuesta-Herranz J, Madero M, Díaz-Perales A. Characterization of IgE epitopes of Cuc m 2, the major melon allergen, and their role in cross-reactivity with pollen profilins. *Clin Exp Allergy.* 2010 Jan;40(1):174-81.
Torrent M, Sunyer J, Muñoz L, Cullinan P, Iturriaga MV, Figueroa C, Vall O, Taylor AN, Anto JM. Early-life domestic aeroallergen exposure and IgE sensitization at age 4 years. *J Allergy Clin Immunol.* 2006 Sep;118(3):742-8.
Towers GH. FAHF-1 purporting to block peanut-induced anaphylaxis. *J Allergy Clin Immunol.* 2003 May;111(5):1140; author reply 1140-1.
Towle A. *Modern Biology.* Austin: Harcourt Brace, 1993.
Trojanová I, Rada V, Kokoska L, Vlková E. The bifidogenic effect of Taraxacum officinale root. *Fitoterapia.* 2004 Dec;75(7-8):760-3.
Troncone R, Caputo N, Florio G, Finelli E. Increased intestinal sugar permeability after challenge in children with cow's milk allergy or intolerance. *Allergy.* 1994 Mar;49(3):142-6.
Trout L, King M, Feng W, Inglis SK, Ballard ST. Inhibition of airway liquid secretion and its effect on the physical properties of airway mucus. *Am J Physiol.* 1998 Feb;274(2 Pt 1):L258-63.
Tsai JC, Tsai S, Chang WC. Comparison of two Chinese medical herbs, Huangbai and Qianniuzi, on influence of short circuit current across the rat intestinal epithelia. *J Ethnopharmacol.* 2004 Jul;93(1):21-5.
Tsong T. Deciphering the language of cells. *Trends in Biochem Sci.* 1989;14:89-92.
Tucker KL, Olson B, Bakun P, Dallal GE, Selhub J, Rosenberg IH. Breakfast cereal fortified with folic acid, vitamin B-6, and vitamin B-12 increases vitamin concentrations and reduces homocysteine concentrations: a randomized trial. *Am J Clin Nutr.* 2004 May;79(5):805-11.
Tulk HM, Robinson LE. Modifying the n-6/n-3 polyunsaturated fatty acid ratio of a high-saturated fat challenge does not acutely attenuate postprandial changes in inflammatory markers in men with metabolic syndrome. *Metabolism.* 2009 Jul 20.
Tunnicliffe WS, Burge PS, Ayres JG. Effect of domestic concentrations of nitrogen dioxide on airway responses to inhaled allergen in asthmatic patients. *Lancet.* 1994 Dec 24-31;344(8939-8940):1733-6.
Tunnicliffe WS, Fletcher TJ, Hammond K, Roberts K, Custovic A, Simpson A, Woodcock A, Ayres JG. Sensitivity and exposure to indoor allergens in adults with differing asthma severity. *Eur Respir J.* 1999 Mar;13(3):654-9.
Tursi A, Brandimarte G, Giorgetti GM, Elisei W. Mesalazine and/or Lactobacillus casei in maintaining long-term remission of symptomatic uncomplicated diverticular disease of the colon. *Hepatogastroenterology.* 2008 May-Jun;55(84):916-20.
U.S. Food and Drug Administration *Guidance for Industry Botanical Drug Products.* CfDEaR. 2000
Uddenfeldt M, Janson C, Lampa E, Leander M, Norbäck D, Larsson L, Rask-Andersen A. High BMI is related to higher incidence of asthma, while a fish and fruit diet is related to a lower- Results from a long-term follow-up study of three age groups in Sweden. *Respir Med.* 2010 Jul;104(7):972-80.
Udupa AL, Udupa SL, Guruswamy MN. The possible site of anti-asthmatic action of Tylophora asthmatica on pituitary-adrenal axis in albino rats. *Planta Med.* 1991 Oct;57(5):409-13.
Ueno H, Yoshioka K, Matsumoto T. Usefulness of the skin index in predicting the outcome of oral challenges in children. *J Investig Allergol Clin Immunol.* 2007;17(4):207-10.
Ueno M, Adachi A, Fukumoto T, Nishitani N, Fujiwara N, Matsuo H, Kohno K, Morita E. Analysis of causative allergen of the patient with baker's asthma and wheat-dependent exercise-induced anaphylaxis (WDEIA). *Arerugi.* 2010 May;59(5):552-7.
Ukabam SO, Mann RJ, Cooper BT. Small intestinal permeability to sugars in patients with atopic eczema. *Br J Dermatol.* 1984 Jun;110(6):649-52.

REFERENCES AND BIBLIOGRAPHY

Ulrich RS, Simons RF, Losito BD, Fiorito E, Miles MA, Zelson M. Stress recovery during exposure to natural and urban environments. J Envir Psychol. 1991;11:201-30.

Unsel M, Sin AZ, Ardeniz O, Erdem N, Ersoy R, Gulbahar O, Mete N, Kokuludağ A. New onset egg allergy in an adult. *J Investig Allergol Clin Immunol.* 2007;17(1):55-8.

Upadhyay AK, Kumar K, Kumar A, Mishra HS. Tinospora cordifolia (Willd.) Hook. f. and Thoms. (Guduchi) - validation of the Ayurvedic pharmacology through experimental and clinical studies. *Int J Ayurveda Res.* 2010 Apr;1(2):112-21.

Urata Y, Yoshida S, Irie Y, Tanigawa T, Amayasu H, Nakabayashi M, Akahori K. Treatment of asthma patients with herbal medicine TJ-96: a randomized controlled trial. *Respir Med.* 2002 Jun;96(6):469-74.

Vally H, Thompson PJ, Misso NL. Changes in bronchial hyperresponsiveness following high- and low-sulphite wine challenges in wine-sensitive asthmatic patients. *Clin Exp Allergy.* 2007 Jul;37(7):1062-6.

van Beelen VA, Roeleveld J, Mooibroek H, Sijtsma L, Bino RJ, Bosch D, Rietjens IM, Alink GM. A comparative study on the effect of algal and fish oil on viability and cell proliferation of Caco-2 cells. *Food Chem Toxicol.* 2007 May;45(5):716-24.

van Elburg RM, Uil JJ, de Monchy JG, Heymans HS. Intestinal permeability in pediatric gastroenterology. *Scand J Gastroenterol Suppl.* 1992;194:19-24.

van Huisstede A, Braunstahl GJ. Obesity and asthma: co-morbidity or causal relationship? *Monaldi Arch Chest Dis.* 2010 Sep;73(3):116-23.

van Kampen V, Merget R, Rabstein S, Sander I, Bruening T, Broding HC, Keller C, Muesken H, Overlack A, Schultze-Werninghaus G, Walusiak J, Raulf-Heimsoth M. Comparison of wheat and rye flour solutions for skin prick testing: a multi-centre study (Stad 1). *Clin Exp Allergy.* 2009 Dec;39(12):1896-902.

van Odijk J, Peterson CG, Ahlstedt S, Bengtsson U, Borres MP, Hulthén L, Magnusson J, Hansson T. Measurements of eosinophil activation before and after food challenges in adults with food hypersensitivity. *Int Arch Allergy Immunol.* 2006;140(4):334-41.

van Zwol A, Moll HA, Fetter WP, van Elburg RM. Glutamine-enriched enteral nutrition in very low birthweight infants and allergic and infectious diseases at 6 years of age. *Paediatr Perinat Epidemiol.* 2011 Jan;25(1):60-6.

Vanderhoof JA. Probiotics in allergy management. *J Pediatr Gastroenterol Nutr.* 2008 Nov;47 Suppl 2:S38-40.

VanHaitsma TA, Mickleborough T, Stager JM, Koceja DM, Lindley MR, Chapman R. Comparative effects of caffeine and albuterol on the bronchoconstrictor response to exercise in asthmatic athletes. *Int J Sports Med.* 2010 Apr;31(4):231-6.

Vanto T, Helppilä S, Juntunen-Backman K, Kalimo K, Klemola T, Korpela R, Koskinen P. Prediction of the development of tolerance to milk in children with cow's milk hypersensitivity. *J Pediatr.* 2004 Feb;144(2):218-22.

Vargas C, Bustos P, Diaz PV, Amigo H, Rona RJ. Childhood environment and atopic conditions, with emphasis on asthma in a Chilean agricultural area. *J Asthma.* 2008 Jan-Feb;45(1):73-8.

Varonier HS, de Haller J, Schopfer C. Prevalence of allergies in children and adolescents. *Helv Paediatr Acta.* 1984;39:129-136.

Varraso R, Fung TT, Barr RG, Hu FB, Willett W, Camargo CA Jr. Prospective study of dietary patterns and chronic obstructive pulmonary disease among US women. *Am J Clin Nutr.* 2007 Aug;86(2):488-95.

Varraso R, Fung TT, Hu FB, Willett W, Camargo CA. Prospective study of dietary patterns and chronic obstructive pulmonary disease among US men. *Thorax.* 2007 Sep;62(9):786-91. 2007 May 15.

Varraso R, Jiang R, Barr RG, Willett WC, Camargo CA Jr. Prospective study of cured meats consumption and risk of chronic obstructive pulmonary disease in men. *Am J Epidemiol.* 2007 Dec 15;166(12):1438-45. 2007 Sep 4. 17785711; .

Vassallo MF, Banerji A, Rudders SA, Clark S, Mullins RJ, Camargo CA Jr. Season of birth and food allergy in children. *Ann Allergy Asthma Immunol.* 2010 Apr;104(4):307-13.

Vempati R, Bijlani RL, Deepak KK. The efficacy of a comprehensive lifestyle modification programme based on yoga in the management of bronchial asthma: a randomized controlled trial. *BMC Pulm Med.* 2009 Jul 30;9:37.

Vendt N, Grünberg H, Tuure T, Malminiemi O, Wuolijoki E, Tillmann V, Sepp E, Korpela R. Growth during the first 6 months of life in infants using formula enriched with Lactobacillus rhamnosus GG: double-blind, randomized trial. *J Hum Nutr Diet.* 2006 Feb;19(1):51-8.

Venkatachalam KV. Human 3'-phosphoadenosine 5'-phosphosulfate (PAPS) synthase: biochemistry, molecular biology and genetic deficiency. *IUBMB Life.* 2003 Jan;55(1):1-11.

Venkatesan N, Punithavathi D, Babu M. Protection from acute and chronic lung diseases by curcumin. *Adv Exp Med Biol.* 2007;595:379-405.

Venter C, Hasan Arshad S, Grundy J, Pereira B, Bernie Clayton C, Voigt K, Higgins B, Dean T. Time trends in the prevalence of peanut allergy: three cohorts of children from the same geographical location in the UK. *Allergy.* 2010 Jan;65(1):103-8.

Venter C, Meyer R. Session 1: Allergic disease: The challenges of managing food hypersensitivity. *Proc Nutr Soc.* 2010 Feb;69(1):11-24.

Venter C, Pereira B, Grundy J, Clayton CB, Arshad SH, Dean T. Prevalence of sensitization reported and objectively assessed food hypersensitivity amongst six-year-old children: A population-based study. *Pediatr Allergy Immunol.* 2006;17: 356-363.

Venter C, Pereira B, Grundy J, Clayton CB, Roberts G, Higgins B, Dean T. Incidence of parentally reported and clinically diagnosed food hypersensitivity in the first year of life. *J Allergy Clin Immunol.* 2006;117: 1118-1124.

Ventura MT, Polimeno L, Amoruso AC, Gatti F, Annoscia E, Marinaro M, Di Leo E, Matino MG, Buquicchio R, Bonini S, Tursi A, Francavilla A. Intestinal permeability in patients with adverse reactions to food. *Dig Liver Dis.* 2006 Oct;38(10):732-6.

Venturi A, Gionchetti P, Rizzello F, Johansson R, Zucconi E, Brigidi P, Matteuzzi D, Campieri M. Impact on the composition of the faecal flora by a new probiotic preparation: preliminary data on maintenance treatment of patients with ulcerative colitis. *Aliment Pharmacol Ther.* 1999 Aug;13(8):1103-8.

Verhasselt V. Oral tolerance in neonates: from basics to potential prevention of allergic disease. *Mucosal Immunol.* 2010 Jul;3(4):326-33.

Verstege A, Mehl A, Rolinck-Werninghaus C, Staden U, Nocon M, Beyer K, Niggemann B. The predictive value of the skin prick test weal size for the outcome of oral food challenges. Clin Exp Allergy. 2005 Sep;35(9):1220-6. Rolinck-Werninghaus C, Staden U, Mehl A, Hamelmann E, Beyer K, Niggemann B. Specific oral tolerance induction with food in children: transient or persistent effect on food allergy? *Allergy.* 2005 Oct;60(10):1320-2.

Vidgren HM, Agren JJ, Schwab U, Rissanen T, Hanninen O, Uusitupa MI. Incorporation of n-3 fatty acids into plasma lipid fractions, and erythrocyte membranes and platelets during dietary supplementation with fish, fish oil, and docosahexaenoic acid-rich oil among healthy young men. *Lipids.* 1997 Jul;32(7):697-705.

Viinanen A, Munhbayarlah S, Zevgee T, Narantsetseg L, Naidansuren Ts, Koskenvuo M, Helenius H, Terho EO. Prevalence of asthma, allergic rhinoconjuctivitis and allergic sensitization in Mongolia. *Allergy.* 2005;60:1370-1377.

Vila R, Mundina M, Tomi F, Furlán R, Zacchino S, Casanova J, Cañigueral S. Composition and antifungal activity of the essential oil of Solidago chilensis. *Planta Med.* 2002 Feb;68(2):164-7.

Viljanen M, Kuitunen M, Haahtela T, Juntunen-Backman K, Korpela R, Savilahti E. Probiotic effects on faecal inflammatory markers and on faecal IgA in food allergic atopic eczema/dermatitis syndrome infants. *Pediatr Allergy Immunol.* 2005 Feb;16(1):65-71.

Viljanen M, Savilahti E, Haahtela T, Juntunen-Backman K, Korpela R, Poussa T, Tuure T, Kuitunen M. Probiotics in the treatment of atopic eczema/dermatitis syndrome in infants: a double-blind placebo-controlled trial. *Allergy.* 2005 Apr;60(4):494-500.

Vinson JA, Proch J, Bose P. MegaNatural((R)) Gold Grapeseed Extract: In Vitro Antioxidant and In Vivo Human Supplementation Studies. *J Med Food.* 2001 Spring;4(1):17-26.

Visitsunthorn N, Pacharn P, Jirapongsananuruk O, Weeravejsukit S, Sripramong C, Sookrung N, Bunnag C. Comparison between Siriraj mite allergen vaccine and standardized commercial mite vaccine by skin prick testing in normal Thai adults. *Asian Pac J Allergy Immunol.* 2010 Mar;28(1):41-5.

Visness CM, London SJ, Daniels JL, Kaufman JS, Yeatts KB, Siega-Riz AM, Liu AH, Calatroni A, Zeldin DC. Association of obesity with IgE levels and allergy symptoms in children and adolescents: results from the National Health and Nutrition Examination Survey 2005-2006. *J Allergy Clin Immunol.* 2009 May;123(5):1163-9, 1169.e1-4.

Visness CM, London SJ, Daniels JL, Kaufman JS, Yeatts KB, Siega-Riz AM, Calatroni A, Zeldin DC. Association of childhood obesity with atopic and nonatopic asthma: results from the National Health and Nutrition Examination Survey 1999-2006. *J Asthma.* 2010 Sep;47(7):822-9.

Vlieg-Boerstra BJ, Dubois AE, van der Helde S, Bijleveld CM, Wolt-Plompen SA, Oude Elberink JN, Kukler J, Jansen DF, Venter C, Duiverman EJ. Ready-to-use introduction schedules for first exposure to allergenic foods in children at home. *Allergy.* 2008 Jul;63(7):903-9.

Vlieg-Boerstra BJ, van der Heide S, Bijleveld CM, Kukler J, Duiverman EJ, Wolt-Plompen SA, Dubois AE. Dietary assessment in children adhering to a food allergen avoidance diet for allergy prevention. *Eur J Clin Nutr.* 2006 Dec;60(12):1384-90.

Voicekovska JG, Orlikov GA, Karpov IuG, Teibe U, Ivanov AD, Baidekalne I, Voicehovskis NV, Maulins E. External respiration function and quality of life in patients with bronchial asthma in correction of selenium deficiency. *Ter Arkh.* 2007;79(8):38-41.

Voĭtsekhovskaia IuG, Skesters A, Orlikov GA, Silova AA, Rusakova NE, Larmane LT, Karpov IuG, Ivanov AD, Maulins E. Assessment of some oxidative stress parameters in bronchial asthma patients beyond add-on selenium supplementation. *Biomed Khim.* 2007 Sep-Oct;53(5):577-84.

Vojdani A. Antibodies as predictors of complex autoimmune diseases. *Int J Immunopathol Pharmacol.* 2008 Apr-Jun;21(2):267-78.

von Berg A, Filipiak-Pittroff B, Krämer U, Link E, Bollrath C, Brockow I, Koletzko S, Grübl A, Heinrich J, Wichmann HE, Bauer CP, Reinhardt D, Berdel D; GINIplus study group. Preventive effect of hydrolyzed infant formulas persists until age 6 years: long-term results from the German Infant Nutritional Intervention Study (GINI). *J Allergy Clin Immunol.* 2008 Jun;121(6):1442-7.

von Berg A, Koletzko S, Grübl A, Filipiak-Pittroff B, Wichmann HE, Bauer CP, Reinhardt D, Berdel D; German Infant Nutritional Intervention Study Group. The effect of hydrolyzed cow's milk formula for allergy prevention in the first year of life: the

REFERENCES AND BIBLIOGRAPHY

German Infant Nutritional Intervention Study, a randomized double-blind trial. *J Allergy Clin Immunol.* 2003 Mar;111(3):533-40.

von Kruedener S, Schneider W, Elstner EF. A combination of Populus tremula, Solidago virgaurea and Fraxinus excelsior as an anti-inflammatory and antirheumatic drug. A short review. *Arzneimittelforschung.* 1995 Feb;45(2):169-71.

von Mutius E, Vercelli D. Farm living: effects on childhood asthma and allergy. *Nat Rev Immunol.* 2010 Dec;10(12):861-8. 2010 Nov 9.

Vulevic J, Drakoularakou A, Yaqoob P, Tzortzis G and Gibson GR; Modulation of the fecal microflora profile and immune function by a novel trans-galactooligosaccharide mixture (B-GOS) in healthy elderly volunteers. *Am J Clin Nutr.* 1988 88;1438-1446.

Waddell L. Food allergies in children: the difference between cow's milk protein allergy and food intolerance. *J Fam Health Care.* 2010;20(3):104.

Wahler D, Gronover CS, Richter C, Foucu F, Twyman RM, Moerschbacher BM, Fischer R, Muth J, Prufer D. Polyphenoloxidase silencing affects latex coagulation in Taraxacum spp. *Plant Physiol.* 2009 Jul 15.

Waite DA, Eyles EF, Tonkin SL, O'Donnell TV. Asthma prevalence in Tokelauan children in two environments. *Clin Allergy.* 1980;10:71-75.

Walders-Abramson N, Wamboldt FS, Curran-Everett D, Zhang L. Encouraging physical activity in pediatric asthma: a case-control study of the wonders of walking (WOW) program. *Pediatr Pulmonol.* 2009 Sep;44(9):909-16.

Walker S, Wing A. Allergies in children. *J Fam Health Care.* 2010;20(1):24-6.

Walker WA. Antigen absorption from the small intestine and gastrointestinal disease. *Pediatr Clin North Am.* 1975 Nov;22(4):731-46.

Walker WA. Antigen handling by the small intestine. *Clin Gastroenterol.* 1986 Jan;15(1):1-20.

Walle UK, Walle T. Transport of the cooked-food mutagen 2-amino-1-methyl-6-phenylimidazo- 4,5-b pyridine (PhIP) across the human intestinal Caco-2 cell monolayer: role of efflux pumps. *Carcinogenesis.* 1999 Nov;20(11):2153-7.

Walsh MG. Toxocara infection and diminished lung function in a nationally representative sample from the United States population. *Int J Parasitol.* 2010 Nov 8.

Walsh SJ, Rau LM: Autoimmune diseases: a leading cause of death among young and middle-aged women in the United States. *Am J Public Health* 2000, 90(9): 1463-1466.

Wang G, Liu CT, Wang ZL, Yan CL, Luo FM, Wang L, Li TQ. Effects of Astragalus membranaceus in promoting T-helper cell type 1 polarization and interferon-gamma production by up-regulating T-bet expression in patients with asthma. *Chin J Integr Med.* 2006 Dec;12(4):262-7.

Wang H, Chang B, Wang B. The effect of herbal medicine including astragalus membranaceus (fisch) bge, codonpsis pilosula and glycyrrhiza uralensis fisch on airway responsiveness. *Zhonghua Jie He He Hu Xi Za Zhi.* 1998 May;21(5):287-8.

Wang J, Lin J, Bardina L, Goldis M, Nowak-Wegrzyn A, Shreffler WG, Sampson HA. Correlation of IgE/IgG4 milk epitopes and affinity of milk-specific IgE antibodies with different phenotypes of clinical milk allergy. *J Allergy Clin Immunol.* 2010 Mar;125(3):695-702, 702.e1-702.e6.

Wang J, Patil SP, Yang N, Ko J, Lee J, Noone S, Sampson HA, Li XM. Safety, tolerability, and immunologic effects of a food allergy herbal formula in food allergic individuals: a randomized, double-blinded, placebo-controlled, dose escalation, phase 1 study. *Ann Allergy Asthma Immunol.* 2010 Jul;105(1):75-84.

Wang J. Management of the patient with multiple food allergies. *Curr Allergy Asthma Rep.* 2010 Jul;10(4):271-7.

Wang JL, Shaw NS, Kao MD. Magnesium deficiency and its lack of association with asthma in Taiwanese elementary school children. *Asia Pac J Clin Nutr.* 2007;16 Suppl 2:579-84.

Wang JS, Hung WP. The effects of a swimming intervention for children with asthma. *Respirology.* 2009 Aug;14(6):838-42.

Wang KY, Li SN, Liu CS, Perng DS, Su YC, Wu DC, Jan CM, Lai CH, Wang TN, Wang WM. Effects of ingesting Lactobacillus- and Bifidobacterium-containing yogurt in subjects with colonized Helicobacter pylori. *Am J Clin Nutr.* 2004 Sep;80(3):737-41.

Wang YH, Yang CP, Ku MS, Sun HL, Lue KH. Efficacy of nasal irrigation in the treatment of acute sinusitis in children. *Int J Pediatr Otorhinolaryngol.* 2009 Dec;73(12):1696-701. 2009 Sep 27.

Wang YM, Huan GX. *Utilization of Classical Formulas.* Beijing, China: Chinese Medicine and Pharmacology Publishing Co, 1998.

Waring G, Levy D. Challenging adverse reactions in children with food allergies. *Paediatr Nurs.* 2010 Jul;22(6):16-22.

Waser M, Michels KB, Bieli C, Flöistrup H, Pershagen G, von Mutius E, Ege M, Riedler J, Schram-Bijkerk D, Brunekreef B, van Hage M, Lauener R, Braun-Fahrländer C; PARSIFAL Study team. Inverse association of farm milk consumption with asthma and allergy in rural and suburban populations across Europe. *Clin Exp Allergy.* 2007 May;37(5):661-70.

Watkins BA, Hannon K, Ferruzzi M, Li Y. Dietary PUFA and flavonoids as deterrents for environmental pollutants. *J Nutr Biochem.* 2007 Mar;18(3):196-205.

Watson R. Preedy VR. Botanical Medicine in Clinical Practice. Oxfordshire: CABI, 2008.

Watzl B, Bub A, Blockhaus M, Herbert BM, Lührmann PM, Neuhäuser-Berthold M, Rechkemmer G. Prolonged tomato juice consumption has no effect on cell-mediated immunity of well-nourished elderly men and women. *J Nutr.* 2000 Jul;130(7):1719-23.

Webber CM, England RW. Oral allergy syndrome: a clinical, diagnostic, and therapeutic challenge. *Ann Allergy Asthma Immunol.* 2010 Feb;104(2):101-8; quiz 109-10, 117.

Webster D, Taschereau P, Belland RJ, Sand C, Rennie RP. Antifungal activity of medicinal plant extracts; preliminary screening studies. *J Ethnopharmacol.* 2008 Jan 4;115(1):140-6.

Wei A, Shibamoto T. Antioxidant activities and volatile constituents of various essential oils. *J Agric Food Chem.* 2007 Mar 7;55(5):1737-42.

Weiler JM, Layton T, Hunt M. Asthma in United States Olympic athletes who participated in the 1996 Summer Games. J Allergy Clin Immunol. 1998 Nov;102(5):722-6. 7.

Weiner MA. *Secrets of Fijian Medicine*. Berkeley, CA: Univ. of Calif., 1969.

Weisgerber M, Webber K, Meurer J, Danduran M, Berger S, Flores G. Moderate and vigorous exercise programs in children with asthma: safety, parental satisfaction, and asthma outcomes. Pediatr Pulmonol. 2008 Dec;43(12):1175-82.

Weiss RF. *Herbal Medicine*. Gothenburg, Sweden: Beaconsfield, 1988.

Wen MC, Huang CK, Srivastava KD, Zhang TF, Schofield B, Sampson HA, Li XM. Ku-Shen (Sophora flavescens Ait), a single Chinese herb, abrogates airway hyperreactivity in a murine model of asthma. *J Allergy Clin Immunol.* 2004;113:218.

Wen MC, Taper A, Srivastava KD, Huang CK, Schofield B, Li XM. Immunology of T cells by the Chinese Herbal Medicine Ling Zhi (Ganoderma lucidum) *J Allergy Clin Immunol.* 2003;111:S320.

Wen MC, Wei CH, Hu ZQ, Srivastava K, Ko J, Xi ST, Mu DZ, Du JB, Li GH, Wallenstein S, Sampson H, Kattan M, Li XM. Efficacy and tolerability of anti-asthma herbal medicine intervention in adult patients with moderate-severe allergic asthma. *J Allergy Clin Immunol.* 2005;116:517-24.

Werbach M. *Nutritional Influences on Illness*. Tarzana, CA: Third Line Press, 1996.

West CE, Hammarström ML, Hernell O. Probiotics during weaning reduce the incidence of eczema. *Pediatr Allergy Immunol.* 2009 Aug;20(5):430-7.

West R. Risk of death in meat and non-meat eaters. *BMJ.* 1994 Oct 8;309(6959):955.

Westerholm-Ormio M, Vaarala O, Tiittanen M, Savilahti E. Infiltration of Foxp3- and Toll-like receptor-4-positive cells in the intestines of children with food allergy. *J Pediatr Gastroenterol Nutr.* 2010 Apr;50(4):367-76.

Wheeler JG, Shema SJ, Bogle ML, Shirrell MA, Burks AW, Pittler A, Helm RM. Immune and clinical impact of *Lactobacillus acidophilus* on asthma. *Ann Allergy Asthma Immunol.* 1997 Sep;79(3):229-33.

White LB, Foster S. The Herbal Drugstore. Emmaus, PA: Rodale, 2000.

Whitfield KE, Wiggins SA, Belue R, Brandon DT. Genetic and environmental influences on forced expiratory volume in African Americans: the Carolina African-American Twin Study of Aging. *Ethn Dis.* 2004 Spring;14(2):206-11.

WHO. *Guidelines for Drinking-water Quality.* 2nd ed, vol. 2. Geneva: World Health Organization, 1996.

WHO. Health effects of the removal of substances occurring naturally in drinking water, with special reference to demineralized and desalinated water. Report on a working group (Brussels, 20-23 March 1978). *EURO Reports and Studies.* 1979;16.

WHO. How trace elements in water contribute to health. *WHO Chronicle.* 1978;32:382-385.

WHO. *INFOSAN Food Allergies. Information Note No. 3.* Geneva, Switzerland: World Health Organization, 2006.

Widdicombe JG, Ernst E. Clinical cough V: complementary and alternative medicine: therapy of cough. *Handb Exp Pharmacol.* 2009;(187):321-42.

Wilkens H, Wilkens JH, Uffmann J, Bövers J, Fröhlich JC, Fabel H. Effect of the platelet-activating factor antagonist BN 52063 on exertional asthma. *Pneumologie.* 1990 Feb;44 Suppl 1:347-8.

Willard T, Jones K. *Reishi Mushroom: Herb of Spiritual Potency and Medical Wonder.* Issaquah, Washington: Sylvan Press, 1990.

Willard T. *Edible and Medicinal Plants of the Rocky Mountains and Neighbouring Territories.* Calgary: 1992.

Willemsen LE, Koetsier MA, Balvers M, Beermann C, Stahl B, van Tol EA. Polyunsaturated fatty acids support epithelial barrier integrity and reduce IL-4 mediated permeability in vitro. *Eur J Nutr.* 2008 Jun;47(4):183-91.

Williams DM. Considerations in the long-term management of asthma in ambulatory patients. *AM J Health Sits Pham.* 2006;63:S14-21.

Wilson D, Evans M, Guthrie N, Sharma P, Baisley J, Schonlau F, Burki C. A randomized, double-blind, placebo-controlled exploratory study to evaluate the potential of pycnogenol for improving allergic rhinitis symptoms. *Phytother Res.* 2010 Aug;24(8):1115-9.

Wilson K, McDowall L, Hodge D, Chetcuti P, Cartledge P. Cow's milk protein allergy. *Community Pract.* 2010 May;83(5):40-1.

Wilson L. *Nutritional Balancing and Hair Mineral Analysis.* Prescott, AZ: LD Wilson, 1998.

Wilson NM, Charette L, Thomson AH, Silverman M. Gastro-oesophageal reflux and childhood asthma: the acid test. *Thorax.* 1985 Aug;40(8):592-7.

REFERENCES AND BIBLIOGRAPHY

Winchester AM. *Biology and its Relation to Mankind.* New York: Van Nostrand Reinhold, 1969.

Wittenberg JS. *The Rebellious Body.* New York: Insight, 1996.

Woessner KM, Simon RA, Stevenson DD. Monosodium glutamate sensitivity in asthma. *J Allergy Clin Immunol.* 1999 Aug;104(2 Pt 1):305-10.

Wöhrl S, Hemmer W, Focke M, Rappersberger K, Jarisch R. Histamine intolerance-like symptoms in healthy volunteers after oral provocation with liquid histamine. *Allergy Asthma Proc.* 2004 Sep-Oct;25(5):305-11.

Wolvers DA, van Herpen-Broekmans WM, Logman MH, van der Wielen RP, Albers R. Effect of a mixture of micronutrients, but not of bovine colostrum concentrate, on immune function parameters in healthy volunteers: a randomized placebo-controlled study. *Nutr J.* 2006 Nov 21;5:28.

Wolverton BC. *How to grow fresh air: 50 houseplants that purify your home or office.* New York: Penguin, 1997.

Wong GWK, Hui DSC, Chan HH, Fox TF, Leung R, Zhong NS, Chen YZ, Lai CKW. Prevalence of respiratory and atopic disorders in Chinese schoolchildren. *Clinical and Experimental Allergy.* 2001;31:1125-1231.

Wong WM, Lai KC, Lam KF, Hui WM, Hu WH, Lam CL, Xia HH, Huang JQ, Chan CK, Lam SK, Wong BC. Prevalence, clinical spectrum and health care utilization of gastro-oesophageal reflux disease in a Chinese population: a population-based study. *Aliment Pharmacol Ther.* 2003 Sep 15;18(6):595-604.

Wood M. *The Book of Herbal Wisdom.* Berkeley, CA: North Atlantic, 1997.

Wood RA, Kraynak J. *Food Allergies for Dummies.* Hoboken, NJ: Wiley Publ, 2007.

Woods RK, Abramson M, Bailey M, Walters EH. International prevalences of reported food allergies and intolerances. Comparisons arising from the European Community Respiratory Health Survey (ECRHS) 1991-1994. *Eur J Clin Nutr* 2001;55:298-304.

Woods RK, Abramson M, Bailey M, Walters EH. International prevalences of reported food allergies and intolerances. Comparisons arising from the European Community Respiratory Health Survey (ECRHS) 1991-1994. *Eur J Clin Nutr.* 2001 Apr;55(4):298-304.

Woods RK, Abramson M, Raven JM, Bailey M, Weiner JM, Walters EH. Reported food intolerance and respiratory symptoms in young adults. *Eur Respir J.* 1998;11: 151-155.

Wouters EF, Reynaert NL, Dentener MA, Vernooy JH. Systemic and local inflammation in asthma and chronic obstructive pulmonary disease: is there a connection? *Proc Am Thorac Soc.* 2009 Dec;6(8):638-47.

Wright A, Lavoie KL, Jacob A, Rizk A, Bacon SL. Effect of body mass index on self-reported exercise-triggered asthma. *Phys Sportsmed.* 2010 Dec;38(4):61-6.

Wright GR, Howieson S, McSharry C, McMahon AD, Chaudhuri R, Thompson J, Donnelly I, Brooks RG, Lawson A, Jolly L, McAlpine L, King EM, Chapman MD, Wood S, Thomson NC. Effect of improved home ventilation on asthma control and house dust mite allergen levels. *Allergy.* 2009 Nov;64(11):1671-80.

Wright RJ. Epidemiology of stress and asthma: from constricting communities and fragile families to epigenetics. *Immunol Allergy Clin North Am.* 2011 Feb;31(1):19-39.

Wu B, Yu J, Wang Y. Effect of Chinese herbs for tonifying Shen on balance of Th1/Th2 in children with asthma in remission stage. *Zhongguo Zhong Xi Yi Jie He Za Zhi.* 2007 Feb;27(2):120-2.

Xiao P, Kubo H, Ohsawa M, Higashiyama K, Nagase H, Yan YN, Li JS, Kamei J, Ohmiya S. kappa-Opioid receptor-mediated antinociceptive effects of stereoisomers and derivatives of (+)-matrine in mice. *Planta Med.* 1999 Apr;65(3):230-3.

Xie JY, Dong JC, Gong ZH. Effects on herba epimedii and radix Astragali on tumor necrosis factor-alpha and nuclear factor-kappa B in asthmatic rats. *Zhongguo Zhong Xi Yi Jie He Za Zhi.* 2006 Aug;26(8):723-7.

Xu X, Zhang D, Zhang H, Wolters PJ, Killeen NP, Sullivan BM, Locksley RM, Lowell CA, Caughey GH. Neutrophil histamine contributes to inflammation in mycoplasma pneumonia. *J Exp Med.* 2006 Dec 25;203(13):2907-17.

Yadav RK, Ray RB, Vempati R, Bijlani RL. Effect of a comprehensive yoga-based lifestyle modification program on lipid peroxidation. *Indian J Physiol Pharmacol.* 2005 Jul-Sep;49(3):358-62.

Yadav VS, Mishra KP, Singh DP, Mehrotra S, Singh VK. Immunomodulatory effects of curcumin. *Immunopharmacol Immunotoxicol.* 2005;27(3):485-97.

Yadzir ZH, Misnan R, Abdullah N, Bakhtiar F, Arip M, Murad S. Identification of Ige-binding proteins of raw and cooked extracts of Loligo edulis (white squid). *Southeast Asian J Trop Med Public Health.* 2010 May;41(3):653-9.

Yang Z. Are peanut allergies a concern for using peanut-based formulated foods in developing countries? *Food Nutr Bull.* 2010 Jun;31(2 Suppl):S147-53.

Yeager S. *The Doctor's Book of Food Remedies.* Emmaus, PA: Rodale Press, 1998.

Yeh CC, Lin CC, Wang SD, Chen YS, Su BH, Kao ST. Protective and anti-inflammatory effect of a traditional Chinese medicine, Xia-Bai-San, by modulating lung local cytokine in a murine model of acute lung injury. *Int Immunopharmacol.* 2006 Sep;6(9):1506-14.

Yu L, Zhang Y, Chen C, Cui HF, Yan XK. Meta-analysis on randomized controlled clinical trials of acupuncture for asthma. *Zhongguo Zhen Jiu.* 2010 Sep;30(9):787-92.

Yu LC. The epithelial gatekeeper against food allergy. *Pediatr Neonatol*. 2009 Dec;50(6):247-54.

Yusoff NA, Hampton SM, Dickerson JW, Morgan JB. The effects of exclusion of dietary egg and milk in the management of asthmatic children: a pilot study. *J R Soc Promot Health*. 2004 Mar;124(2):74-80.

Zanjanian MH. The intestine in allergic diseases. *Ann Allergy*. 1976 Sep;37(3):208-18.

Zarkadas M, Scott FW, Salminen J, Ham Pong A. Common Allergenic Foods and Their Labelling in Canada. *Can J Allerg Clin Immun*. 1999; 4:118-141.

Zeiger RS, Heller S. The development and prediction of atopy in high-risk children: follow-up at age seven years in a prospective randomized study of combined maternal and infant food allergen avoidance. *J Allergy Clin Immunol*. 1995 Jun;95(6):1179-90.

Zhang T, Srivastava K, Wen MC, Yang N, Cao J, Busse P, Birmingham N, Goldfarb J, Li XM. Pharmacology and immunological actions of a herbal medicine ASHMI on allergic asthma. *Phytother Res*. 2010 Jul;24(7):1047-55.

Zhang Z, Lai HJ, Roberg KA, Gangnon RE, Evans MD, Anderson EL, Pappas TE, Dasilva DF, Tisler CJ, Salazar LP, Gern JE, Lemanske RF Jr. Early childhood weight status in relation to asthma development in high-risk children. *J Allergy Clin Immunol*. 2010 Dec;126(6):1157-62. 2010 Nov 4.

Zhao FD, Dong JC, Xie JY. Effects of Chinese herbs for replenishing shen and strengthening qi on some indexes of neuro-endocrino-immune network in asthmatic rats. *Zhongguo Zhong Xi Yi Jie He Za Zhi*. 2007 Aug;27(8):715-9.

Zhao J, Bai J, Shen K, Xiang L, Huang S, Chen A, Huang Y, Wang J, Ye R. Self-reported prevalence of childhood allergic diseases in three cities of China: a multicenter study. *BMC Public Health*. 2010 Sep 13;10:551.

Zheng M. Experimental study of 472 herbs with antiviral action against the herpes simplex virus. *Zhong Xi Yi Jie He Za Zhi*. 1990 Jan;10(1):39-41, 6.

Zhou Q, Zhang B, Verne GN. Intestinal membrane permeability and hypersensitivity in the irritable bowel syndrome. *Pain*. 2009 Nov;146(1-2):41-6.

Zhu HH, Chen YP, Yu JE, Wu M, Li Z. Therapeutic effect of Xincang Decoction on chronic airway inflammation in children with bronchial asthma in remission stage. *Zhong Xi Yi He Xue Bao*. 2005 Jan;3(1):23-7.

Ziaei Kajbaf T, Asar S, Alipoor MR. Relationship between obesity and asthma symptoms among children in Ahvaz, Iran: A cross sectional study. *Ital J Pediatr*. 2011 Jan 6;37(1):1.

Zielen S, Kardos P, Madonini E. Steroid-sparing effects with allergen-specific immunotherapy in children with asthma: a randomized controlled trial. *J Allergy Clin Immunol*. 2010 Nov;126(5):942-9. 2010 Jul 10.

Ziment I, Tashkin DP. Alternative medicine for allergy and asthma. *J Allergy Clin Immunol*. 2000 Oct;106(4):603-14.

Ziment I. Alternative therapies for asthma. *Curr Opin Pulm Med*. 1997 Jan;3(1):61-71.

Zizza, C. The nutrient content of the Italian food supply 1961-1992. *Euro J Clin Nutr*. 1997;51: 259-265.

Zoccatelli G, Pokoj S, Foetisch K, Bartra J, Valero A, Del Mar San Miguel-Moncin M, Vieths S, Scheurer S. Identification and characterization of the major allergen of green bean (Phaseolus vulgaris) as a non-specific lipid transfer protein (Pha v 3). *Mol Immunol*. 2010 Apr;47(7-8):1561-8.

Index

(Herbs, foods and other natural solutions are too numerous to index)

abdominal pain, 78, 79, 80, 82
absorption, 66, 68, 69, 75, 86, 179, 192
acetaminophen, 113, 114, 138
Acetobacter aceti, 185
Acetobacter xylinoides, 185
Acetobacter xylinum, 185
acetylcholine, 37, 113, 160
acid, 104, 203
acid reflux (GERD), 10, 26, 28, 42, 51, 53, 54, 55, 56, 57, 58, 59, 122, 159, 165, 173
acidolin, 68
acidosis, 14, 205
Actinomyces sp., 61
actinomycin, 61
adherens junctions, 87
adhesion, 72, 74, 88
aerobic, 103
agave, 192
AIDS, 66, 72
airway remodeling, 45, 51, 52
alcohol, 35, 99, 101, 117, 207, 223, 242
algae, 103, 104
allergic contact dermatitis, 127, 128
allergic rhinitis, 38, 111, 166, 176, 221, 235
allergies, 71, 84, 86, 88
alveoli, 13, 14, 15, 26, 45, 51, 120, 121, 233
amasake, 181
aminoglycoside, 138
ammonia, 104
anaerobic, 103
anaphylaxis, 200
antibiotics, 41, 113, 138, 180, 187, 191
antibodies, 69
antigen, 84
antigens, 18, 19, 20, 30, 32, 33, 36
antihistamines, 34
anxiety, 42, 219, 220, 236
appetite, 156
arachidonic acid, 112, 140, 170, 200, 208, 210, 211, 212, 213

aromatic hydrocarbons, 125
arthritis, 88, 107
artificial colors, 117
asbestos, 122, 129, 130, 238, 242, 243
asparagus, 192
Aspergillus oryzae, 184
aspirin, 112, 113, 115, 140, 141, 143, 144, 145, 147
asthma, 71, 88, 113, 115
atherosclerosis, 74
atopic dermatitis, 28, 66, 73, 83, 84, 85, 89
Ayurveda, 148
azoreductase, 206
Bacillus subtilis, 80
bacterial translocation, 86
bacteroides, 84, 94
Bacteroides fragilis, 85
basophils, 47, 48, 51
B-cells, 22, 23, 24, 34
Belgian endive, 192
benzene, 125, 127
benzophenone-3, 127
beta-amyloid, 203
beta-carotene, 149
beta-glucosidase, 72
beta-glucuronidase, 206
beta-lactoglobulin, 187, 188
bifidobacteria, 191
Bifidobacterium animalis, 79, 81, 83
Bifidobacterium bifidum, 92
Bifidobacterium infantis, 80, 81
Bifidobacterium lactis, 76, 82, 84, 88, 89
Bifidobacterium longum, 79, 82, 83, 85, 88, 91, 92
bile acids, 179
biotin, 179
bloating, 80, 81, 82
blood pressure, 114
Borrelia burgdorferi, 63, 106, 107
boswellia, 151

breastfeeding, 169, 174
breast-feeding, 65, 67
bronchitis, 13, 26, 70, 120, 126, 153, 155, 157, 159, 160, 162, 163, 167, 168
brush barrier, 17, 18, 28, 29, 87, 181
bulgarican, 74
burn, 73
butter, 181, 183
buttermilk, 181, 183, 184
cadmium, 102, 122, 125, 134
calcium, 69, 70, 75, 106, 179, 192
Campylobacter jejuni, 110, 191
cancer, 71, 89, 127, 128, 140, 146, 147
Candida albicans, 67, 68, 69, 71, 78, 88, 90, 93, 95, 109
carbon dioxide, 5, 11, 14, 15, 17, 42, 118
carbon monoxide, 119, 120, 123, 124, 125, 131, 134, 236
carcinogens, 127
carcinomatous peritonitis, 71
carotenoids, 149
cayenne, 149, 150
celecoxib, 144
cheese, 65, 70, 75, 77, 183
chicory, 192
chlorine, 10, 26, 42, 109, 119, 226
chlorofluorocarbons (CFCs), 118, 129
cholera, 106
cholesterol, 66, 69, 71, 73, 75, 147, 181
chronic fatigue, 150
cilia, 10, 11, 15, 16, 26, 42, 52, 121, 123, 232
cimetidine, 138
clostridia, 78, 107, 110
Clostridium difficile, 61, 66, 71, 72, 73, 110
Clostridium perfringens, 61
Clostridium tetani, 61
cobalamine, 179
cockroaches, 134
cold weather, 10, 16, 26, 42, 50, 225, 228, 230, 237, 239, 243, 244, 245
colic, 66, 68, 73
colitis, 69, 81, 82, 91
colon, 16, 190, 191, 206
colon cancer, 71, 72

colonic, 79
common cold, 13, 26, 52, 108, 152, 153, 168, 169, 229, 235
conjunctiva, 61, 62, 63
constipation, 71, 72
COPD, 120, 132
copper, 105, 179
cortisol, 59, 153, 157, 236
Corynebacterium diphtheriae, 61
Corynebacterium sp., 61
cottage cheese, 181, 183
coughing, 43, 45, 47, 54, 126, 156, 160, 162, 165, 168, 170, 173
COX-1, 111, 114, 115, 144
COX-2, 111, 114, 115, 144, 146
C-reactive protein (CRP), 51, 70, 93, 166, 213
Crohn's disease, 51, 213
curcumin, 150
cyclooxygenase (COX), 58, 101, 111, 112, 113, 114, 115, 116, 139, 140, 144, 146, 148, 151, 166, 171
cytokines, 32, 36, 67, 77, 80, 81, 85, 91, 102, 154, 158, 176, 211, 219
cytomegalovirus, 108
degranulation, 19
dehydration, 149
depression, 220
dermatitis, 33, 85
desmosomes, 87
detergents, 104
detoxification, 139, 140, 141, 150
diabetes, 150
diaphragm, 231, 232
diarrhea, 33, 65, 66, 67, 69, 71, 74, 79, 110, 114, 115, 116, 147
diphtheria, 61
diverticular disease, 70
diverticulitis, 89
dust mites, 39, 48, 124, 238, 239, 243
dyspepsia, 67, 69, 78
ear infection, 72, 96, 110
eczema, 33, 67, 68, 72, 73, 82, 83, 84, 85, 86, 113, 144
elastin, 147

INDEX

electrocardiogram, 21
emphysema, 15, 126
endocrine, 139
endothelium-derived relaxing factor (EDRF), 47
endotoxins, 78, 87, 105, 111, 134, 193, 206, 238, 241
Enterococcus faecalis, 62
eosinophil cationic protein (ECP), 44, 45
eosinophilia, 97
epinephrine, 37, 152
epithelium, 21, 87
Escherichia coli, 62, 67, 68, 69, 75, 78, 84, 90, 106, 107, 110, 192
esophagus, 111, 114
essential fatty acids, 180
exercise-induced asthma, 40
extrinsic asthma, 37
fever, 106, 114, 139, 143, 144
fibrin, 148
flatulence, 67, 74, 80
flavonoids, 192
floating, 104
folic acid, 179
food allergies, 37, 40, 41, 49, 55, 156
forced expiratory flow (FEF), 158
forced expiratory volume (FEV), 41, 124, 154, 158, 166, 168, 176
forests, 103
formaldehyde, 40, 99, 119, 122, 130, 131, 133, 134, 242
fragrances, 126, 127, 240
free radicals, 128, 141, 144, 147
fructooligosaccharides, 191
fructooligosachharides, 191
fucoidan, 202
fungi, 78, 95, 110, 141, 184, 186
galactooligosaccharide, 191
galactooligosaccharides (GOS), 188
gallbladder, 150
garlic, 184, 192
gas, 21
gastrin, 9, 26, 42, 90, 111
gastritis, 113, 141, 147

gastroenteritis, 66
German Commission E, 147
ginger, 138, 139, 148, 149, 150, 151
gingivitis, 65, 67, 68, 75, 76, 77, 107
Glucobacter bluconicum, 185
glucose, 72, 87
glutathione, 34, 141
glutathione peroxidase, 215
glycoproteins, 17, 18, 19, 28, 29
goblet cells, 9, 10, 13, 26, 42
golf, 230
gums, 75, 76, 77, 107
H. pylor, 148
Haemophilus influenzae, 62
hay fever, 13, 26, 162
headaches, 114, 115, 116, 143, 148
heart disease, 115
Helicobacter pylori, 66, 67, 68, 69, 71, 72, 75, 78, 90, 91, 92, 93, 107
hemoglobin, 17, 123
Heomonphilus influenzae, 96
hepatitis, 106, 108, 147, 148, 150, 151
Herpes simplex, 74
herpes simplex virus-1, 108
high-density lipoproteins (HDL), 66, 69, 71
histamine, 34, 35, 36, 38, 47, 48, 49, 51, 88, 109, 113, 153, 154, 155, 159, 160, 161, 164, 166, 171, 200, 218, 221
HIV, 67, 72, 74
hives, 38, 49, 163
homosalate, 127
hormones, 181
human rhinovirus (HRV), 108
hydroxyl radical, 123
hypertension, 114
hystocompatibility complex class II, 48
ibuprofen, 114
IgA, 5, 11, 37, 156, 194
IgE, 23, 25
imidacloprid, 103
immunity, 139
immunoglobulins, 5, 34, 37, 46, 49, 50
immunosuppression, 102
inflammation, 77, 78, 82, 91

influenza, 52, 68, 71, 72, 229
interferon, 71, 85, 97
interleukin, 36, 71, 74, 79, 80, 85, 91, 102, 153
intestines, 78, 89, 91, 95, 110, 181
intrinsic asthma, 38
inulin, 97, 191, 192
iron, 179
irritable bowel syndrome, 78, 79, 80, 81, 88, 151
irritable bowel syndrome (IBS), 33
Japanese cedar pollen allergies, 83
Jerusalem artichoke, 192
kefir, 181, 183
kelp, 202
keratoconjunctivitis, 69
kidney disease, 107
kidney infections, 62
kidney stones, 66, 74, 75, 147
kim chi, 73
koji, 184
kombucha, 181, 185
lactase, 33
lactic acid, 66, 67, 70, 78, 179, 182, 183
Lactobacillus acidophilus, 67, 68, 69, 79, 80, 81, 82, 83, 86, 88, 92, 93, 94, 95, 96, 97, 182, 187
Lactobacillus brevis, 75, 76, 92, 93
Lactobacillus bulgaricus, 74, 77, 88, 182
Lactobacillus casei, 70, 72, 77, 84, 85, 86, 90, 91, 92, 96, 97
Lactobacillus coryniformis, 88
Lactobacillus gasseri, 88
Lactobacillus GG, 96
Lactobacillus helveticus, 70, 81
Lactobacillus plantarum, 73, 79, 80, 89, 97
Lactobacillus reuteri, 67, 76, 77, 78, 79, 82, 89, 92, 94, 95
Lactobacillus rhamnosus, 72, 77, 78, 79, 80, 81, 83, 84, 85, 86, 89, 94, 95, 96
Lactobacillus salivarius, 66
lactocidin, 68
lactolin, 73
lactose, 65, 66, 68, 69, 75, 183, 192

lactulose, 33
lassi, 181, 185
LDL cholesterol, 198
lead, 42, 57, 102, 122, 123, 131, 207, 226, 240
leeks, 192
leptin, 74
leukotrienes, 34, 35, 38, 39, 46, 47, 48, 49, 51, 158, 161, 164, 166, 167, 200, 210, 218
lignans, 192
limbic system, 21
lipid, 147
lipopolysaccharides, 107
liver, 51, 71, 73, 88, 100, 103, 107, 113, 114, 115, 116, 121, 137, 138, 139, 141, 147, 148, 150, 151, 171, 172, 179, 198, 201, 209, 211, 212, 213, 222, 227
liver damage, 113, 114, 138, 147
liver disease, 107
liver enzymes, 138, 147
low-back pain, 144, 146, 150
low-density lipoproteins (LDL), 66, 69, 73, 75
lozenges, 76, 93
lung cancer, 71
lung capacity, 16, 120, 122, 129, 167, 230, 231, 233
lung infection, 96
lung infections, 121, 227, 229
lutein, 203
luteolin, 150
lyme, 106
lymphocytes, 66, 71
lysine, 73
macromolecules, 18, 19, 20, 30, 35
macrophages, 34
magnesium, 179
manganese, 179
mango, 185
mannitol, 33, 153
mast cells, 34, 36, 44, 47, 48, 49, 51, 161, 167, 200
mattresses, 129
meadowsweet, 112, 140, 141, 144, 146, 147, 148

melanoma, 128
memory, 42
mercury, 102, 119, 122, 134, 180, 211
metapneumovirus (hMPV), 108
methacholine, 41, 56
methicillin-resistant *Staphylococcus aureus*, 106, 110
methyl-benzylidene camphor, 127
microflora, 66, 92, 94
microorganism, 65
microvilli, 9, 13, 17, 18, 19, 26, 28, 29, 30, 87
milk, 65, 66, 69, 70, 71, 72, 75, 77, 82, 83, 84, 85, 88, 91, 96, 182, 183, 192
milk allergies, 36
milk allergy, 188
miso, 181, 184
mold, 40, 105, 108, 109, 131, 132, 134, 193, 229, 239, 242, 243, 245
monocytes, 71, 74, 79
monosodium glutamate (MSG), 117, 118
mother, 75, 82, 83
MSM (methylsulfonylmethane), 221
mucin, 4, 9, 10, 11, 13, 17, 26, 28, 42
mucopolysaccharides, 4, 11, 17, 18, 19, 28, 29, 58, 90, 168
mucosa, 21, 72, 83, 85
mucosal membrane, 18, 19, 28, 29, 67, 90
mucous membranes, 5, 6, 7, 9, 10, 11, 12, 13, 15, 16, 25, 26, 37, 42, 57, 59, 100, 101, 121, 123, 159, 162, 165, 168, 172, 190, 216, 234, 235, 237, 238
muscles, 114
mutation, 106
Mycoplasma pneumoniae, 62
Mycoplasmas, 106
nanobacteria, 106
naproxen, 114, 138
nasal, 96
nausea, 67, 74, 82, 113, 114, 115, 116, 139, 147, 148, 149
necrotizing fascitis, 107
negative ions, 238
Neisseria meningitides, 62
neonicotinoid, 103

neuropathic, 150
neutrophils, 34, 44, 46, 47, 48, 51
niacin, 179
nitrate, 76
nitric oxide, 35
nitric oxide (NO), 47, 48, 155, 167, 207
nitrogen, 5, 11, 118, 119, 120, 124, 125, 134
nitroreductase, 206
NSAIDs, 87, 111, 114, 116, 148
nutrition, 87, 88, 192
occupational asthma, 40
octyl-dimethyl-PABA, 127
octylmethoxycinnamate, 127
oil, 103, 128
olfactory, 21
oligosaccharides, 191, 192
oral plaque, 64, 65, 68
organic foods, 187, 200, 221
oxybenzone, 127
oxygen, 66, 68, 71, 103, 185
ozone, 119, 120, 121, 134, 236, 237, 239
pancreatitis, 89
pantothenic acid, 179
parathyroid hormone, 70
particulates, 118, 119, 121, 237, 238, 239, 245
pasteurization, 182
pathobiotic, 181
peak expiratory flow, 157, 238
Pediococcus pentosaceus, 97
periodontal disease, 64, 67, 75
pesticides, 78, 87
pharmaceutical, 86, 87
pharmaceuticals, 68, 103
phenol, 140
phospholipids, 90
photo-contact allergy, 127
photosensitivity, 114
phytanic acid, 134, 206
phytonutrients, 193
Picha fermentans, 185
pneumonia, 13, 26, 70, 74, 96, 106, 132, 169
polarity, 21
pollen, 38, 48, 134, 166, 194, 199, 233

polyphenols, 144, 179, 192
polyps, 89
polysaccharide, 202
Porphyromonas gingivalis, 75, 107
posture, 232
potassium, 140
prebiotics, 84, 97, 184, 191, 192
preservatives, 116
Prevotella intermedia, 75
propellants, 129, 240
Propionibacterium freudenreichii, 79, 80, 81, 84
prostaglandins, 34, 35, 38, 46, 47, 48, 51, 52, 111, 112, 113, 140, 141, 144, 163, 210
proteinuria, 203
Proteus sp., 62
Pseudomonas aeruginosa, 62, 71, 72, 97
psoriasis, 88
psychophiles, 106
psyllium, 92
pyridoxine, 77, 179
quercetin, 149
reactive oxygen species, 44, 177, 178
refined sugars, 101, 188, 216
refractory asthma, 41
reservatrol, 192
Reye's Syndrome, 113
rhinomanometer, 21
rhinorrhea, 83
Rhizopus oligosporus, 185
Rhyzopus oryzae, 185
riboflavin, 179
rivers, 103
rofecoxib, 144, 146
root canals, 107
rotavirus, 65, 67, 69, 71, 72, 74, 75
running, 230
Saccharomyces boulardii, 79, 91, 92
Saccharomyces cerevisiae, 193
Saccharomycodes Ludwigii, 185
salicin, 112, 140, 141, 143, 144, 145, 147
saliva, 76, 77, 85, 89
salivaricin, 65
salmonella, 191

Salmonella sp., 67, 68
sauerkraut, 73, 181
Schizosaccharomyces pombe, 185
sepsis, 74, 97
septic arthritis, 62
septum, 21
shigella, 191
shoyu, 184
side-effects, 68
sigmoidoscopy, 91
sinus, 21
sinusitis, 13, 26, 41, 49, 51, 59, 88, 122, 153, 159, 165, 173, 234, 235
skin cancer, 128
skin prick test, 32
sleep, 70
smoke, 38, 39, 40, 45, 50, 59, 119, 125, 126, 175, 211, 233, 236
smooth muscles, 37, 43, 52, 161, 163, 167, 170, 226, 227
sodium benzoate, 116
soil, 103
soot, 119
sour, 181, 182
sourness, 70, 73
soy, 176, 181, 182, 184, 185, 188, 208, 220
spirochete bacteria, 63
Staphylococcus aureus, 63, 66, 96, 107
Staphylococcus epidermidis, 63
Streptococcus mitis, 63
Streptococcus mutans, 64, 66, 67, 73, 75, 76, 77, 107
Streptococcus pneumoniae, 64, 66, 96
Streptococcus pyogenes, 75, 107
Streptococcus pyrogenes, 63
Streptococcus salivarius, 64, 65, 190
Streptococcus thermophilus, 28, 65, 77, 84, 88, 92, 96
stress, 35, 69, 82, 137
sulfites, 117
sulfuric acid, 104
sulphur dioxide, 118, 119, 120, 121
sun, 141
sunburn, 128

INDEX

sunscreen, 127, 128
superbugs, 106, 110
swimming, 119, 224, 230, 231
synbiotics, 93
syncytial virus (RSV), 108
tablets, 76, 77, 92
tamari, 181, 182
Tannerella forsynthensis, 75, 107
tannins, 192
tar, 16, 125
T-cells, 24, 34, 35, 68, 69, 72
teeth, 75, 107
teeth enamel, 64
tempeh, 181, 185
temperature, 183, 184, 185, 186
Th1, 73, 80, 85
Th2, 73, 83
T-helper cells-1 (Th1), 154, 156, 158
T-helper cells-2 (Th2), 154, 156, 158
thermophiles, 106
thiamin, 179
thiobarbituric acid-reactive products (TBARs), 44
thrombosis, 112
thromboxanes, 111, 112, 113, 140
thymus, 230
thyroid, 103
thyroid gland, 103
tight junctions, 17, 18, 19, 29, 30, 32, 87
tonsillitis, 69
toxemia, 205
toxic chemicals, 78, 138
toxins, 18, 19, 28, 30, 34, 35, 180
transcellular pathway, 19
transgalactooligosaccharides, 191
transgalactooligosaccharides (TOS), 188
Treponema pallidum, 63
triglycerides, 69, 71, 75, 181
tuberculosis, 106

tumor necrosis factor, 154, 159, 163, 164
turbinate, 21
turbinates, 16, 233
turmeric, 150, 151
ulcer, 72, 81
ulcerative colitis, 35, 65, 66, 67, 79, 81, 89, 90, 91, 92
ulcers, 114, 115, 116, 139, 141, 147, 148, 149, 151
ultraviolet
UV-A, 128
UV-B, 128
uncertainty, 192
urban areas, 120
uric acid, 147
urinary tract, 68, 93, 143, 146
urine, 66, 116, 143
uritica, 49
vagina, 66, 67, 68, 93, 94, 95
vaginitis, 69, 93, 94
vaginosis, 69, 71, 72, 94, 95
virus, 69
vitamin C, 140
vitamin K, 179
vitamins, 202, 203
volatile organic compounds (VOCs), 118, 124, 125, 129, 131, 133, 238, 240, 242, 243
vomiting, 82
walking, 149
water, 106, 184, 186
wheat, 184, 192
wheezing, 117
willow, 112, 140, 141, 143, 144, 145, 146
xenoestrogens, 104
yeasts, 108, 109
yogurt, 65, 79, 82, 85, 88, 92, 94, 95, 96, 97, 181, 182, 185, 192
zeaxanthin, 203

Made in the USA
Lexington, KY
03 May 2015